Atlas of Visual Fields

Atlas of Visual Fields

Donald L. Budenz, M.D.
Bascom Palmer Eye Institute
Department of Ophthalmology
University of Miami School of Medicine
Miami, Florida

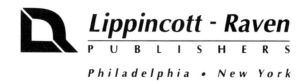
Lippincott - Raven
P U B L I S H E R S
Philadelphia • New York

Manufacturing Manager: Dennis Teston
Production Manager: Lawrence Bernstein
Production Editor: Lawrence Bernstein
Cover Designer: Karen K. Quigley
Indexer: Victoria Boyle
Compositor: Maryland Composition
Printer: Quebecor Kingsport

Library of Congress Cataloging-in-Publication Data

Budenz, Donald L.
    Atlas of visual fields / Donald L. Budenz.
      p. cm.
    Includes bibliographical references and index.
    ISBN 0-397-51741-6
    1. Perimetry—Atlases.   2. Visual fields—Atlases.   3. Eye—
Diseases—Diagnoses—Atlases. I. Title.
    [DNLM: 1. Visual Fields—atlases.   2. Perimetry—methods—atlases.
    3. Eye Diseases—diagnosis—atlases.   WW 145 B927a   1997]
RE79.P4B83   1997
617.7'15—dc21
DNLM/DLC
for Library of Congress

To my wife, Susan, a Proverbs 31 woman.

Contents

Contributors

Donald L. Budenz, M.D.
Bascom Palmer Eye Institute
Department of Ophthalmology
University of Miami School of Medicine
900 N.W. 17th Street
Miami, Florida 33136

Steven J. Gedde, M.D.
Bascom Palmer Eye Institute
Department of Ophthalmology
University of Miami School of Medicine
900 N.W. 17th Street
Miami, Florida 33136

R. Michael Siatkowski, M.D.
Bascom Palmer Eye Institute
Department of Ophthalmology
University of Miami School of Medicine
900 N.W. 17th Street
Miami, Florida 33136

Preface

This book is designed to help ophthalmologists, optometrists, and neurologists learn how to interpret automated visual fields. As an atlas, it is primarily pictorial in nature, presenting visual fields from actual patients that illustrate teaching points in analyzing visual fields. Each field is accompanied by a brief clinical history, interpretation, and explanation. The purpose of this book is to teach a systematic approach to reading automated fields as well as to develop pattern recognition for the majority of visual fields encountered in clinical practice.

Measurement of the visual field is the most commonly performed ancillary test in eye care. Automated static perimetry has, for the most part, replaced manual kinetic perimetry in clinical practice for several reasons. Automated perimetry is more sensitive to early visual field change than manual kinetic perimetry.[1-3] Kinetic perimetry is an art that few take the time to master and the results are highly operator-dependent. Because it is computerized, the testing procedure in automated perimetry is standardized and less dependent on who performs the test. Complex statistical analyses can be performed on the results obtained with automated perimetry that cannot be performed with manual perimetry. Fields can be performed in different offices with comparable machines, thus facilitating the sharing of important historical clinical information as well as permitting statistical analysis to judge change over time.

I have no financial interest in the company that manufactures or sells the Humphrey Visual Field Analyzer. I have selected the Humphrey Visual Field Analyzer primarily because it is the field analyzer with which I have the most familiarity. The analyzer also happens to be the one most commonly used in clinical practice.

References

1. Krieglstein GK, Schrems W, Gramer E, Leydhecker W. Detectability of early glaucomatous field defects: a controlled comparison of Goldmann versus Octopus perimetry. *Doc Ophthal Proc Ser* 1981;26:19.
2. Beck RW, Bergstrom TJ, Lichter PR. A clinical comparison of visual field testing with a new automated perimeter, the Humphrey field analyzer, and the Goldmann perimeter. *Ophthalmology* 1985;92:77.
3. Katz J, Tielsch JM, Quigley HA, Sommer A. Automated perimetry detects visual field loss before manual Goldmann perimetry. *Ophthalmology* 1995;102:21.

Acknowledgments

I am greatly indebted to my mentor, Douglas R. Anderson, M.D., who first stimulated my interest in automated perimetry and provided editorial assistance for chapters 1 and 5. Many of the ideas presented in this book are Dr. Anderson's and can be found in more detail in his comprehensive textbook, *Automated Static Perimetry* (Mosby-Yearbook, 1992). I would also like to acknowledge Alexander J. Brucker, M.D., to whom I owe the idea for this book. Dr. Brucker also kindly provided editorial assitance for chapters 1, 2, and 4. I am grateful to V. Michael Patella, O.D. who kindly provided help with some of the figures and the appendix. I would also like to thank Joe Ettleson, Cherylee Whyly, Marlen Miguel, Marcia Anderson, and Kelly Roland of the Bascom Palmer Eye Institute for their assistance in obtaining visual fields.

Donald L. Budenz, MD

1

Introduction to Automated Perimetry

Donald L. Budenz

WHAT DOES AUTOMATED PERIMETRY MEASURE?

Automated static perimetry provides a map of the visual field by projecting stimuli of various light intensities, sizes, and colors onto a bowl-shaped screen (Fig. 1-1) which also may vary in light, intensity, and color. Unlike kinetic perimeters, which use a moving test object, static perimeters project stationary stimuli in various locations in the visual field. The measure of light intensity used in automated perimetry is the decibel, which is actually a measure of attenuation of light. Automated perimeters have a single light bulb for projecting stimuli, which, if unattenuated, has an intensity of 0 dB (10,000 apostilbs on the Humphrey Field Analyzer and 1,000 or 4,000 apostilbs on the Octopus perimeter). The intensity of the stimulus is decreased using neutral-density filters. As the attenuation of the light (measured in decibels) is increased, the intensity (measured in apostilbs) decreases. The dimmest stimulus seen by the patient 50% of the time is recorded as the threshold on the visual field printout in decibels. Therefore, the higher the number recorded on the visual field printout, the dimmer the stimulus seen and the better the retinal sensitivity at a particular point.

HOW DOES THE AUTOMATED PERIMETER MEASURE THE VISUAL FIELD?

The full threshold program of the Humphrey perimeter, which is the most commonly performed test, proceeds as follows. The perimetrist first enters the patient's demographic and clinical characteristics. The test to be performed is then selected. If the central 30° or less is being tested, the patient's best corrected refraction plus age-appropriate reading add is placed in the trial lens holder. The eye that is not being tested is occluded. The patient is comfortably seated at the perimeter bowl with his or her chin in the chin rest and forehead positioned against the bar and is given the response button. The patient's head is centered so that the eye to be tested is directly opposite the central fixation light and is not tilted, in any plane. The room lights are dimmed and the trial lens holder is

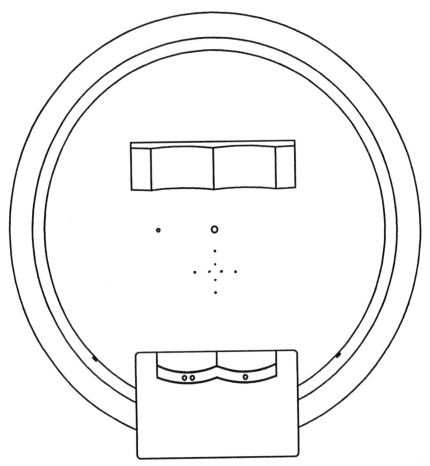

Figure 1-1. Inside of Humphrey perimeter bowl. The illustration shows the central fixation light and the small and large diamonds of lights, just below the fixation light. The central fixation light is used for most patients, although those with central scotomas may not be able to fixate on this target. These patients may be tested by using the center of the small or large diamond of lights (depending on the size of the scotoma), which are below the central fixation light. If the center of one of the triangles is used for fixation, then the perimeter projects stimuli in locations based on this alternate location for central fixation. The small triangle of lights is also used when determining the sensitivity of the fovea. The black spot to the left of the central fixation light is part of the gaze tracking system of the new Humphrey perimeters. (Courtesy of K. Aviantas, Humphrey Instruments)

positioned just in front of the lashes. Instructions, as outlined on the video screen, are read to the patient. It is important to tell the patient that he or she is not expected to see all of the lights. For patients taking an automated field for the first time, a 1-minute demonstration program may be performed at this time.

For measurement of foveal threshold, which we perform on all threshold tests, the patient is first asked to look in the center of the small diamond consisting of four lights below the central fixation light (see Fig. 1-1). The foveal sensitivity is then measured. After this, the patient is instructed to look at the central yellow fixation light throughout the remainder of the test.

The computer then presents stimuli at four locations 9° from the horizontal and vertical meridians. These "primary points" are determined twice, as are the six other points used to calculate short-term fluctuation (see Fig. 1-15) and any points that are 5 dB higher or lower than the expected value in the age-matched normal population. As a starting point for the four cardinal points, the computer uses expected values from age-matched normal subjects. With the patient fixating at the central fixation light, the location of the physiologic blind spot is determined by the perimeter projecting a single suprathreshold size III stimulus in the expected location of the blind spot, 15° temporal to fixation, and slightly inferior to the horizontal meridian. If the patient responds to the stimulus presented at this location, the blind spot is assumed to be here. If the patient does not respond, the perimeter locates the blind spot by presenting suprathreshold stimuli in the area around the expected location of the physiologic blind spot until the blind spot is localized. The sensitivity at individual points in the remainder of the visual field are then determined by a preselected strategy. The different strategies for determining threshold are reviewed in the Appendix. During the course of the test, the computer also tests patient fixation, false positive rate, and false negative rate as described later. After the completion of the test, the perimetrist prints out the results.

WHAT TEST SHOULD I ORDER?

Because the novice perimetrist may be confused by the number of different tests available on automated perimeters and the variables that can be changed within an individual test, the following guidelines are given. For the work-up of visual loss of unknown cause, we perform a full-threshold test of the central 24° or 30° in both eyes with a size III (approximately 4 mm²) white stimulus projected onto a white background. This should pick up the majority of problems affecting central acuity and help with developing a differential diagnosis of the cause of the visual loss.

Depending on the disease process, the visual field in retinal disease may be tested in a variety of ways. Diseases that affect the retina diffusely or primarily in the retinal periphery (such as retinitis pigmentosa, CMV retinitis, retinal detachment, or retinoschisis) should be tested using Goldmann perimetry or a full field threshold-related suprathreshold 120 point test. The latter tests the central and peripheral field extending out to 60° in each meridian, using stimuli 6 dB more intense than the value expected for an individual patient (calculated based on full-thresholding of four points at the beginning of the test). Following progression in these types of retinal diseases involves documentation of enlargement of the visual field defect rather than deepening of the defect, so suprathreshold testing is adequate and much faster. On the other hand, macular diseases (such as drug toxicity or age-related macular degeneration) should be evaluate with central 10°, 24°, or 30° full-threshold tests, which maximize detection of defects centrally and provide the ability to follow disease progression. Figure 4-1 shows the anatomic relationship between the retina and visual field tested with various visual field tests.

For the work-up of the patient with suspected glaucoma, a central 24° or 30° field is used with a size III (provided the vision is not less than 20/80) white stimulus on a white background. More specifically, we prefer the 24-2 program of the Humphrey perimeter, which tests 54 points spaced 6° apart within 24° of fixation, except nasally, which is measured out to 30°. A central 30° field (program 30-2) is acceptable, although the peripheral rim of points is often ignored due to the prevalence of edge or lens rim artifact (Figs. 2-2 through 2-6) and the variability in responses in this peripheral group of points. Figure 1-2 shows the difference between the 24-2 and 30-2 test point locations. Full-threshold or abbreviated threshold (eg, FASTPAC) programs should be used to determine individual sensitivities for the diagnosis of glaucoma, rather than screening suprathreshold programs, which lack the sensitivity needed to diagnose early disease[1] as well as the ability to follow-up disease over time.[2] (As of this writing, the glaucoma hemifield test is not available with the FASTPAC program. This is a disadvantage of substituting this abbreviated testing strategy for the full-threshold strategy, particularly in evaluating those with suspected glaucoma. Chapter 5 reviews the use of the glaucoma hemifield test for evaluating glaucoma suspects as well as alternate criteria for determining whether an early glaucoma defect is present.) For judging progression in glaucoma, the full-threshold or FASTPAC[2] strategies should be employed consistently until an adequate baseline has been established. The patient should then be followed-up using a similar strategy of thresholding or a baseline-related suprathreshold program,[3] which uses answers from the patient's baseline visual field(s) to determine whether individual points have changed. In severe visual field loss from glaucoma, there may only be a small central island remaining. To increase the likelihood of detecting progression in these such patients, the central 5° or 10° may be tested, which increases the number of points that can be followed, as described in chapter 5.

With rare exception (see chapter 8), screening for neurologic diseases that effect the visual pathways may be performed using an age-related central 30° suprathreshold test (central 76-point test).[4] This program tests the same points as the 30-2 program (Fig. 1-2) but presents stimuli that are 6 dB more intense than expected in an age-matched normal population. If the subject sees the stimulus, the point is counted as normal. If the subject does not see the stimulus, the point is retested to confirm that the subject did not see it. The advantage of using the suprathreshold test is that it takes only one fourth of the time, without reducing the sensitivity of determining the presence of neuro-ophthalmic defects.[4] Full-threshold testing of the central 24° or 30° is most appropriate for following known neurologic disease, since deepening of an existing defect would be missed on suprathreshold testing.[5]

A special suprathreshold test, called the blepharoplasty/ptosis screening test, is used in the evaluation of ptosis. This test (Fig. 10-1) maps the superior visual field with and without the upper eyelid taped to document the degree to which ptosis is affecting the

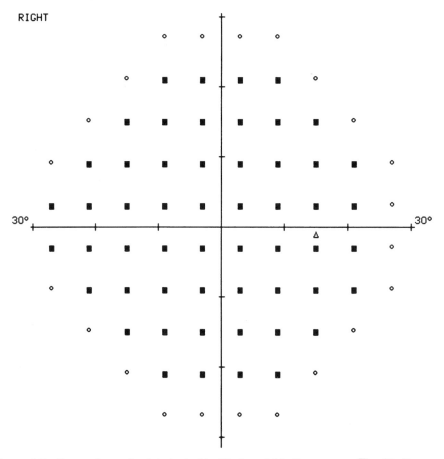

Figure 1-2. Comparison of points tested in 30–2 and 24–2 programs. The 30–2 program tests all 76 points shown above (squares and circles); whereas the 24–2 program tests the 54 points within the central 24° (squares only). Edge artifact and lens rim artifact are difficult to distinguish and are exceedingly common, particularly when testing out to the peripheral 30°. In fact, this artifact is so common that the edge points of the 30° field are largely ignored in interpretation and many clinicians have switched to testing the 24° field, which eliminates the outer edge of points (open circles) except for the two points straddling the horizontal nasal meridian. These two points are tested in the 24–2 program because of the clinical utility of looking for a nasal step in glaucoma suspects. (See chapter 5) (Used with permission from Anderson DR. Automated static perimetry. St. Louis: Mosby–Year Book, 1992:163).

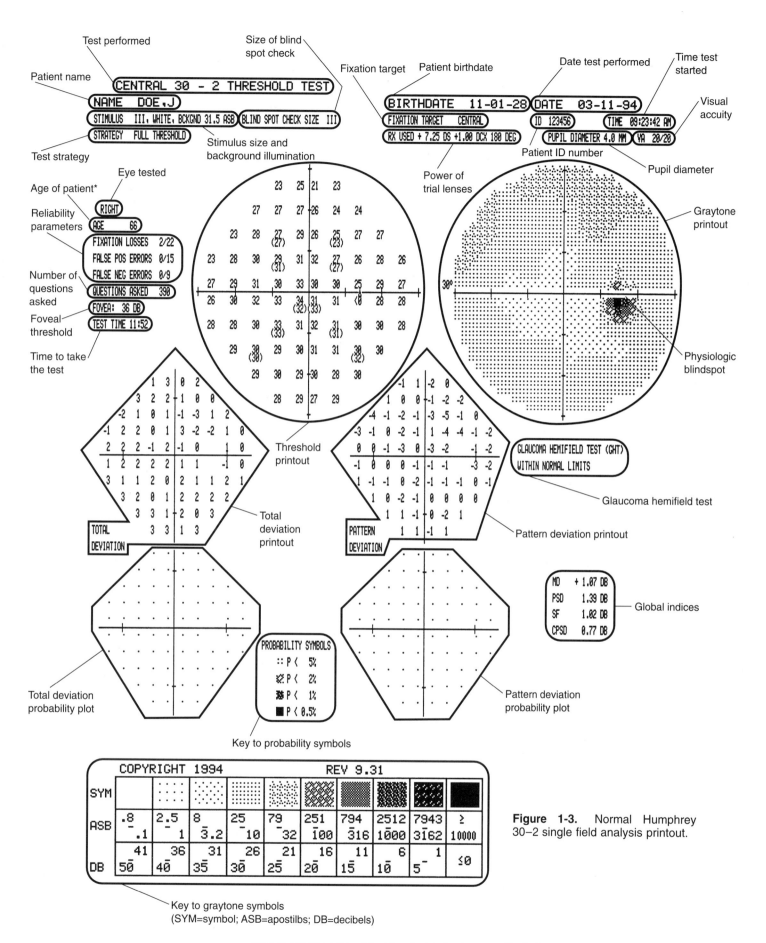

Figure 1-3. Normal Humphrey 30–2 single field analysis printout.

*Age of patient on the printout is calculated using year of test minus year of birth and does not take into account the month.

visual field. Finally, visual disability may be assessed using monocular or binocular suprathreshold testing in which functionally important areas of the visual field (central and inferior to fixation) are weighted more heavily than other areas. This visual field program is called the Esterman test and is described in detail in chapter 11.

If the threshold sensitivities are exceedingly low (<15 dB), or the visual acuity poor, (for example, worse than 20/80) consider increasing the size of the stimulus to size V (approximately 64 mm^2). This will increase the range of points to follow because the new values will have better sensitivities. Patients with a central scotoma and poor visual acuity can still be tested with a size III test object if a different fixation target is used (see Fig. 1-9).

SYSTEMATIC INTERPRETATION OF THE VISUAL FIELD

Like any complex test in medicine, the automated visual field should be interpreted in a systematic fashion. In visual field analysis, it is helpful to organize the approach by answering the following questions as the visual field printout is reviewed:

1. What *type of visual field test* was performed?
2. What are the *patient demographics and clinical characteristics*?
3. How *reliable* is the visual field?
4. Is the visual field *abnormal*?
5. What is the *pattern* of the abnormality?
6. Is the field *worsening*?
7. Is the abnormality or worsening due to *disease or artifact*?

All of this information is available from the printout and every visual field should be interpreted in this systematic fashion so that important information is not overlooked. Finally, the visual field should always be interpreted using as much clinical information as possible. Thus, the visual field is used as an adjunct to a thorough clinical examination of the visual system.

The most commonly performed test in automated perimetry is the 30-2 or 24-2 full threshold test. For orientation, a single field analysis printout is shown and explained in Figure 1-3.

Figure 1-4 shows the equivalent visual field printout of the Octopus perimeter.

Figure 1-4. Normal Octopus Seven-in-One printout. Printout of the Octopus G1X program, which tests 59 points within the central 30°. The location of the points tested is different in the Octopus glaucoma threshold and screening programs (G1, G1X, G2, STX, and ST) than the original Octopus perimeter program 32 or the Humphrey 30−2 program. This pattern of test locations concentrates more on the paracentral and nasal step regions by presenting more points in these areas. The seven-in-one printout provides similar information to the single field analysis printout of the Humphrey perimeter. The *demographic, clinical, test information, and reliability parameters* (catch trials) are contained at the top of the printout. The *mean diffuse depression* (MDD) is a measurement of the amount of lens opacification as measured by a lens opacity meter. The *grayscale of values* and *threshold values* are located just under this. The *threshold printout* gives the sensitivity, in decibels, at each test location as well as the mean sensitivity (MS) in each of the four quadrants, which can be used for comparison with follow-up fields. The *comparison printout* and *probability plot*, in the lower left, are similar to the *total deviation printout* and *total deviation probability plots* on the Humphrey single field analysis printout described below. The *corrected comparison printout* and *probability plot*, in the lower center, are similar to the pattern deviation printout and probability plot of the Humphrey single field analysis printout. The graph in the lower right is a *defect (Bebie) curve*, which is a graph of the sensitivities of the subject compared with age-matched controls. The *global indices*, found in the lower right corner of the printout, give the MS of the entire field, mean defect (MD, similar to mean deviation), loss variance (LV, similar to pattern standard deviation), corrected loss variance (CLV, similar to corrected pattern standard deviation), short-term fluctuation (SF), and reliability factor (RF). The reliability factor is based on the false positive and false negative errors in the catch trials; values from 0% to 15% are considered acceptable. (Courtesy of Tom Tomasso, Interzeag)

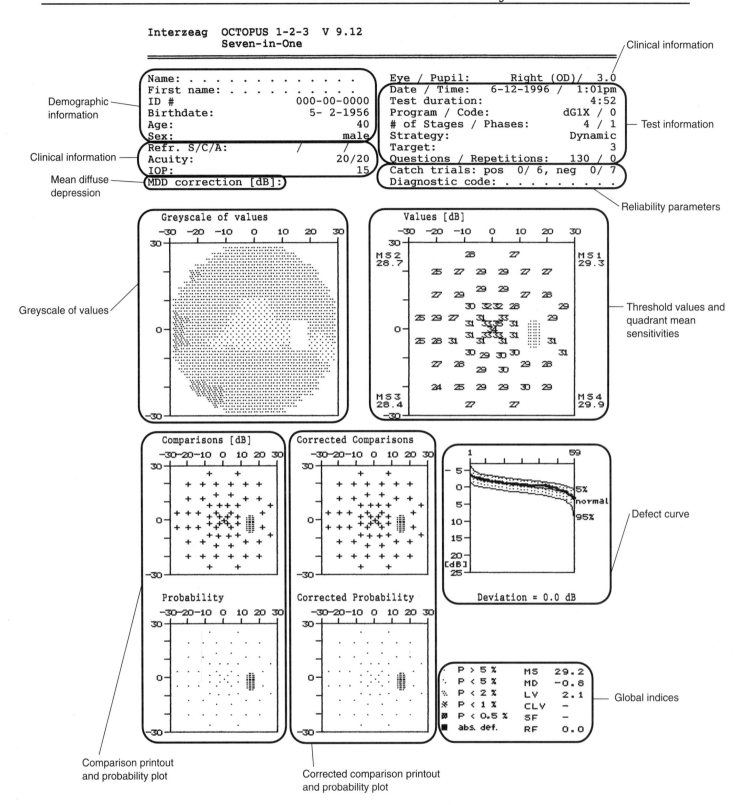

WHAT TYPE OF VISUAL FIELD TEST WAS PERFORMED?

The following information related to the type of test and testing parameters is contained at the top of the visual field printout: region of the visual field tested, pattern of stimuli tested,* stimulus size, stimulus color, intensity of background illumination, size of the stimulus used to map the blind spot, and testing strategy used to determine the threshold values. The fixation target used is typically central, although patients with central scotomas who may have difficulty fixating on the central target can be tested by looking in the central region of four fixation lights arranged in a diamond. All of the above parameters can be modified in particular testing situations as outlined in the Humphrey Field Analyzer Owner's Manual. (Allergan Humphrey, San Leandro, CA)

WHAT ARE THE PATIENT CHARACTERISTICS?

Important demographic and clinical information is available at the top of the printout, including the patient's name, birth date, date of the visual field, patient identification number (ID), time the test was started, corrective lenses used in testing the patient, pupil diameter, visual acuity, eye tested, and age of the patient. In addition, the time it took the patient to take the test (test time) and the number of questions asked are recorded.

HOW RELIABLE IS THE VISUAL FIELD?

The Humphrey perimeter has multiple measures of reliability built in to the test procedure. These include measurements of fixation loss rate, false positive rate, false negative rate, and short-term fluctuation.

Fixation Loss Rate

The fixation loss rate is quantified to get a rough estimate of the percentage of the time the patient fails to look at the central fixation light. It is determined by projecting approximately 5% of the stimuli within the patient's blind spot, which is located at the beginning of the test, as previously described. The ratio of fixation losses/fixation loss trials is recorded in the upper left corner of the single field analysis printout (see Fig. 1-3). The fixation loss trials are concentrated toward the beginning of the test so that the perimetrist can determine early in the course of the test whether a problem with fixation exists. If fixation losses are high, it may mean that the patient is not looking straight ahead a good portion of the time. Fixation losses greater than 20% produce an ''xx'' next to the proportion of fixation losses, along with the message ''low patient reliability.'' Figures 1-5 and 1-6 are examples of patients with high fixation losses from poor reliability.

A high fixation loss rate is very common and usually underestimates visual field loss in glaucoma patients but not normals.[6] Because fixation losses are determined by projecting a target in the presumed location of the blind spot, two other explanations for high fixation losses are that the blind spot was determined incorrectly (Fig. 1-7) or that the patient has a high false positive rate (Figs.1-10, 1-11).[7] Such instances are very common, perhaps more common than actual instances of poor fixation.[8] For this reason, we generally accept a fixation loss rate of up to 33% before declaring a field unreliable.

Incorrect determination of the blind spot (Fig. 1-7) is suspected during the test when the fixation alarm sounds (prompted by 2 out of 5 fixation losses) but the patient appears

(text continues on page 12)

---

* The notation 24-2 denotes that the central 24° is tested and the central points tested are offset from the horizontal and vertical meridians. Testing these points is not considered clinically useful in testing the visual field in diseases of the visual pathways because of the importance of determining whether visual field defects respect the vertical or horizontal meridians.

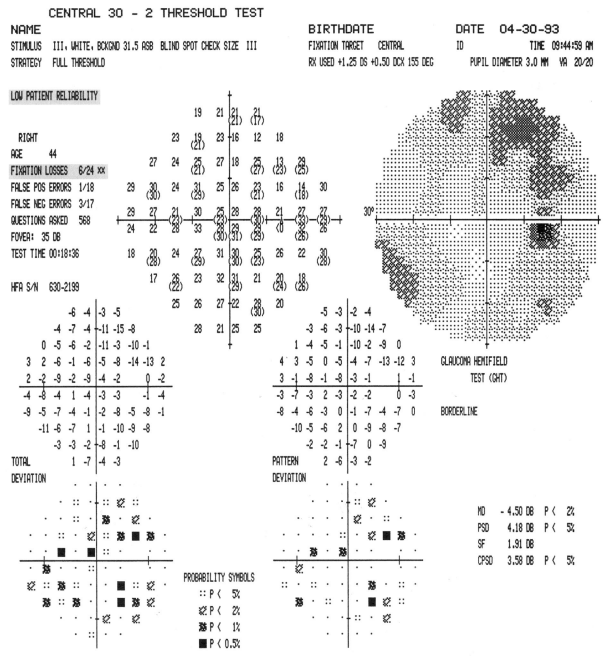

Figure 1-5. High fixation losses. Central 30° field of the right eye of a 44-year-old patient with unexplained visual complaints following corneal foreign body removal. The visual field shows reduction of sensitivity in all quadrants with no localizing pattern. Note high fixation losses and "low patient reliability" message. The perimetrist's comment of "poor patient fixation" confirmed the suspicion that the high fixation loss rate was real, rather than artifactual.

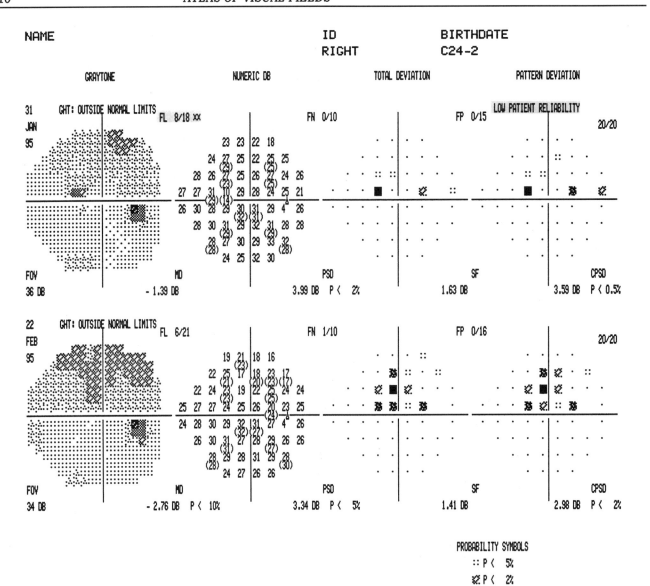

Figure 1-6. High fixation losses. Serial 24° fields of a 70-year-old glaucoma patient. The initial field obtained (*top*) had a high fixation loss rate, which prompted the "low patient reliability" message. The repeat field, which contained fewer fixation losses, is slightly worse. These fields show how high fixation losses can underestimate the severity of visual field loss in glaucoma patients.

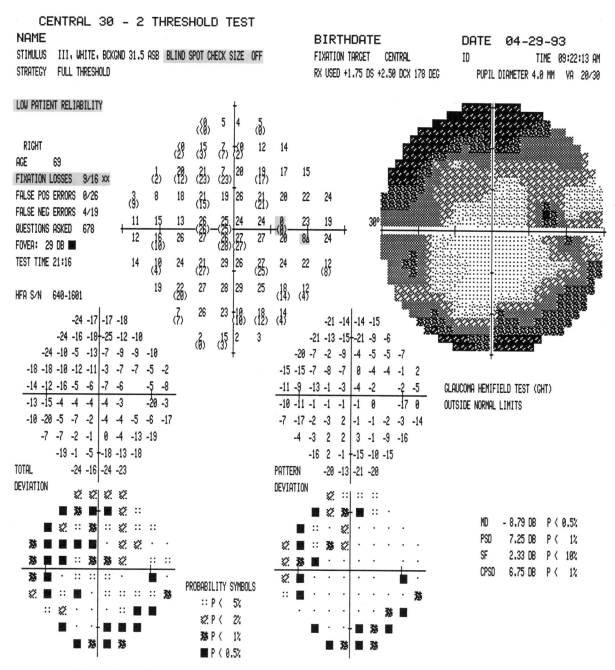

Figure 1-7. High fixation loss from incorrect blind spot localization. Central 30–2 full threshold visual field of the right eye of a 69-year-old glaucoma suspect. The field is abnormal, showing superior and inferior defects that are worst superonasally. However, the fixation loss rate is over 20%, prompting the "xx" notation and the "low patient reliability" message (*highlighted*). In addition, the blind spot check size reads "off," indicating that the perimetrist decided to stop checking for fixation losses after 16 trials, because the patient demonstrated such poor fixation. Note that in the threshold printout, the blind spot was originally mapped to the location given by the small triangle, but later, a sensitivity of 8 dB was obtained in this location. The patient's true blind spot is probably located 15° temporal to fixation, a location that has an isolated absolute scotoma (0 dB and < 0 dB).

to be looking at the central fixation target (as determined by the perimetrist's observation through the video eye monitor or telescope). When this happens, either the blind spot can be replotted or the size of the blind spot check size can be reduced. If the blind spot cannot be plotted, then the blind spot check can be turned off, which will discontinue the fixation loss part of the program. In this case, the perimetrist must monitor fixation visually and comment on fixation using direct observation (which is how fixation was measured during the ''olden days'' of Goldmann perimetry).

The new Humphrey perimeters have a built-in gaze tracking system, which uses a continuous infrared sensor to detect deviation of the eye from central fixation. Eyelid or eyelash ptosis interferes with the sensor, but taping the upper eyelid open (which probably should be done on these patients anyway) allows the gaze tracking system to function. Figure 1-8 is an example of a visual field performed with the new gaze tracking device.

Patients may have poor fixation for physiologic reasons, such as poor vision or a central scotoma (Figure 1-9). Patients with a central scotoma may have difficulty fixating on the central fixation target. If this is the cause of high fixation losses, the central target may be replaced by a small or large diamond of lights (depending on the size of the central scotoma). Figure 1-1 shows the location of these alternate fixation locations.

If the patient is responding to the noise of the machine setting up to deliver a stimulus, rather than the visual stimulus, or is ''trigger-happy'' and pushes the response button frequently when stimuli are not presented, a false positive rate will accompany the high fixation loss rate (Figures 1-10 and 1-11).

False Positive Errors

False positive errors are determined by the analyzer setting up to project a stimulus (with all the accompanying mechanical noises and appropriate time delay) but then not projecting one. If the patient presses the response button in this situation, a false positive response is counted. The ratio of false positives to false positive trials is noted in the upper left of the single field analysis printout. If the false positive rate exceeds 33%, an ''xx'' appears next to the number of false positives and the ''low patient reliability'' message appears above the reliability parameters. In all likelihood, the field becomes unreliable long before 33% false positives are measured, and even two false positive responses should create doubts as to the reliability of the test.

A high false positive rate may indicate a ''trigger happy'' patient (one who is so eager to respond to the next stimulus that he responds to the time delay or sounds before the stimulus is actually presented), a patient who does not understand the test instructions, or a patient who is unable to maintain fixation. Patients with high false positive responses almost always have a high fixation loss message. This happens for one of two reasons. Most commonly, patients who are ''trigger happy'' may respond to stimuli presented in the blind spot despite good fixation. Alternatively, if the primary problem is poor fixation, the patient will see the stimuli presented in the location determined at the beginning of the test to represent the physiologic blind spot. The visual field technician's comments regarding fixation are the key to differentiating these two circumstances. A high false positive rate combined with high fixation losses generally produces an artificially good visual field and causes difficulty with interpretation in following visual field defects.

Sometimes the patient is operating with the mind-set that the automated field test is like a game show and that he or she needs to press the button quickly, maybe before the stimulus (which shines for 0.2 seconds), goes off (ie, pressing the button twice in response to a single stimulus). The patient should be instructed that a deliberate, accurate response is necessary, and that there is an ample interval after the light is shown during which the machine waits to see if there is a response.

(text continues on page 17)

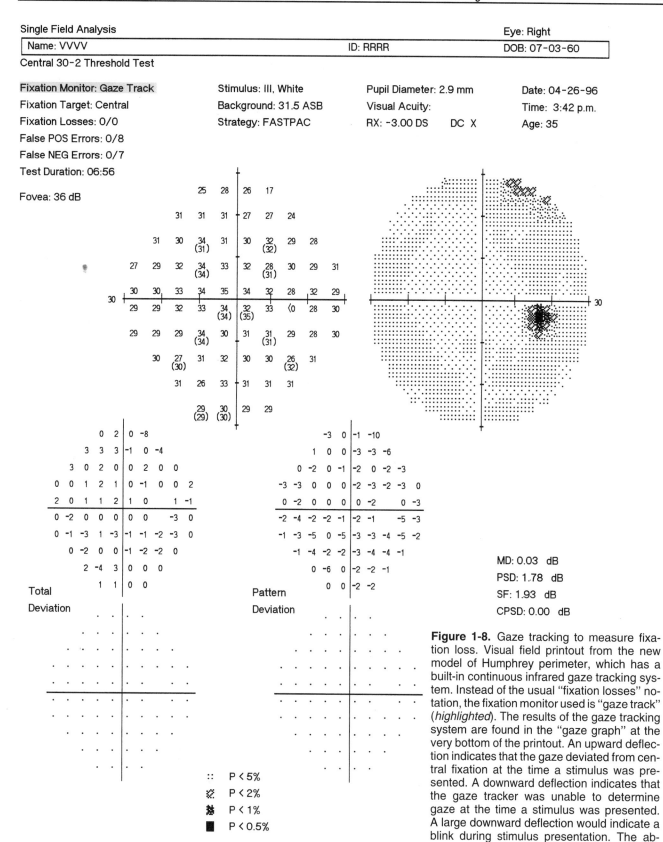

Single Field Analysis

Eye: Right

| Name: VVVV | ID: RRRR | DOB: 07-03-60 |

Central 30-2 Threshold Test

Fixation Monitor: Gaze Track

Fixation Target: Central

Fixation Losses: 0/0

False POS Errors: 0/8

False NEG Errors: 0/7

Test Duration: 06:56

Fovea: 36 dB

Stimulus: III, White

Background: 31.5 ASB

Strategy: FASTPAC

Pupil Diameter: 2.9 mm

Visual Acuity:

RX: -3.00 DS   DC X

Date: 04-26-96

Time: 3:42 p.m.

Age: 35

Total Deviation

Pattern Deviation

MD: 0.03 dB

PSD: 1.78 dB

SF: 1.93 dB

CPSD: 0.00 dB

:: P < 5%

⸬ P < 2%

P < 1%

■ P < 0.5%

Figure 1-8. Gaze tracking to measure fixation loss. Visual field printout from the new model of Humphrey perimeter, which has a built-in continuous infrared gaze tracking system. Instead of the usual "fixation losses" notation, the fixation monitor used is "gaze track" (*highlighted*). The results of the gaze tracking system are found in the "gaze graph" at the very bottom of the printout. An upward deflection indicates that the gaze deviated from central fixation at the time a stimulus was presented. A downward deflection indicates that the gaze tracker was unable to determine gaze at the time a stimulus was presented. A large downward deflection would indicate a blink during stimulus presentation. The absence of any markings indicates central fixation. Note three periods during this test when gaze was poor, as indicated by upward deflections in the gaze graph.

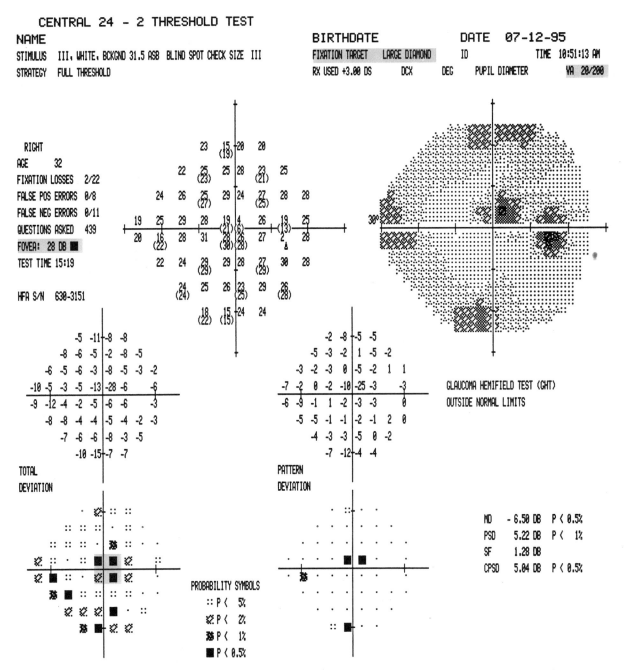

CENTRAL 24 - 2 THRESHOLD TEST

NAME   BIRTHDATE   DATE 07-12-95
STIMULUS III, WHITE, BCKGND 31.5 ASB BLIND SPOT CHECK SIZE III   FIXATION TARGET LARGE DIAMOND   ID   TIME 10:51:13 AM
STRATEGY FULL THRESHOLD   RX USED +3.00 DS   DCX   DEG PUPIL DIAMETER   VA 20/200

RIGHT
AGE   32
FIXATION LOSSES   2/22
FALSE POS ERRORS 0/8
FALSE NEG ERRORS 0/11
QUESTIONS ASKED   439
FOVEA: 28 DB ■
TEST TIME 15:19

HFA S/N 630-3151

TOTAL
DEVIATION

PATTERN
DEVIATION

GLAUCOMA HEMIFIELD TEST (GHT)
OUTSIDE NORMAL LIMITS

PROBABILITY SYMBOLS
:: P < 5%
▨ P < 2%
▩ P < 1%
■ P < 0.5%

MD   - 6.50 DB   P < 0.5%
PSD   5.22 DB   P < 1%
SF   1.28 DB
CPSD   5.04 DB   P < 0.5%

Figure 1-9. Poor fixation from central scotoma. Central 24° field from a patient with a central scotoma secondary to dominant optic atrophy. The foreal threshold and visual acuity are reduced and the central scotoma is seen best on the total deviation plot. Because of the central scotoma, the patient had poor central fixation and this field was performed using the large diamond for fixation. Patients with poor central acuity from a central scotoma can still undergo testing with a size III stimulus, if the fixation target is changed to the small or large diamond, depending on the size of the central scotoma.

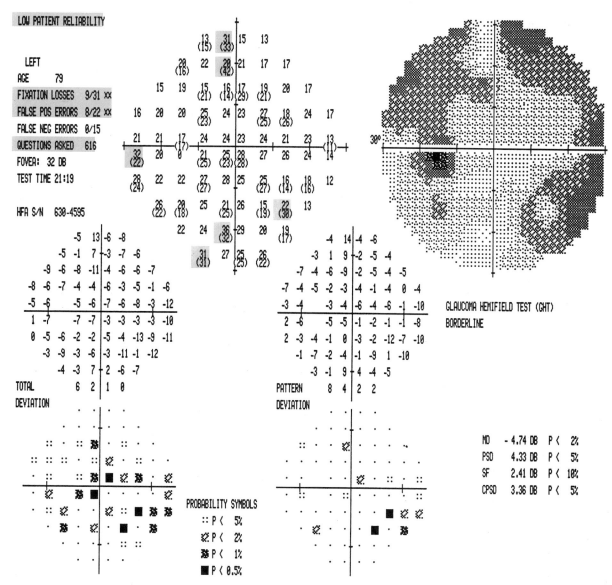

Figure 1-10. High false positive rate and fixation losses. This Central 30° field of the left eye. The visual field shows scattered areas of depression with perhaps a localized defect inferonasally on the pattern deviation plot. There is a high rate of fixation losses and false positive errors, both of which generate the message "low patient reliability." Results of this field are suspect, particularly because the false positive rate is so high. Repeat field testing with reinstruction is indicated. Also note the high number of questions asked (over 600, compared with the usual 400 to 450) and the long time it took to complete the test in this eye (21 minutes, compared with approximately 14 minutes). This is related to the great variability of responses given by this patient, as well as the increased number of double-determined points due to abnormally high thresholds at many points from false positive responses. (Highlighted in threshold printout.)

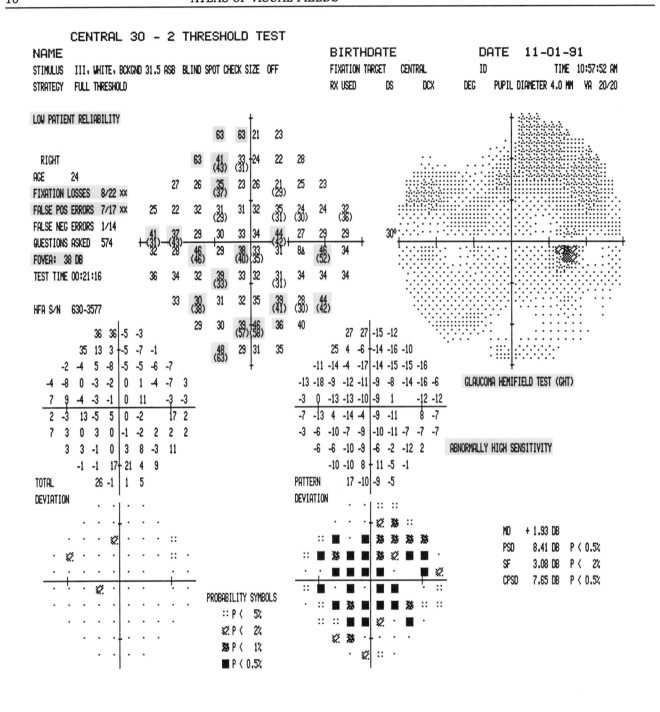

CENTRAL 30 - 2 THRESHOLD TEST

NAME

STIMULUS   III, WHITE, BCKGND 31.5 ASB   BLIND SPOT CHECK SIZE   OFF

STRATEGY   FULL THRESHOLD

BIRTHDATE   DATE 11-01-91

FIXATION TARGET CENTRAL   ID   TIME 10:57:52 AM

RX USED   DS   DCX   DEG   PUPIL DIAMETER 4.0 MM   VA 20/20

LOW PATIENT RELIABILITY

RIGHT

AGE   24

FIXATION LOSSES 8/22 xx

FALSE POS ERRORS 7/17 xx

FALSE NEG ERRORS 1/14

QUESTIONS ASKED   574

FOVEA: 38 DB

TEST TIME 00:21:16

HFA S/N   630-3577

GLAUCOMA HEMIFIELD TEST (GHT)

ABNORMALLY HIGH SENSITIVITY

MD   + 1.93 DB

PSD   8.41 DB   P < 0.5%

SF   3.08 DB   P < 2%

CPSD 7.65 DB   P < 0.5%

TOTAL DEVIATION

PATTERN DEVIATION

PROBABILITY SYMBOLS

:: P < 5%

▨ P < 2%

▨ P < 1%

■ P < 0.5%

GRAYTONE SYMBOLS						REV AK			
SYM	:·:	·:·	:::	▦	▨	▨	▩	▨	■
ASB	.8 .1	2.5 1	8 3.2	25 10	79 32	251 100	794 316	2512 1000	7943 3162	≥ 10000
DB	41 50	36 40	31 35	26 30	21 25	16 20	11 15	6 10	1 5	≤0

BASCOM PALMER EYE INST.

4TH. FLOOR

GLAUCOMA

COMMENTS...............

HUMPHREY INSTRUMENTS

A CARL ZEISS COMPANY

False Negative Errors

False negative errors are determined when the perimeter presents suprathreshold stimuli in locations that have previously been determined to have better sensitivities than the suprathreshold stimulus. If the patient fails to respond, a false negative error is recorded. If the number of false negative responses exceeds 33%, an ''xx'' appears next to the number of false negatives and the ''low patient reliability'' message appears above the reliability parameters. A high number of false negative responses may indicate inattentiveness (Figure 2-12), poor fixation (Figure 1-13), fatigue (Figure 2-14), or malingering (Figures 1-14 and 9-1) and produces an artificially poor visual field. It is also possible for false negative responses to occur in fields with broad areas of relative abnormality. This occurs because, with fatigue, a stimulus that was previously visible may become invisible as test time increases (see figure 2-15 and accompanying legend).

Short-Term Fluctuation

Short-term fluctuation is a measure of normal physiologic variation and intratest reliability. It is measured when the analyzer double-determines 10 preselected points during the course of the test session. The location of these points is important to keep in mind when differentiating the causes of high short-term fluctuation (Figure 1-15). The short-term fluctuation appears at the lower right of the single field analysis printout, along with the global indices and is the standard deviation of the threshold values obtained with repeat determination. Short-term fluctuation is a continuum and is recorded in decibels. The probability that the patient's short-term fluctuation would be found in the normal population is given as a *P* value. High short-term fluctuation may be caused by poor test taking (Figure 1-15), poor fixation (Figure 1-16), high false positive errors (Figure 1-17), or a scotoma which either encompasses, or is adjacent to, one or more of the 10 points used to determine short-term fluctuation (Figure 1-18). Short-term fluctuation is also used in calculating the corrected pattern standard deviation and is taken into account when judging progression of the visual field in glaucoma (Chapter 5).

IS THE VISUAL FIELD ABNORMAL?

Having determined that the visual field is reliable, the next step is to determine whether the field is normal or abnormal. Information about the normality of the visual field may be obtained by looking at the threshold printout, foveal threshold, graytone printout total deviation printout and probability plot, mean deviation, and glaucoma hemifield test.

(text continues on page 25)

Figure 1-11. High false positive rate and fixation losses. Sometimes a high false positive rate will produce a "supranormal" visual field, as evidenced by "white scotomas" on the graytone printout and the message "abnormally high sensitivity" on the glaucoma hemifield test. This visual field demonstrates this phenomenon. The graytone symbols, at the bottom of the printout, are included to demonstrate the fact that the white areas of the visual field represent area with sensitivities of greater than 40 dB, which is nonphysiologic. The total deviation plot is normal because almost all of the patients responses exceed the sensitivities of age-matched controls, as evidenced by the fact that all the numbers in the total deviation plot are positive integers. The pattern deviation plot appears abnormal because the normal points seem depressed relative to the supranormal points, which are highlighted in the threshold printout. Any time you can identify points in the threshold printout that have higher sensitivity than the foveal threshold (except in patients with a central scotoma), chances are those sensitivities are artificially high owing to false positive responses.

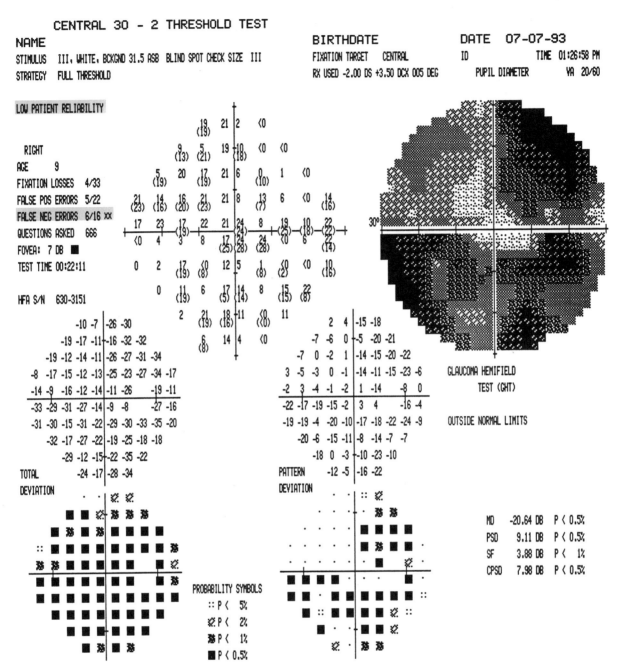

Figure 1-12. High false negative rate. Visual field of a 9-year-old girl with glaucoma secondary to Axenfeld-Reiger's syndrome. Note the high false negative rate, which has prompted the "low patient reliability" message.

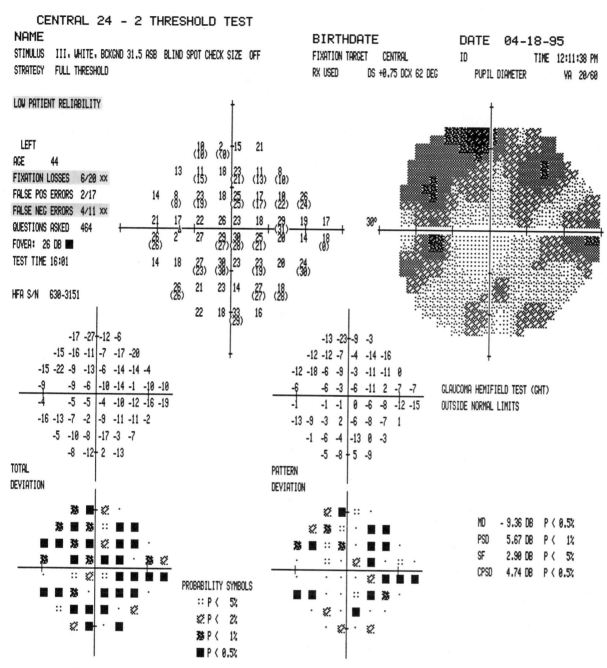

```
CENTRAL 24 - 2 THRESHOLD TEST
NAME                                        BIRTHDATE           DATE  04-18-95
STIMULUS  III, WHITE, BCKGND 31.5 ASB  BLIND SPOT CHECK SIZE  OFF    FIXATION TARGET   CENTRAL      ID              TIME 12:11:38 PM
STRATEGY   FULL THRESHOLD                   RX USED      DS +0.75 DCX 62 DEG   PUPIL DIAMETER          VA  20/60

LOW PATIENT RELIABILITY


   LEFT
AGE     44
FIXATION LOSSES   6/20 xx
FALSE POS ERRORS  2/17
FALSE NEG ERRORS  4/11 xx
QUESTIONS ASKED   464
FOVEA: 26 DB ■
TEST TIME 16:01

HFA S/N   630-3151
```

TOTAL
DEVIATION

PATTERN
DEVIATION

PROBABILITY SYMBOLS
:: P < 5%
※ P < 2%
▩ P < 1%
■ P < 0.5%

GLAUCOMA HEMIFIELD TEST (GHT)
OUTSIDE NORMAL LIMITS

MD   - 9.36 DB   P < 0.5%
PSD   5.67 DB   P < 1%
SF   2.90 DB   P < 5%
CPSD   4.74 DB   P < 0.5%

Figure 1-13. High false negative errors from poor fixation. Patients who have poor fixation may not be fixating centrally at the time the suprathreshold stimuli are presented in the determination of false negative errors. If the stimulus falls on an area of the retina that is less sensitive because of poor fixation, a false negative error will be recorded. This visual field shows a high fixation loss rate and high false negative errors, which prompted the "low patient reliability" message.

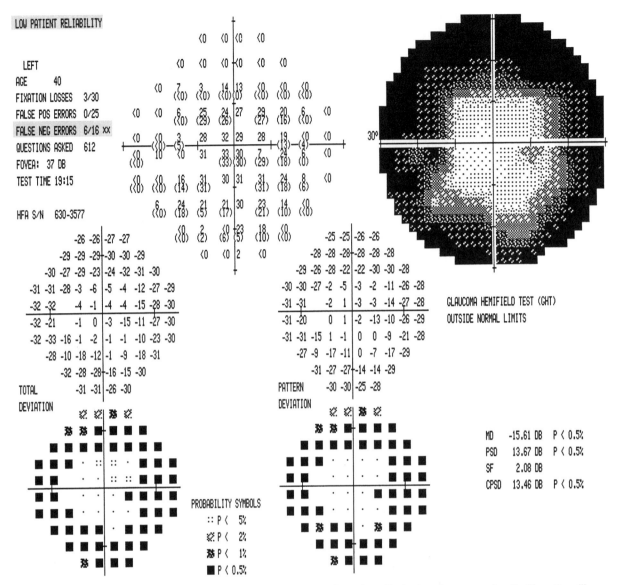

Figure 1-14. High false negative errors from malingering. Patients who present with "functional" or nonphysiologic visual field defects often present with constricted visual fields, as did the patient shown above. The patient's visual field abnormality was out of proportion to the findings on examination, which prompted Tangent screen testing at 1 and 3 meters. The visual field did not expand and the patient was diagnosed to be malingering. The high false negative rate is from the patient intentionally not responding to suprathreshold stimuli.

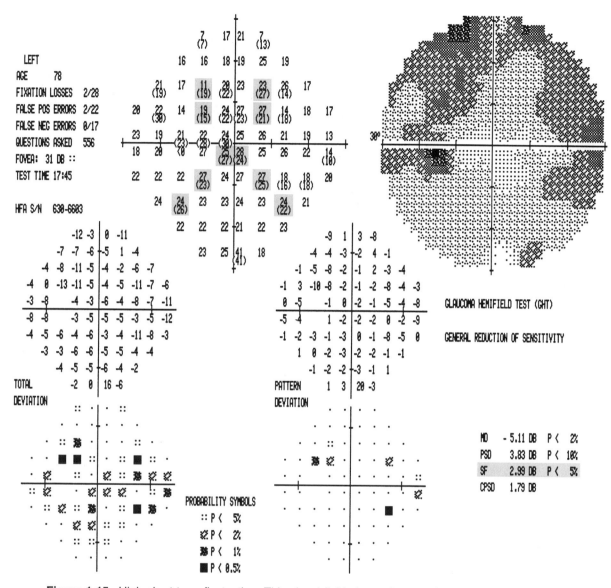

Figure 1-15. High short-term fluctuation. This visual field shows the 10 points that are double-determined for the calculation of short-term fluctuation. In this case, the short-term fluctuation is 2.99 dB, which would be expected in less than 5% percent of the population.

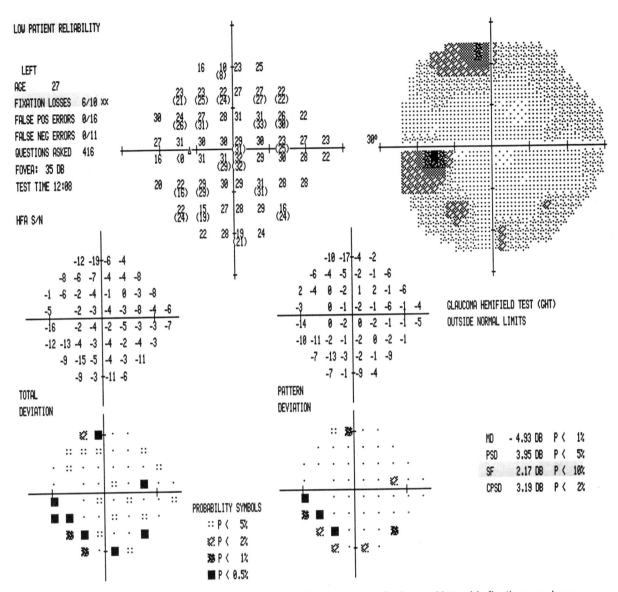

LOW PATIENT RELIABILITY

LEFT
AGE   27
FIXATION LOSSES   6/10 xx
FALSE POS ERRORS 0/16
FALSE NEG ERRORS 0/11
QUESTIONS ASKED   416
FOVEA: 35 DB
TEST TIME 12:08

HFA S/N

16   10 23   25
        (8)
    23 23 22 27 27 22
    (21)(25)(24)   (27)(22)
30 24 27 28 31 31 26 22
    (26)(31)   (33)(30)
27 31 30 30 29 30 23 27 23   30°
16 (0 31 31 31   (25)28 22
            (29)(32)
20 22 23 30 29 31 28 28
    (16)(29)   (31)
    22 15 27 28 29 16
    (24)(19)   (24)
        22 28 19 24
                (21)

TOTAL DEVIATION

-12 -19 -6 -4
 -8 -6 -7 -4 -4 -8
 -1 -6 -2 -4 -1 0 -3 -8
 -5   -2 -3 -4 -3 -8 -4 -6
-16   -2 -4 -2 -5 -3 -3 -7
-12 -13 -4 -3 -4 -2 -4 -3
 -9 -15 -5 -4 -3 -11
     -9 -3 -11 -6

PATTERN DEVIATION

-10 -17 -4 -2
 -6 -4 -5 -2 -1 -6
  2 -4   0 -2 1   2 -1 -6
 -3   0 -1 -2 -1 -6 -1 -4
-14   0 -2 0 -2 -1 -1 -5
-10 -11 -2 -1 -2   0 -2 -1
 -7 -13 -3 -2 -1 -9
     -7 -1 -9 -4

GLAUCOMA HEMIFIELD TEST (GHT)
OUTSIDE NORMAL LIMITS

PROBABILITY SYMBOLS
:: P < 5%
⊠ P < 2%
▩ P < 1%
■ P < 0.5%

MD   - 4.93 DB   P < 1%
PSD   3.95 DB   P < 5%
SF   2.17 DB   P < 10%
CPSD   3.19 DB   P < 2%

Figure 1-16. High short-term fluctuation with high fixation losses. Patients with trouble fixating may have high short-term fluctuation. When the 10 points used to determine short-term fluctuation are checked the second time, the two points will differ if the patient is not fixating in the same location as the first check. This field shows a slightly elevated short-term fluctuation, possibly as a result of a high fixation loss rate. When the 10 points used to determine short-term fluctuation are checked the second time, the two points will differ if the patient is not fixating in the same location as the first check.

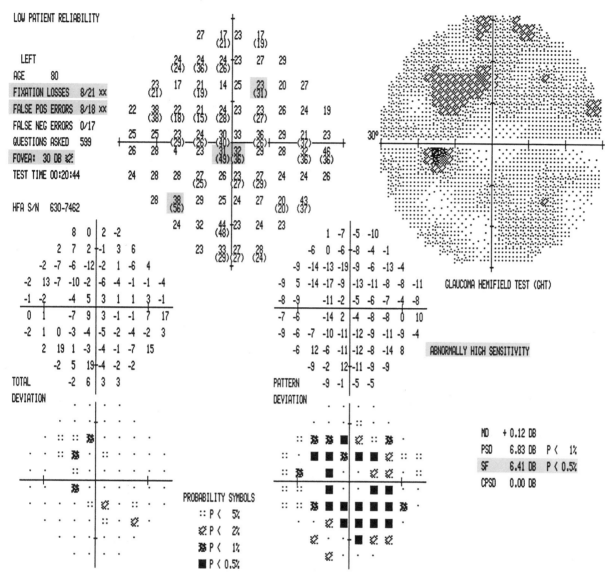

Figure 1-17. High short-term fluctuation from high false positive rate. High short-term fluctuation, which is a measure of intratest variability in responses, may be found in the "trigger-happy" patient, who responds to stimuli that are not really seen, as reflected in the false positive errors. In this field, the thresholds of many of the 10 points used to calculate short-term fluctuation vary widely. Some reflect high intratest difference, but others (*highlighted*) are higher than the foveal threshold, which is physiologically impossible (in the absence of a central scotoma). They are high because the patient is responding to the noise of the machine setting up to present the stimuli or pressing the response button too soon, as described under the false positive section, above. The glaucoma hemifield test has revealed that many of the patient's responses are higher than physiologically expected and declares that the field has an "abnormally high sensitivity." Fixation losses are also high because the patient is responding, inappropriately, to stimuli presented in the blind spot. Typical of patients with a high false positive rate, there are numerous "white scotomas" on the graytone printout.

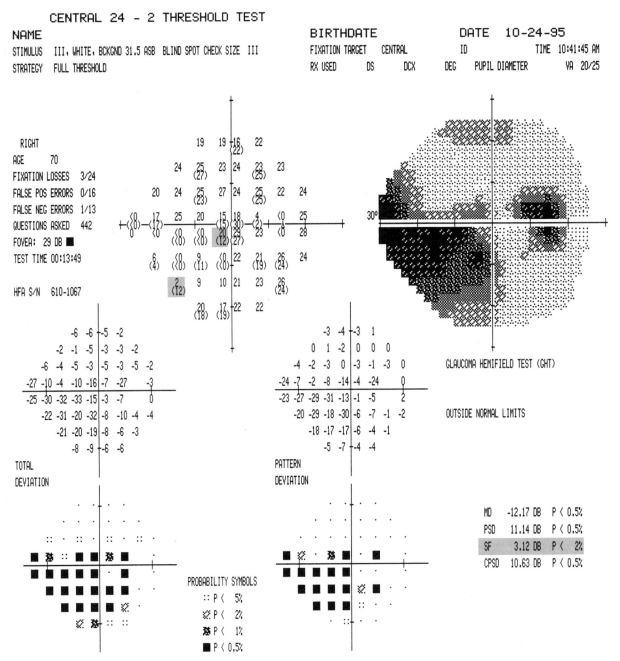

Figure 1-18. High short-term fluctuation from physiologic variability. Responses in automated perimetry are known to be highly variable within or adjacent to a relative scotoma. This visual field from a patient with glaucoma, shows a nasal visual field defect. The short-term fluctuation is high. Note how most of the short-term fluctuation is due to two points that are within the scotoma (*highlighted*), whereas repeat determinations of the other eight points used in determining short-term fluctuation in the more normal areas of the field show good reproducibility. The high short-term fluctuation, therefore, is not due to poor reliability but physiologic variability of points that are tested in areas of the field with reduced sensitivity.

Threshold Printout

The raw data that is obtained by the perimeter is contained in the threshold plot, located at the center of the upper part of the single field analysis printout (see figure 1-3).The sensitivity of the retina at a given location is recorded in decibels (dB), which is a measure of attenuation of light. The higher the decibel reading, the dimmer the stimulus presented. The lower the decibel reading, the brighter the stimulus presented, to a maximum of 0 dB attenuation. A threshold reading of < 0 indicates that the subject could not see the brightest stimulus presented. It is, in fact, rarely necessary to review the information contained in the threshold plot. Exceptions include determination of the cause of high short-term fluctuation and point-wise determination of visual field progression.

Foveal Threshold

Foveal threshold, which measures foveal sensitivity, is determined at the beginning of the test as the patient looks in the center of four lights located inferior to the central fixation light within the perimetry bowl (see figure 1-1). The foveal threshold is measured twice and is recorded in the upper left of the single field printout (see figure 1-3) but not in the threshold printout. If the foveal threshold differs from age-matched controls, a symbol representing the P value is given next to it, denoting the probability that a similar foveal threshold would be found in the normal age-matched population. If significantly abnormal, the patient has some disease process affecting foveal sensitivity, which could be due to media opacification (corneal, lens, or vitreous disease), retinal, optic nerve, or, rarely, chiasmal or diseases posterior to the chiasm. Clinical correlation is necessary to determine the cause of the decreased sensitivity.

Graytone Printout

The graytone printout presents information regarding the abnormality and pattern of the visual field. This printout, in the upper right-hand side of the single field analysis, translates the threshold values into different densities of dots according to the graytone symbol legend at the bottom of the printout (see Figures 1-3, 1-11, and 1-20). The darker the graytone shading appears the deeper the visual field defect.

Total Deviation Printout and Probability Plot

The total deviation printout and probability plot are most useful in determining whether a visual field is abnormal. This consists of two representations of the visual field located at the lower left of the single field printout (see Figure 1-3). The upper of these two printouts is a calculation of the difference, in decibels, between the patient's threshold values and age-corrected normal values at each point measured. If a point has been double-determined, the average of the two values is used to calculate the total deviation. The lower plot is a probability map, which gives a shaded box symbol representing a P value at each point. The key for the probability symbols is to the right of this plot. The P values are interpreted as the likelihood that a specific value would be seen in a normal age-matched population.

Mean Deviation

Mean deviation (MD), one of the global indices listed at the bottom right hand corner of the single field printout, gives the average difference between the patient's overall sensitivity and that of age-matched controls. It is a weighted arithmetic mean of the values contained in the total deviation printout. MD can be negative, indicating below average sensitivity, or positive, indicating above average sensitivity. A P value is provided if the

MD differs significantly from that of age-matched controls. Although the MD provides useful information concerning overall abnormality of a single field and information regarding the worsening or improvement of fields over time, it does not help determine the pattern of the abnormality.

WHAT IS THE PATTERN OF THE ABNORMALITY?

Once the visual field has been declared reliable and abnormal, the pattern of the visual field loss should be characterized. Pattern recognition is an important aspect of visual field interpretation. The visual field provides the opportunity to localize problems with the visual pathways with considerable accuracy. For an outstanding introduction to the topographic analysis of the visual field, the reader is encouraged to read Trobe and Glaser's book, *The Visual Field Manual: A Practical Guide to Testing and Interpretation* (Gainesville: Triad Publishing, 1983).

There are four pieces of information on the single field analysis printout that help determine the pattern of visual field loss: graytone printout, pattern deviation plot, glaucoma hemifield test, and corrected pattern standard deviation.

Graytone Printout

The graytone printout, which has been previously described, may provide information as to the pattern of the visual field defect (Figures 1-20 through 1-22). It is very tempting to interpret the graytone printout in isolation from the rest of the visual field printout because it is visual rather than numeric. However, the graytone printout does not factor in the expected normative data from age-matched controls or the normal decrease in sensitivity as one gets further away from fixation. In addition, the graytone printout does not take into account the phenomenon that localized defects can be superimposed on diffuse depression since it does not adjust for overall depression (or elevation) of the visual field, as does the pattern deviation plot. Examples of the dangers of relying on the graytone printout for pattern interpretation are presented in Figures 1-23 and 1-26.

(text continues on page 34)

Figure 1-19. Diffuse depression of visual field. Visual field of the left eye of a patient with a cataract. The threshold printout is abnormal but is not of any value unless the expected values in the age-matched normal population have been memorized. The foveal threshold is markedly depressed at 25 dB. The black box next to this is a probability symbol. The probability symbol legend, near the bottom of the printout, indicates that this value would be expected to occur in less than 0.5% of age-matched normal subjects. The graytone printout shows the expected black area representing the physiologic blind spot to the left of fixation, diffuse moderate to severe graying of the peripheral field, and a central whiter area. The graytone symbols, at the bottom of the printout, provide the apostilb and decibel values that correspond to the different shades of gray in the graytone printout. The total deviation printout demonstrates that the patient's responses at each location tested differ from the responses of expected age-matched control subjects by -6 to -13 dB. The total deviation probability plot indicates the probability that each of these differences would be found in the normal age-matched population. The mean deviation is -9.97 dB, indicating that, on average, the patients responses differ from those of expected age-matched controls by 9.97 dB. The P value next to the mean deviation indicates that less than 0.5% of the normal age-matched population would be expected to have this mean deviation. The glaucoma hemifield test gives the "general reduction of sensitivity" message, confirming that the field is abnormal and providing information on the pattern of abnormality.

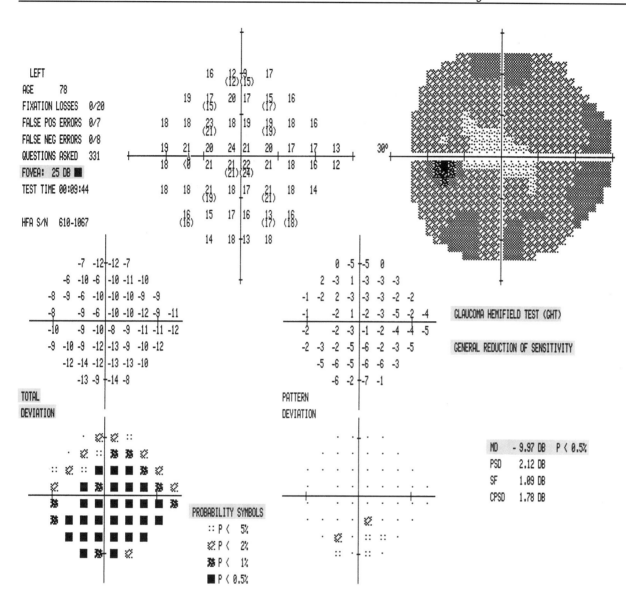

LEFT

AGE   78

FIXATION LOSSES   0/20

FALSE POS ERRORS 0/7

FALSE NEG ERRORS 0/8

QUESTIONS ASKED   331

FOVEA: 25 DB ■

TEST TIME 00:09:44

HFA S/N   610-1067

		16	12 (12)	9 (15)	17		
	19	17 (15)	20	17	15 (17)	16	
	18	18	23 (21)	18	19	19 (19)	18	16
19	21	20	24	21	20	17	17	13
18	(0)	21	21 (21)	22 (24)	21	18	16	12
	18	18	21 (19)	18	17	21 (21)	18	14
	16 (18)	15	17	16	13 (17)	16 (18)	
		14	18	13	18		

30°

TOTAL DEVIATION

		-7	-12	-12	-7		
	-6	-10	-6	-10	-11	-10	
-8	-9	-6	-10	-10	-9	-9	
-8	-9	-6	-10	-10	-12	-9	-11
-10	-9	-10	-8	-9	-11	-11	-12
-9	-10	-9	-12	-13	-9	-10	-12
	-12	-14	-12	-13	-13	-10	
		-13	-9	-14	-8		

PATTERN DEVIATION

		0	-5	-5	0		
	2	-3	1	-3	-3	-3	
-1	-2	2	-3	-3	-3	-2	-2
-1	-2	1	-2	-3	-5	-2	-4
-2	-2	-3	-1	-2	-4	-4	-5
-2	-3	-2	-5	-6	-2	-3	-5
	-5	-6	-5	-6	-6	-3	
		-6	-2	-7	-1		

GLAUCOMA HEMIFIELD TEST (GHT)

GENERAL REDUCTION OF SENSITIVITY

MD   - 9.97 DB   P < 0.5%

PSD   2.12 DB

SF   1.09 DB

CPSD   1.78 DB

PROBABILITY SYMBOLS

:: P < 5%

▨ P < 2%

▩ P < 1%

■ P < 0.5%

GRAYTONE SYMBOLS					REV 6.3				
SYM	⠿	⣿	▦	⣿	▨	▓	▨	▨	■
ASB	.8 – .1	2.5 – 1	8 – 3.2	25 – 10	79 – 32	251 – 100	794 – 316	2512 – 1000	7943 – 3162	≥ 10000
DB	41 50	36 40	31 35	26 30	21 25	16 20	11 15	6 10	1 5	≤0

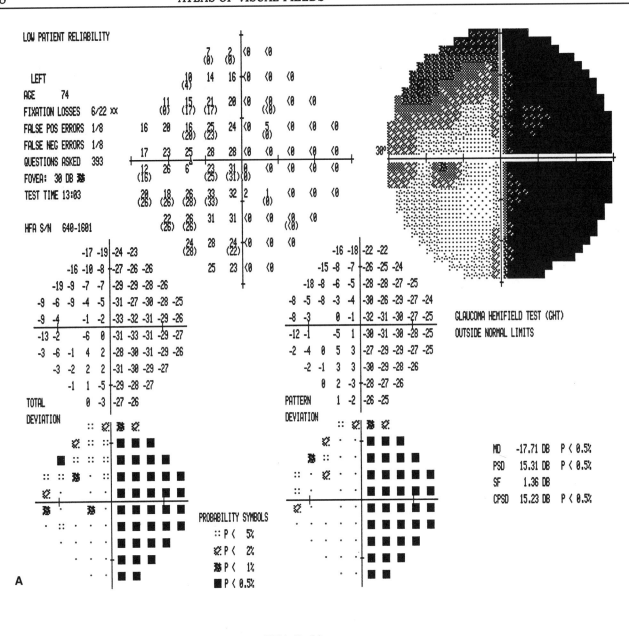

Figure 1-20. Graytone printout. The graytone printout can be helpful in suggesting a particular pattern of field loss. For example, these fields are from the left **(A)** *(continued)*

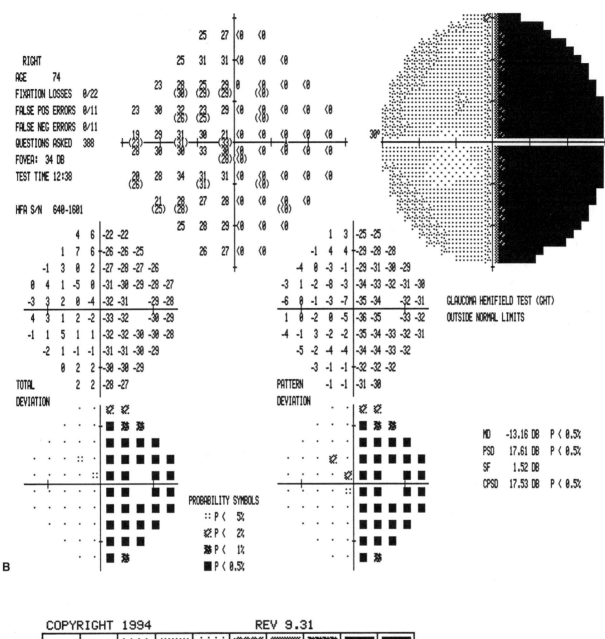

Figure 1-20. *Continued.* and right **(B)** eyes of a patient with encephalomalacia affecting the left parietal and occipital lobes. The graytone printouts show a right complete hemianopic defect. This information could also be obtained by looking at the threshold printout, which shows absolute scotomas (thresholds < 0 dB) on the right side of the fields in both eyes, as well as the total and pattern deviation printouts and their associated plots.

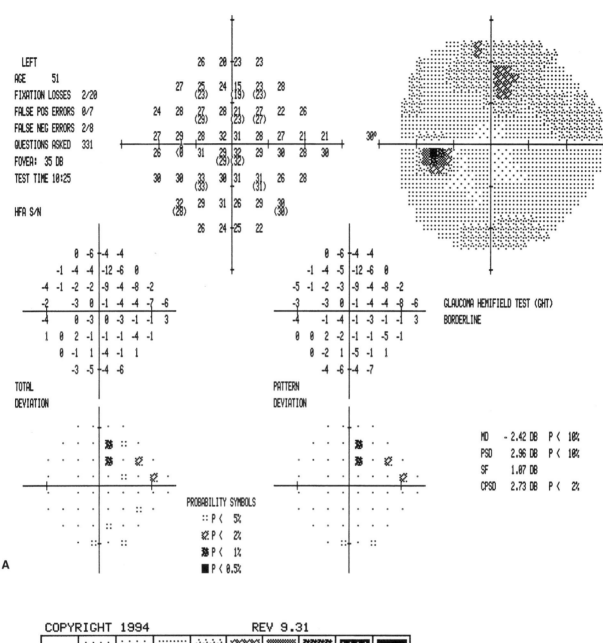

LEFT

AGE   51

FIXATION LOSSES   2/20

FALSE POS ERRORS 0/7

FALSE NEG ERRORS 2/8

QUESTIONS ASKED   331

FOVEA: 35 DB

TEST TIME 10:25

HFA S/N

```
                        26   20 +23  23

                    27   25  24 |15  23  28
                        (23)    (19)(23)

                24  28   27  28 |21  27  22  26
                        (29)    (23)(27)

                27  29   28  32 |31  28  27  21  21      30°

                26  (0   31  29 |32  29  30  28  30
                            (29)(32)

                30  30   33  30 |31  31  26  28
                        (33)        (31)

                    32   29  31 |26  29  30
                    (28)              (30)

                        26   24 +25  22
```

```
          0  -6 +-4  -4                        0  -6 +-4  -4
       -1  -4  -4 |-12 -6   0                -1  -4  -5 |-12 -6   0
    -4  -1  -2  -2 |-9  -4  -8  -2         -5  -1  -2  -3 |-9  -4  -8  -2
    -2      -3   0 |-1  -4  -4  -7  -6         -3      -3   0 |-1  -4  -4  -8  -6
   -4      0  -3 |0   -3  -1  -1   3        -4      -1  -4 |-1  -3  -1  -1   3
    1   0   2  -1 |-1  -1  -4  -1           0   0   2  -2 |-1  -1  -5  -1
       0  -1   1 |-4  -1   1                 0  -2   1 |-5  -1   1
          -3  -5 +-4  -6                        -4  -6 +-4  -7
```

GLAUCOMA HEMIFIELD TEST (GHT)

BORDERLINE

TOTAL
DEVIATION

PATTERN
DEVIATION

PROBABILITY SYMBOLS

:: P < 5%

▨ P < 2%

▩ P < 1%

■ P < 0.5%

MD   - 2.42 DB   P < 10%

PSD   2.96 DB   P < 10%

SF   1.07 DB

CPSD   2.73 DB   P < 2%

A

COPYRIGHT 1994   REV 9.31

SYM									
ASB	.8 – .1	2.5 – 1	8 – 3.2	25 – 10	79 – 32	251 – 100	794 – 316	2512 – 1000	7943 – 3162	≥ 10000
DB	41 50	36 40	31 35	26 30	21 25	16 20	11 15	6 10	1 5	≤0

Figure 1-21. Graytone printout. It is important to look at the graytone printout from both eyes, particularly to look for features suggesting bilateral field defects that may respect the vertical meridian. These fields are from a 50-year-old patient who was followed-up for presumed glaucoma in the right eye for 7 years. The visual field in the right eye *(continued)*

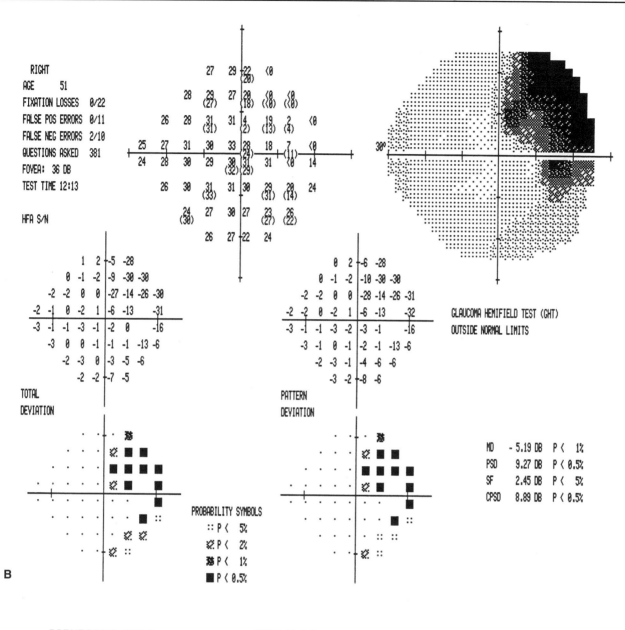

Figure 1-21. *Continued.* **(B)** shows a superior defect that appears to originate at the blind spot but does not cross the vertical meridian. Careful examination of the graytone printout of the left eye **(A)** shows a subtle superior defect, which also lines up along the vertical meridian. An MRI demonstrates an old parenchymal lesion of the left temporal lobe.

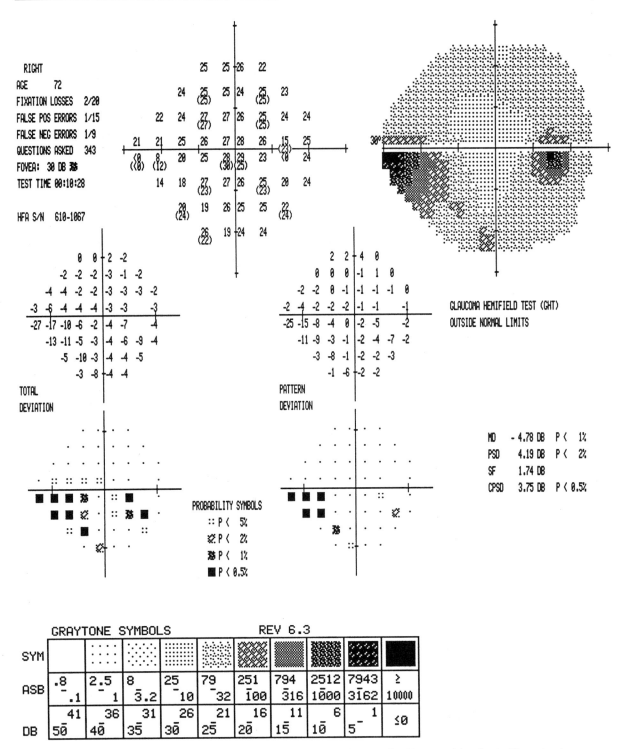

Figure 1-22. Graytone printout. Visual field of the right eye of a 72-year-old patient with early glaucoma. The graytone printout demonstrates the pattern typical of a nasal step in early glaucoma.

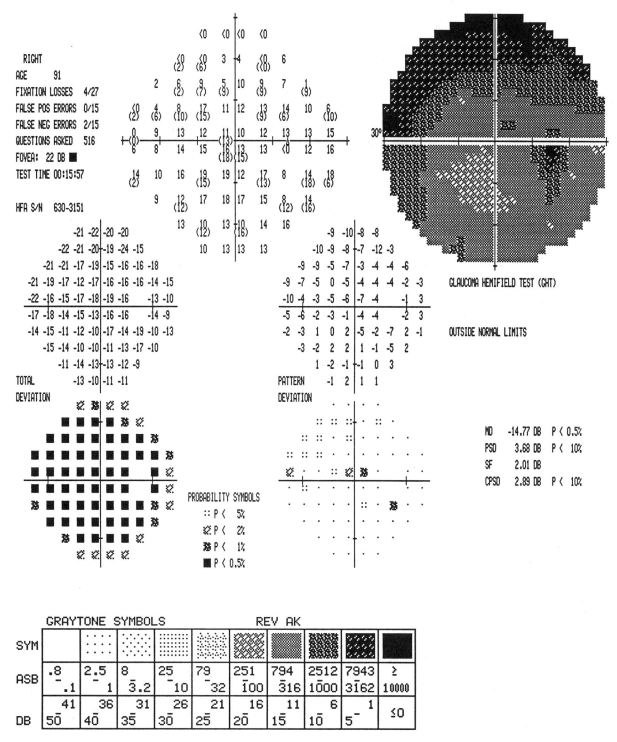

Figure 1-23 data panel:

```
                                    <0   <0 <0   <0
    RIGHT                          <0   <0   3  -4  <0   6
                                   (2)  (6)          (8)
    AGE      91
    FIXATION LOSSES   4/27       2   6   9   5  10  9   7   1
                                   (2) (7) (9)     (9)    (9)
    FALSE POS ERRORS  0/15
    FALSE NEG ERRORS  2/15     <0  4   8  17  11 12  13  14  10  6
                               (2) (6) (10)(15)     (9) (6)    (10)
    QUESTIONS ASKED   516        0   9  13  12  11 10  12  13  13  15
                               (0)              (13)
    FOVEA:  22 DB ■               6   8  14  15  13 13  <0  12  16
                                              (18)(15)
    TEST TIME 00:15:57          14  10  16  19  19 12  17   8  14  18
                               (2)         (15)      (13)   (18)(6)

    HFA S/N   630-3151           9  12  17  18  17 15   8   14
                                   (12)                  (12) (16)

                                13  10  13  10  14  16
                                   (12)    (16)
```

TOTAL DEVIATION

```
        -21 -22 -20 -20
      -22 -21 -20 -19 -24 -15
    -21 -21 -17 -19 -15 -16 -16 -18
  -21 -19 -17 -12 -17 -16 -16 -16 -14 -15
  -22 -16 -15 -17 -18 -19 -16     -13 -10
  -17 -18 -14 -15 -13 -16 -16     -14 -9
  -14 -15 -11 -12 -10 -17 -14 -19 -10 -13
    -15 -14 -10 -10 -11 -13 -17 -10
      -11 -14 -13 -13 -12 -9
TOTAL    -13 -10 -11 -11
DEVIATION
```

PATTERN DEVIATION

```
                      -9 -10 -8 -8
                  -10 -9  -8 -7 -12 -3
              -9 -9 -5 -7 -3 -4 -4 -6
          -9 -7 -5  0 -5 -4 -4 -4 -2 -3
         -10 -4 -3 -5 -6 -7 -4    -1  3
          -5 -6 -2 -3 -1 -4 -4    -2  3
          -2 -3  1  0  2 -5 -2 -7  2 -1
            -3 -2  2  2  1 -1 -5  2
               1 -2 -1 -1  0  3
PATTERN     -1  2  1  1
DEVIATION
```

GLAUCOMA HEMIFIELD TEST (GHT)

OUTSIDE NORMAL LIMITS

MD	-14.77 DB	P < 0.5%
PSD	3.68 DB	P < 10%
SF	2.01 DB	
CPSD	2.89 DB	P < 10%

PROBABILITY SYMBOLS
∷ P < 5%
▨ P < 2%
▩ P < 1%
■ P < 0.5%

GRAYTONE SYMBOLS   REV AK

SYM	··	··	▒	▒	▨	▓	▨	■	■
ASB	.8 - .1	2.5 - 1	8 - 3.2	25 - 10	79 - 32	251 - 100	794 - 316	2512 - 1000	7943 - 3162	≥ 10000
DB	41 - 50	36 - 40	31 - 35	26 - 30	21 - 25	16 - 20	11 - 15	6 - 10	1 - 5	≤0

Figure 1-23. Problem with graytone printout. The graytone printout, if used for interpretation without reviewing the pattern deviation plot, can be misleading. If this field were interpreted using the graytone printout alone, it might be concluded that the patient had generalized depression (from media opacity or diffuse retinal disease) with a superimposed dense superior arcuate nerve fiber bundle defect (from retinal or optic nerve disease). However, after correcting for the patient's age (91) and location of the depression (far superior, which has a higher upper limit for abnormality than more central areas[9]) the field does not appear to contain a significant localized defect in the superior periphery. In fact, the patient had diffuse corneal disease causing the diffuse depression, and cystoid macular edema. The corneal edema was causing the diffuse depression, which is seen on the total deviation plot. Once the computer subtracts the effect of this diffuse depression on the visual field in calculating the pattern deviation plot, a central scotoma is seen, which is due, in this case, to cystoid macular edema.

Pattern Deviation Printout and Probability Plot

The pattern deviation printout and probability plot are the most helpful part of the visual field printout for determining the pattern of a localized abnormality. It is derived from the total deviation plot and subtracts out the effect of diffuse depression of sensitivity or diffuse elevation of sensitivity, thereby making localized defects more apparent. The computer does this by performing a general height adjustment, the details of which may be found in reference 10. The numerical printout shows the deviation of the subject's responses to those of age-matched controls after the effect of diffuse depression or elevation of the visual field has been taken into account. The probability plot indicates the statistical significance at each point and is the part of the visual field which may be relied upon for determining the pattern of visual field abnormality. Examples of the usefulness of the pattern deviation printout and probability plot may be found in Figures 1-24 through 1-27.

Glaucoma Hemifield Test

The glaucoma hemifield test is primarily designed "to identify fields with localized field defects as abnormal."[11] Results of the test are determined by a comparison of five zones in the upper hemifield with five corresponding zones in the lower hemifield (Figure 1-28). Despite the name of the glaucoma hemifield test, not all results of "outside normal limits" are due to glaucoma. Clinical correlation is always recommended to ascertain the cause of the field abnormality. The glaucoma hemifield test also provides information on diffuse depression or elevation of the hill of vision by analyzing the most sensitive points in the total deviation printout.

In the old Humphrey single field analysis printout, one of five messages appears underneath the graytone plot: "within normal limits" (see Figure 1-3), "outside normal limits" (see Figure 1-23), "borderline" (see Figure 1-10), "general reduction of sensitivity" (see Figure 1-20), or "abnormally high sensitivity" (see Figure 1-11). In the new version of Statpac, the relative positivity of the glaucoma hemifield test is also given as a continuum. Fields 1-30 through 1-34 demonstrate the possible results of the glaucoma hemifield test and are presented in this new format.

Corrected Pattern Standard Deviation

The corrected pattern standard deviation (CPSD) is a measure of the degree of localized depression (as opposed to diffuse depression) of the visual field corrected for the patient's age and short-term fluctuation. The higher the CPSD, the greater the chance that a localized area of abnormality exists. If the CPSD is abnormal, a *P* value is provided that gives the percentage of the normal population expected to have that value for CPSD. A high short-term fluctuation (SF) causes a reduction CPSD. In this case, it must be determined, using point-wise analysis of the numeric format printout, whether the high SF is due to physiologic variation in and around scotomas or to poor reliability. If the high SF is due to physiologic variability rather than poor intratest reproducibility, then the CPSD may be artificially low. Figures 1-18, 1-22, 1-24, 1-27, 1-29, and 1-33 are all example of elevated CPSD from localized abnormalities.

ARE THE ABNORMALITIES DUE TO DISEASE OR ARTIFACT?

Once a field has been declared reliable and abnormal, one must ask the important question of whether the abnormality is real or due to testing artifact. Testing artifacts are so common in visual field testing and of such varied types that the entirety of chapter 2 is devoted to the topic.

(text continues on page 45)

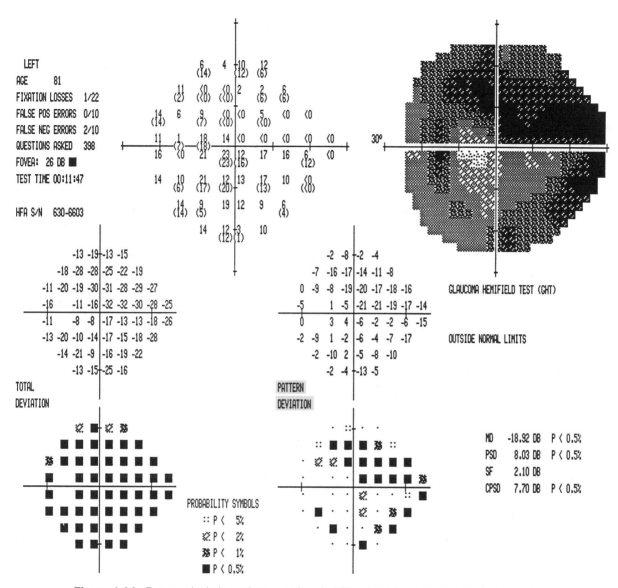

LEFT

AGE   81

FIXATION LOSSES   1/22

FALSE POS ERRORS   0/10

FALSE NEG ERRORS   2/10

QUESTIONS ASKED   398

FOVEA: 26 DB ■

TEST TIME 00:11:47

HFA S/N   630-6603

TOTAL
DEVIATION

PATTERN
DEVIATION

PROBABILITY SYMBOLS

∷ P < 5%

▨ P < 2%

▩ P < 1%

■ P < 0.5%

GLAUCOMA HEMIFIELD TEST (GHT)

OUTSIDE NORMAL LIMITS

MD   -18.92 DB   P < 0.5%

PSD   8.03 DB   P < 0.5%

SF   2.10 DB

CPSD   7.70 DB   P < 0.5%

Figure 1-24. Pattern deviation printout and probability plot. Visual field of the left eye of a glaucoma patient who also has a cataract. The total deviation probability plot is markedly abnormal in all locations and is not helpful in interpreting the pattern of the visual field loss. When the effect of diffuse depression caused by cataract is factored out, the pattern deviation probability plot reveals a dense superior arcuate defect breaking into a nasal step, as well as some possible inferior localized defects, all from glaucoma. In this case, the graytone plot gives essentially the same information.

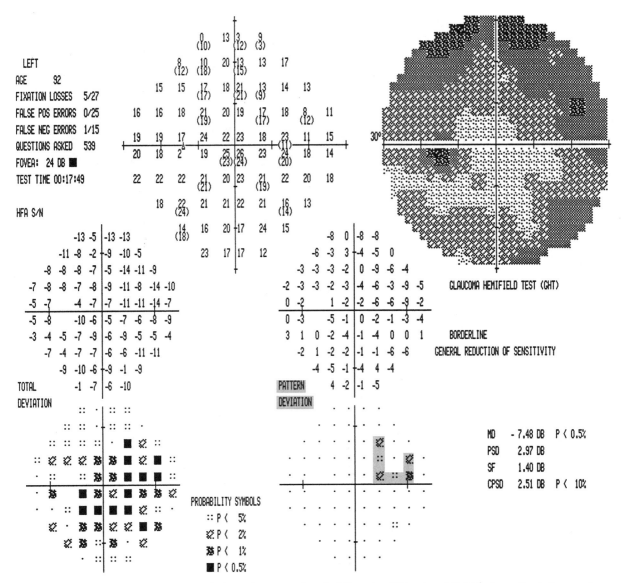

LEFT

AGE   92

FIXATION LOSSES 5/27

FALSE POS ERRORS 0/25

FALSE NEG ERRORS 1/15

QUESTIONS ASKED 539

FOVEA: 24 DB ■

TEST TIME 00:17:49

HFA S/N

TOTAL DEVIATION

PATTERN DEVIATION

PROBABILITY SYMBOLS

∷ P < 5%

▨ P < 2%

▩ P < 1%

■ P < 0.5%

GLAUCOMA HEMIFIELD TEST (GHT)

BORDERLINE

GENERAL REDUCTION OF SENSITIVITY

MD   - 7.48 DB   P < 0.5%

PSD   2.97 DB

SF   1.40 DB

CPSD   2.51 DB   P < 10%

Figure 1-25. Pattern deviation printout and probability plot. This visual field is from the left eye of a patient with diffuse corneal epithelial erosions from radiation keratopathy. She also has elevated intraocular pressure and a larger cup to disc ratio in this eye. The graytone and total deviation printouts show diffuse depression and are not helpful in deciding whether a localized defect from glaucoma might be present. In the pattern deviation probability plot, an early superonasal step can be appreciated (*highlighted*) that fits the criteria for minimal abnormality in diagnosing a localized visual field abnormality (Table 5-1).

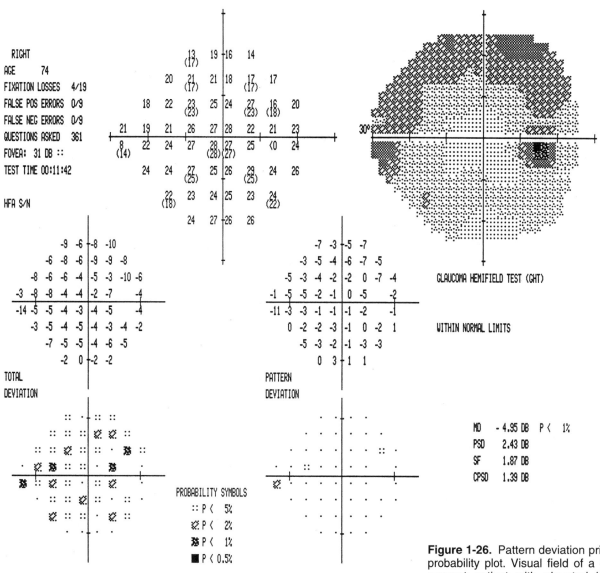

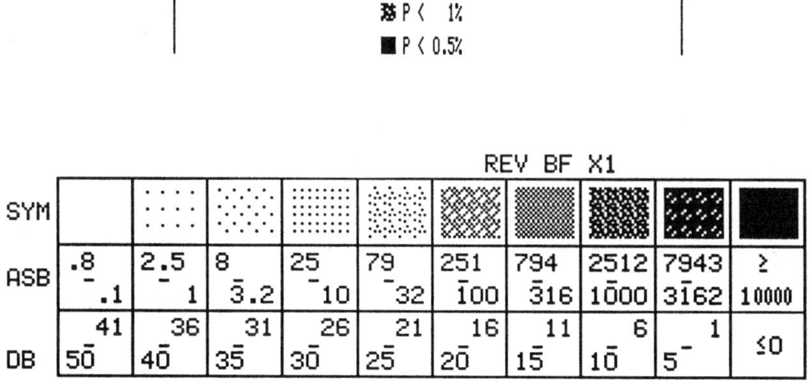

RIGHT

AGE   74

FIXATION LOSSES   4/19

FALSE POS ERRORS   0/9

FALSE NEG ERRORS   0/9

QUESTIONS ASKED   361

FOVEA: 31 DB ::

TEST TIME 00:11:42

HFA S/N

```
                    13   19  16   14
                   (17)
              20    21   21  18   17    17
                   (17)           (17)
        18    22    23   25  24   27   16   20
                   (23)           (23) (18)
  21   19    21    26   27  28   22   21   23
   8   22    24    27   28  27   25  <0   24
  (14)                  (28)(27)
        24    24    27   25  26   29   24   26
                   (25)           (25)
              22    23   24  25   23   24
             (18)                (22)
                    24   27  26   26
```

```
           -9  -6  -8  -10
        -6 -8  -6  -9  -9  -8
     -8 -6  -6  -4  -5  -3 -10 -6
  -3 -8  -8  -4  -4  -2  -7     -4
 -14 -5  -5  -4  -3  -4  -5     -4
  -3 -5  -4  -5  -4  -3  -4  -2
     -7 -5  -5  -4  -6  -5
        -2   0  -2  -2
```

TOTAL
DEVIATION

```
           -7  -3  -5  -7
        -3 -5  -4  -6  -7  -5
     -5 -3  -4  -2  -2   0  -7  -4
  -1 -5  -5  -2  -1   0  -5     -2
 -11 -3  -3  -1  -1  -1  -2     -1
   0 -2  -2  -3  -1   0  -2   1
     -5 -3  -2  -1  -1  -3  -3
        0   3   1   1
```

PATTERN
DEVIATION

GLAUCOMA HEMIFIELD TEST (GHT)

WITHIN NORMAL LIMITS

MD   - 4.95 DB   P < 1%

PSD   2.43 DB

SF   1.87 DB

CPSD   1.39 DB

PROBABILITY SYMBOLS

:: P < 5%

� P < 2%

▨ P < 1%

■ P < 0.5%

Figure 1-26. Pattern deviation printout and probability plot. Visual field of a glaucoma suspect patient with elevated intraocular pressure and cup:disc asymmetry in the right eye. The graytone plot looks rather convincingly like a superior arcuate defect emanating from the blind spot. The inexperienced visual field interpreter might look just at the graytone plot and use this as a basis for treating the patient. The total deviation probability plot shows generalized depression, and the pattern deviation probability plot fails to show any significant localized abnormality.

REV BF X1

SYM									
ASB	.8 .1	2.5 1	8 3.2	25 10	79 32	251 100	794 316	2512 1000	7943 3162	≥ 10000
DB	41 50	36 40	31 35	26 30	21 25	16 20	11 15	6 10	1 5	≤0

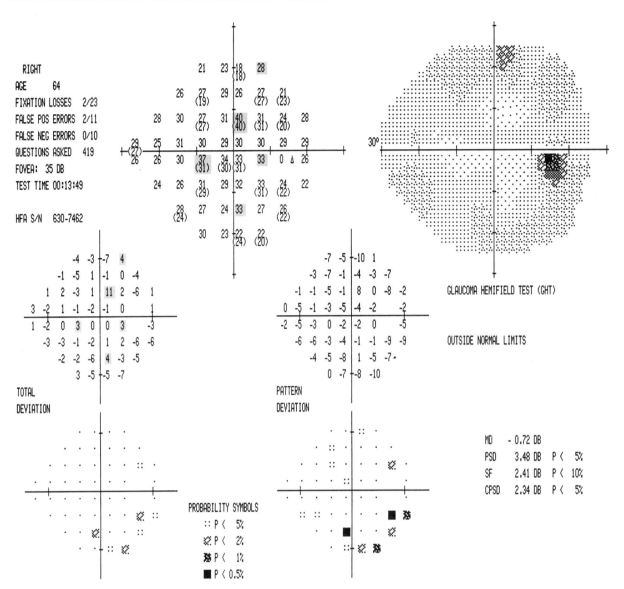

RIGHT

AGE   64

FIXATION LOSSES   2/23

FALSE POS ERRORS 2/11

FALSE NEG ERRORS 0/10

QUESTIONS ASKED   419

FOVEA: 35 DB

TEST TIME 00:13:49

HFA S/N   630-7462

TOTAL
DEVIATION

PATTERN
DEVIATION

GLAUCOMA HEMIFIELD TEST (GHT)

OUTSIDE NORMAL LIMITS

MD   - 0.72 DB

PSD   3.48 DB   P < 5%

SF   2.41 DB   P < 10%

CPSD 2.34 DB   P < 5%

PROBABILITY SYMBOLS

:: P < 5%

▨ P < 2%

▩ P < 1%

■ P < 0.5%

Figure 1-27. Pattern deviation probability plot. This visual field has an abnormality on the pattern deviation probability plot, despite a normal appearing graytone printout and total deviation probability plot. In this case, there is a generalized elevation of the hill of vision due to a few supranormal points, which are highlighted. The supranormal points are usually the result of false positive errors. When the general height adjustment corrects for the elevated hill of vision, the pattern deviation probability plot reveals some areas that are depressed relative to the remainder of the field. The patient has glaucoma with elevated intraocular pressure and a larger cup in this eye compared with the left eye.

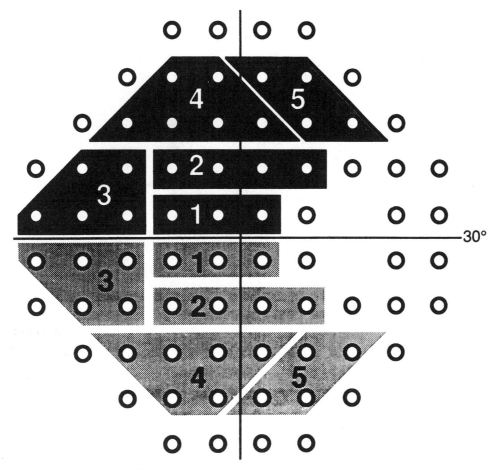

Figure 1-28. Glaucoma hemifield test. In the glaucoma hemifield test, results in five zones in the upper hemifield (which correspond to nerve fiber layer patterns in normal subjects) are compared with results in five mirror image zones in the lower hemifield. If the difference between the mirror image zones would be expected in less than 1% of the normal age-matched population, the glaucoma hemifield test results will be positive. If both mirror image zones are depressed more or less equally, but to a degree found in fewer than 0.5% of the normal age-matched population, the test will also be positive. (From Heijl A, Lindgren G, Lindgren A, Olsson J, Åsman P, Myers S, Patella M. Extended empirical statistical package for evaluation of single and multiple fields in glaucoma: Statpac 2. In Mills RP and Heijl A, eds. Perimetry update 1990/91. Amsterdam: Kugler publications, 1991,303.)

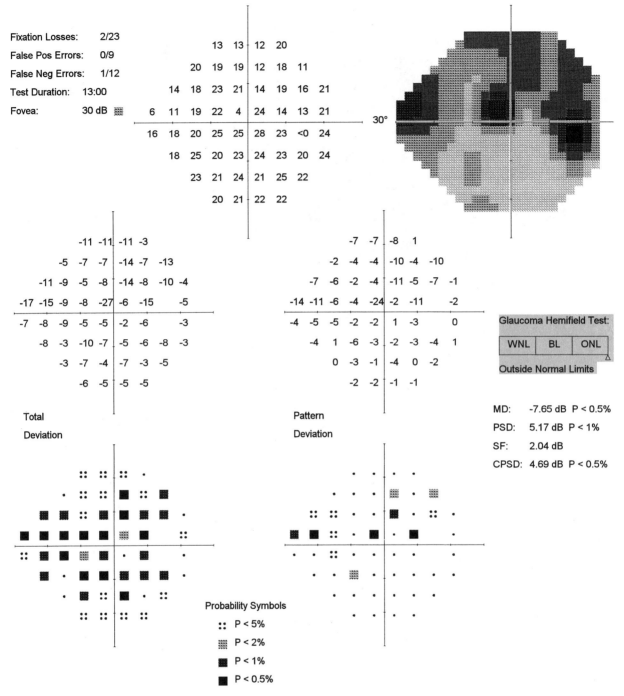

Fixation Losses: 2/23
False Pos Errors: 0/9
False Neg Errors: 1/12
Test Duration: 13:00
Fovea: 30 dB

```
                        13  13 | 12  20
                    20  19  19 | 12  18  11
                14  18  23  21 | 14  19  16  21
        6   11  19  22  4 | 24  14  13  21
    16  18  20  25  25 | 28  23  <0  24        30°
    18  25  20  23 | 24  23  20  24
            23  21  24 | 21  25  22
                20  21 | 22  22
```

```
        -11  -11  -11  -3
    -5   -7   -7  -14  -7  -13
-11  -9   -5   -8  -14  -8  -10  -4
-17 -15  -9   -8  -27  -6  -15      -5
-7  -8   -9   -5   -5 | -2  -6      -3
    -8   -3  -10  -7  -5  -6  -8  -3
        -3   -7   -4  -7  -3  -5
            -6   -5  -5  -5
```

```
                -7   -7 | -8   1
            -2   -4   -4 | -10  -4  -10
        -7   -6   -2   -4 | -11  -5  -7  -1
    -14 -11  -6   -4  -24 | -2  -11      -2
-4  -5   -5   -2   -2 | 1   -3      0
    -4   1   -6   -3 | -2  -3  -4  1
        0   -3   -1 | -4   0  -2
            -2   -2 | -1  -1
```

Total
Deviation

Pattern
Deviation

Glaucoma Hemifield Test:

WNL	BL	ONL

Outside Normal Limits

MD: -7.65 dB P < 0.5%
PSD: 5.17 dB P < 1%
SF: 2.04 dB
CPSD: 4.69 dB P < 0.5%

Probability Symbols

∷   P < 5%
▦   P < 2%
▨   P < 1%
■   P < 0.5%

Figure 1-29. Glaucoma hemifield test: outside normal limits. Normal tension glaucoma patient with superior visual field defects and diffuse depression. The total deviation probability plot shows diffuse central depression. The pattern deviation probability plot reveals localized areas of abnormality superiorly that are not found inferiorly. The glaucoma hemifield test results are highly positive and the message "outside normal limits" appears, indicating a difference between the upper and lower zones that would be found in less than 1% of the normal population.[12] As a single criterion, the message "outside normal limits" on the glaucoma hemifield test may be the most accurate indicator of abnormality.[13,14]

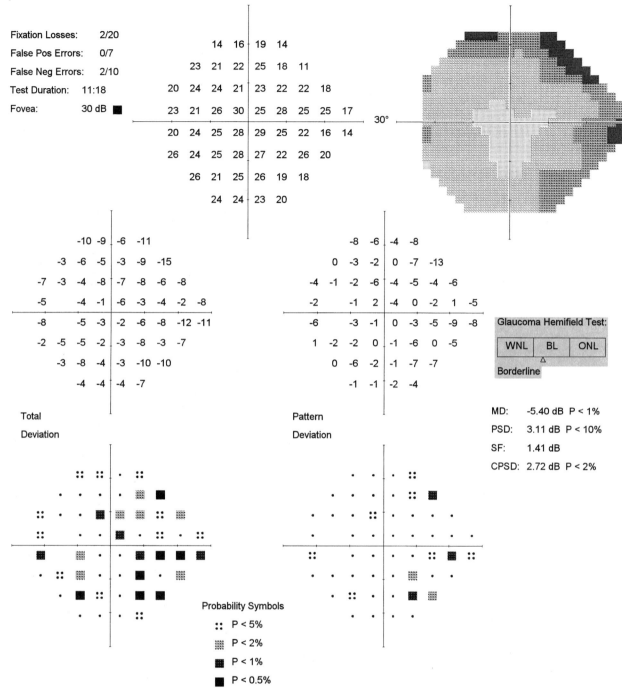

Fixation Losses: 2/20
False Pos Errors: 0/7
False Neg Errors: 2/10
Test Duration: 11:18
Fovea: 30 dB ■

```
              14  16 │ 19  14
          23  21  22 │ 25  18  11
      20  24  24  21 │ 23  22  22  18
      23  21  26  30 │ 25  28  25  25  17      30°
      20  24  25  28 │ 29  25  22  16  14
      26  24  25  28 │ 27  22  26  20
          26  21  25 │ 26  19  18
              24  24 │ 23  20
```

```
         -10  -9 │ -6  -11
      -3  -6  -5 │ -3  -9  -15
  -7  -3  -4  -8 │ -7  -8  -6  -8
  -5      -4  -1 │ -6  -3  -4  -2  -8
  -8      -5  -3 │ -2  -6  -8  -12  -11
  -2  -5  -5  -2 │ -3  -8  -3  -7
      -3  -8  -4 │ -3  -10  -10
          -4  -4 │ -4  -7
```

Total
Deviation

```
              -8  -6 │ -4  -8
           0  -3  -2 │  0  -7  -13
      -4  -1  -2  -6 │ -4  -5  -4  -6
      -2      -1   2 │ -4   0  -2   1  -5
      -6      -3  -1 │  0  -3  -5  -9  -8
   1  -2  -2   0 │ -1  -6   0  -5
           0  -6  -2 │ -1  -7  -7
              -1  -1 │ -2  -4
```

Pattern
Deviation

Glaucoma Hemifield Test:

WNL	BL	ONL
	△	

Borderline

MD: -5.40 dB P < 1%
PSD: 3.11 dB P < 10%
SF: 1.41 dB
CPSD: 2.72 dB P < 2%

Probability Symbols

∷ P < 5%

▦ P < 2%

▨ P < 1%

■ P < 0.5%

Figure 1-30. Glaucoma hemifield test: borderline. Visual field of a glaucoma suspect with a "borderline" glaucoma hemifield test. The pattern deviation plot contains some depressed points that could be caused by early glaucoma. A message of "borderline" on the glaucoma hemifield test indicates a result that is expected in less than 3% but greater than or equal to 1% of the normal population.[12]

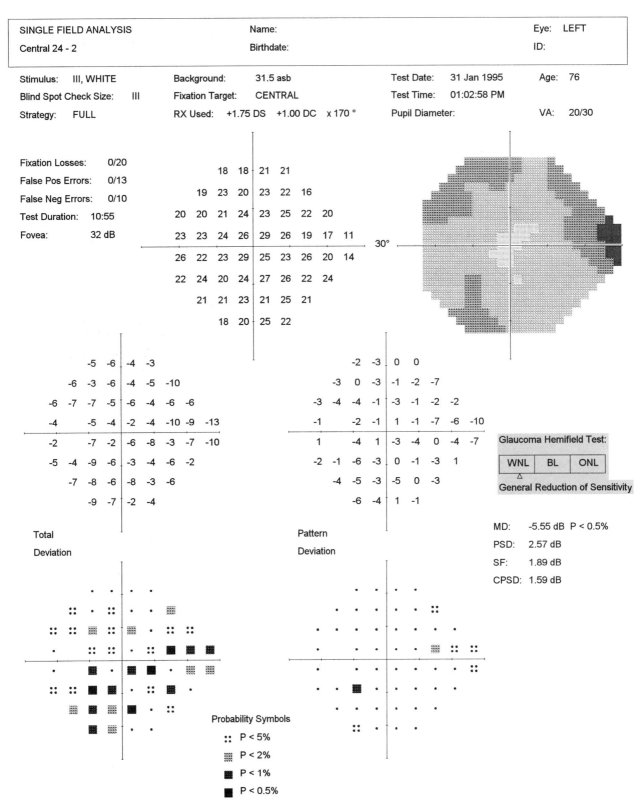

Figure 1-31. Glaucoma hemifield test: general reduction of sensitivity. This visual field from the left eye of a patient with a cataract, shows scattered depressed points in the total deviation probability plot but no cluster of depressed points on the pattern deviation probability plot. The message "general reduction of sensitivity" appears when the criteria for a localized defect are absent and the general height adjustment yields a result in which the best part of the field is depressed to a degree that would be expected in fewer than 0.5% of the age-matched normal population.[15] If this is the only message present and the corrected pattern standard deviation is normal, media opacity or diffuse retinal disease should be suspected as the cause of the abnormal field.

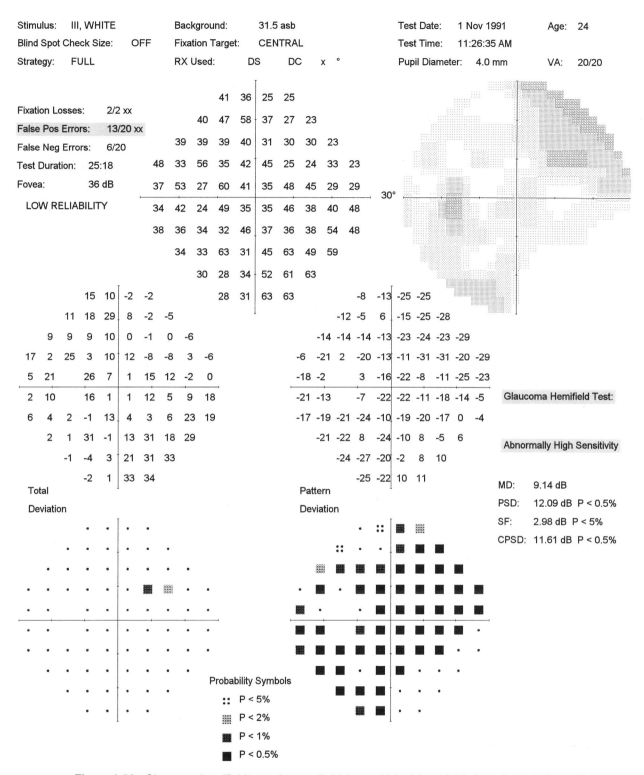

			41	36	25	25			
		40	47	58	37	27	23		
	39	39	39	40	31	30	30	23	
48	33	56	35	42	45	25	24	33	23
37	53	27	60	41	35	48	45	29	29
34	42	24	49	35	35	46	38	40	48
38	36	34	32	46	37	36	38	54	48
	34	33	63	31	45	63	49	59	
		30	28	34	52	61	63		
			28	31	63	63			

Stimulus: III, WHITE

Blind Spot Check Size: OFF

Strategy: FULL

Background: 31.5 asb

Fixation Target: CENTRAL

RX Used: DS   DC   x °

Test Date: 1 Nov 1991   Age: 24

Test Time: 11:26:35 AM

Pupil Diameter: 4.0 mm   VA: 20/20

Fixation Losses: 2/2 xx

False Pos Errors: 13/20 xx

False Neg Errors: 6/20

Test Duration: 25:18

Fovea: 36 dB

LOW RELIABILITY

30°

Total Deviation

		15	10	-2	-2				
	11	18	29	8	-2	-5			
	9	9	9	10	0	-1	0	-6	
17	2	25	3	10	12	-8	-8	3	-6
5	21		26	7	1	15	12	-2	0
2	10		16	1	1	12	5	9	18
6	4	2	-1	13	4	3	6	23	19
	2	1	31	-1	13	31	18	29	
		-1	-4	3	21	31	33		
			-2	1	33	34			

Pattern Deviation

				-8	-13	-25	-25			
			-12	-5	6	-15	-25	-28		
		-14	-14	-14	-13	-23	-24	-23	-29	
-6	-21	2	-20	-13	-11	-31	-31	-20	-29
-18	-2		3	-16	-22	-8	-11	-25	-23
-21	-13		-7	-22	-22	-11	-18	-14	-5
-17	-19	-21	-24	-10	-19	-20	-17	0	-4
	-21	-22	8	-24	-10	8	-5	6	
		-24	-27	-20	-2	8	10		
			-25	-22	10	11			

Glaucoma Hemifield Test:

Abnormally High Sensitivity

MD: 9.14 dB

PSD: 12.09 dB P < 0.5%

SF: 2.98 dB P < 5%

CPSD: 11.61 dB P < 0.5%

Probability Symbols

::   P < 5%

▦   P < 2%

▨   P < 1%

■   P < 0.5%

Figure 1-32. Glaucoma hemifield test: abnormally high sensitivity. Visual field of a patient who has a high false positive rate, which causes an artificially supranormal visual field. The message "abnormally high sensitivity" is generated by the glaucoma hemifield test. This message appears when the general height adjustment is performed in the derivation of the pattern deviation plot and the best part of the field is more sensitive than 99.5% of the age-matched normal population.[15] Typical areas of "white scotomas" are seen on the graytone printout.

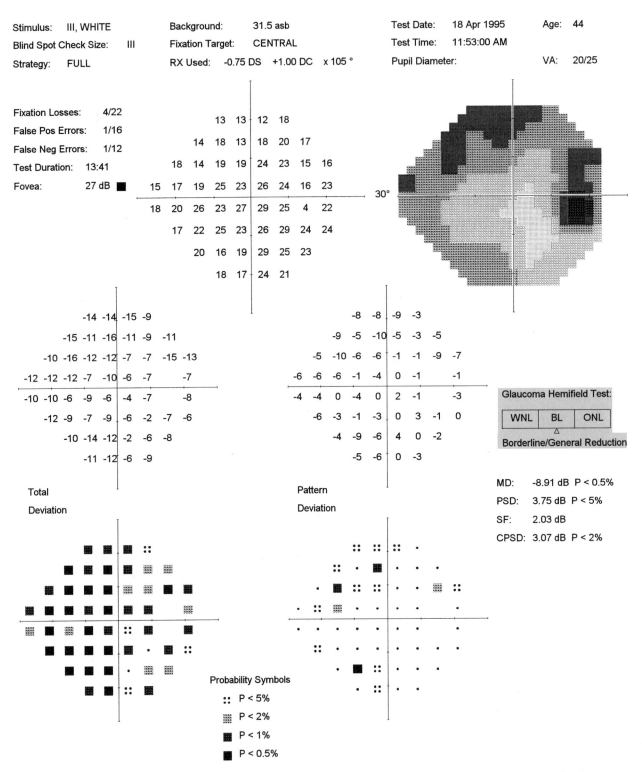

Stimulus: III, WHITE
Blind Spot Check Size: III
Strategy: FULL

Background: 31.5 asb
Fixation Target: CENTRAL
RX Used: -0.75 DS   +1.00 DC   x 105 °

Test Date: 18 Apr 1995   Age: 44
Test Time: 11:53:00 AM
Pupil Diameter: VA: 20/25

Fixation Losses: 4/22
False Pos Errors: 1/16
False Neg Errors: 1/12
Test Duration: 13:41
Fovea: 27 dB

```
              13  13 | 12  18
          14  18  13 | 18  20  17
      18  14  19  19 | 24  23  15  16
  15  17  19  25  23 | 26  24  16  23
  18  20  26  23  27 | 29  25   4  22
  17  22  25  23 | 26  29  24  24
      20  16  19 | 29  25  23
          18  17 | 24  21
```

30°

Total Deviation
```
      -14 -14 -15  -9
  -15 -11 -16 -11  -9 -11
  -10 -16 -12 -12  -7  -7 -15 -13
-12 -12 -12  -7 -10  -6  -7     -7
-10 -10  -6  -9  -6  -4  -7     -8
  -12  -9  -7  -9  -6  -2  -7  -6
  -10 -14 -12  -2  -6  -8
      -11 -12  -6  -9
```

Pattern Deviation
```
       -8  -8  -9  -3
    -9  -5 -10  -5  -3  -5
 -5 -10  -6  -6  -1  -1  -9  -7
-6 -6  -6  -1  -4   0  -1     -1
-4 -4   0  -4   0   2  -1     -3
 -6  -3  -1  -3   0   3  -1   0
    -4  -9  -6   4   0  -2
       -5  -6   0  -3
```

Glaucoma Hemifield Test:

WNL	BL	ONL

△
Borderline/General Reduction

MD: -8.91 dB P < 0.5%
PSD: 3.75 dB P < 5%
SF: 2.03 dB
CPSD: 3.07 dB P < 2%

Probability Symbols

∷ P < 5%
▦ P < 2%
▨ P < 1%
■ P < 0.5%

Figure 1-33. Glaucoma hemifield test: two messages. The messages "borderline" and "general reduction of sensitivity" may appear together under the glaucoma hemifield test. This patient's cataract produced general reduction of sensitivity, seen best on the total deviation probability plot. In addition, glaucoma is suspected with possible localized defects in the superonasal quadrant noted on the pattern deviation probability plot.

IS THE VISUAL FIELD CHANGING OVER TIME?

Judging progression and improvement of the visual field remains largely subjective. Large magnitudes of improvement or worsening are easy to determine, whereas more subtle changes are not. The Humphrey field analyzer comes with several programs that help document change and provide statistical analysis as to the significance of change. These are reviewed in Chapter 5 in the section entitled "Judging Glaucomatous Progression." In addition, multiple examples of fields that are changing over time are included throughout the atlas.

References

1. Katz J, Tielsch JM, Quigley HA, Javitt J, Witt K, Sommer A. Automated suprathreshold screening for glaucoma: the Baltimore Eye Survey. Invest Ophthalmol Vis Sci 1993;34:3271.
2. Mills RP, Barnebey HS, Migliazzo CV, Li Y. Does saving time using FASTPAC or suprathreshold testing reduce quality of visual fields? Ophthalmology 1994;101:1596.
3. Siatkowski RM, Lam BL, Anderson DR, Feuer WJ, Halikman AB. Automated suprathreshold static perimetry screening for detecting neuro-ophthalmologic disease. Ophthalmology 1996;103:907.
4. Araujo ML, Feuer WJ, Anderson DR. Evaluation of baseline-related suprathreshold testing for quick determination of visual field nonprogression. Arch Ophthalmol 1993;111:365.
5. Mills RP. Automated perimetry in neuro-ophthalmology. Int Ophthalmol Clin 1991;31:51.
6. Katz J, Sommer A. Screening for glaucomatous visual field loss. Ophthalmology 1990;97:1032.
7. Katz J, Sommer A. Reliability indexes of automated perimetric tests. Arch Ophthalmol 1988;106:1252.
8. Sanabria O, Feuer WJ, Anderson DR. Pseudo-loss of fixation in automated perimetry. Ophthalmology 1991; 98:76.
9. Heijl A, Lindgren G, Olsson J. Normal variability of static perimetric threshold values across the central visual field. Arch Ophthalmol 1987;105:1544.
10. Anderson, DR. Automated static perimetry. St. Louis: Mosby-Year Book, 1992:82.
11. Humphrey field analyzer owner's manual. San Leandro, CA: Allergan Humphrey 1991:10–16.
12. Anderson, DR. Automated static perimetry. St. Louis: Mosby-Year Book, 1992:88.
13. Katz J, Tielsch JM, Quigley HA, Sommer A. Automated perimetry detects visual field loss before manual Goldmann perimetry. Ophthalmology 1995;102:21
14. Anderson, DR. Automated static perimetry. St. Louis: Mosby-Year Book, 1992:123.
15. Anderson, DR. Automated static perimetry. St. Louis: Mosby-Year Book, 1992:90.

2

Artifacts in Automated Perimetry

Donald L. Budenz

Once an abnormality has been detected by automated perimetry, it is important to determine whether the abnormality is real or if it is due to testing artifact. The rule of thumb that any abnormal test in medicine should be confirmed through a second test before being acted on is generally true in visual field testing, although obvious abnormalities in the appropriate clinical context probably do not need confirmation with a second test. Poor reliability is the most common cause of artifact in automated perimetry and is covered in Chapter 1. This chapter explores artifacts found on automated perimetry that are not related to reliability, in hopes that the reader will recognize them and not be fooled into thinking an abnormality is real when it is artifactual.

Figures 2.1–2.22 follow on pages 48–76.

References appear on page 77.

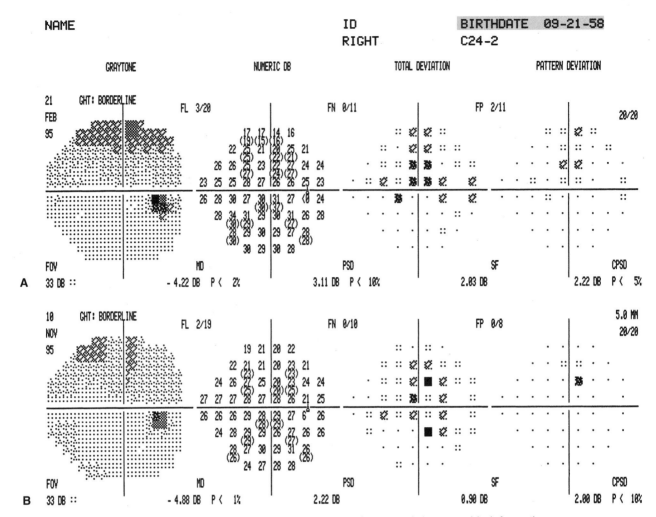

Figure 2-1. Effect of incorrect date of birth. Incorrectly entered demographic information can cause artifacts in visual fields and lead to erroneous interpretation. This series of visual fields are from a 67-year-old with suspected glaucoma. Fields **A** and **B** were analyzed using an incorrect birthdate (09-21-28). The computer assumed the patient was 37-years-old* and compared her responses with those of control subjects 30 years her junior, producing artificially unfavorable mean deviations and total deviation plots. All of these parameters depend, either directly or indirectly, on the correct date of birth being entered. In addition, the foveal threshold (33 dB) in fields A and B is statistically abnormal in a 37-year-old at the *P* < 5% level.

* When calculating the age of the patient, the statistical package of the Humphrey perimeter does not take into account the day or month of the patient's date of birth or date the field was obtained. The age of the patient is calculated by subtracting the year of the birthdate from the year the test was performed. This is the age printed in the upper left-hand corner of the single field analysis.

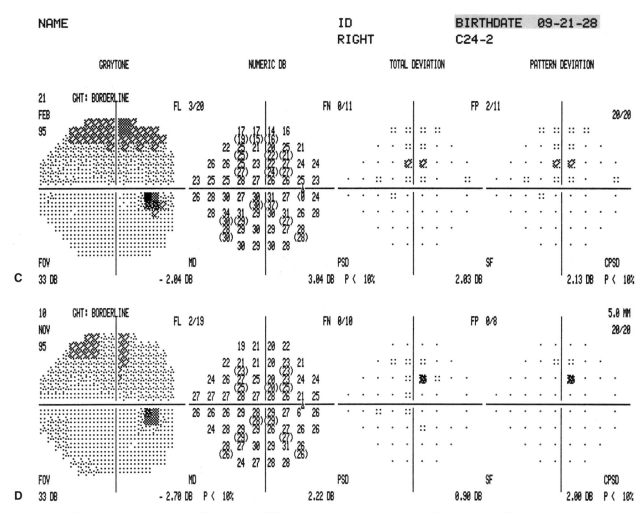

Figure 2-1. *Continued.* Fields **C** and **D** are a recalculation of the field data using the correct date of birth (09-21-28). The mean deviations and total deviation plots in fields C and D are much less abnormal and less worrisome clinically. The foveal threshold is not statistically abnormal in the patient's actual age group, so no *P* value is associated with the foveal threshold in fields C and D.

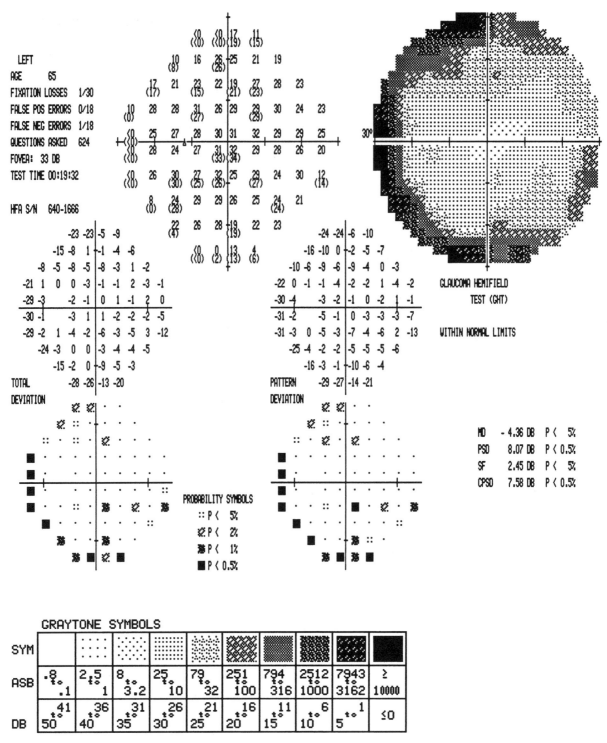

Figure 2-2. Lens rim artifact. If the corrective lens and lens holder are placed too far away from the eye or not centered properly, a dense ring scotoma may appear in the periphery of the field,[1] as in this patient. Ring scotomas from lens rim artifact are usually absolute (ie, sensitivities of < 0 dB) and may mimic arcuate scotomas in found glaucoma and nonglaucomatous optic neuropathies or ring scotomas found in retinitis pigmentosa. Using the thinner wire rimmed trial lenses rather than the thick rimmed trial lenses and proper lens positioning minimize this artifact. (Courtesy of Karen Joos, MD)

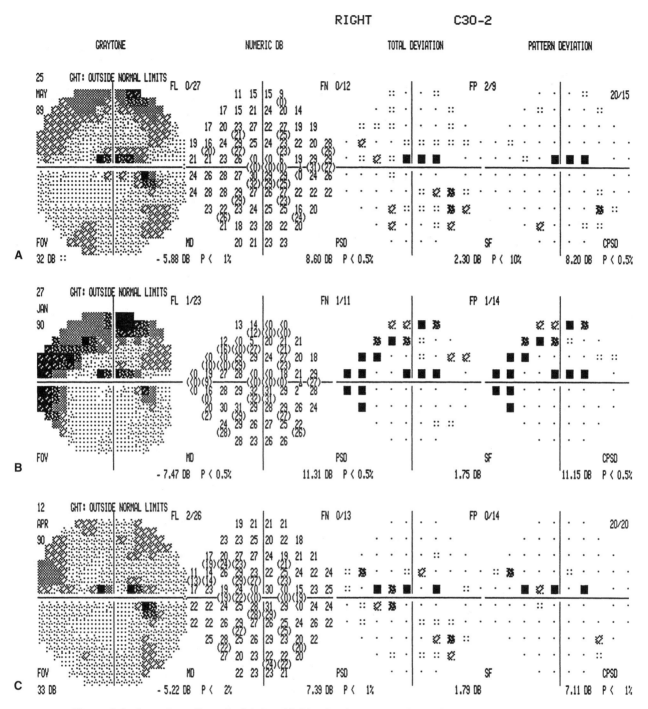

Figure 2-3. Lens rim artifact. Serial visual fields of a glaucoma patient referred for worsening glaucoma. Field **A** shows a dense superior arcuate scotoma splitting fixation. Field **B**, performed just 8 months later, shows worsening mean deviation, a new superior arcuate scotoma, and a new inferonasal step. This was interpreted as worsening of glaucomatous visual field. Because these changes occurred rather rapidly and were not in keeping with the remainder of the clinical findings, the field was repeated. The repeat visual field (field **C**), performed with proper lens positioning, was more similar to the baseline visual field and the changes in field B were attributed to lens rim artifact. Although usually manifesting at the edge of the visual field, the lens may be so displaced that a pseudoarcuate scotoma is produced. (Adapted with permission from Anderson DR. Automated static perimetry. St. Louis: Mosby–Year Book, 1992:139.)

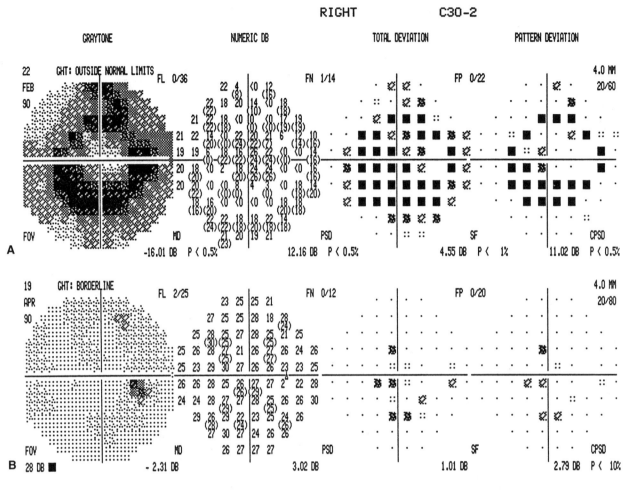

Figure 2-4. Lens rim artifact. Visual field **A** shows a ring scotoma in the graytone printout and pattern deviation plots that resemble glaucomatous visual field loss or perhaps late-onset retinitis pigmentosa. However, on repeat testing with proper lens positioning, fundus findings were normal and the visual field contained only nonspecific generalized depression (field **B**). This extreme example of lens rim artifact is produced by the trial frame holder and lens being positioned too far forward, away from the eye being tested. This and the previous two fields demonstrate the importance of repeating visual fields that appear to be worsening or are out of keeping with the clinical appearance of the patient. (Adapted with permission from Anderson DR. Automated static perimetry. St. Louis: Mosby–Year Book, 1992:142).

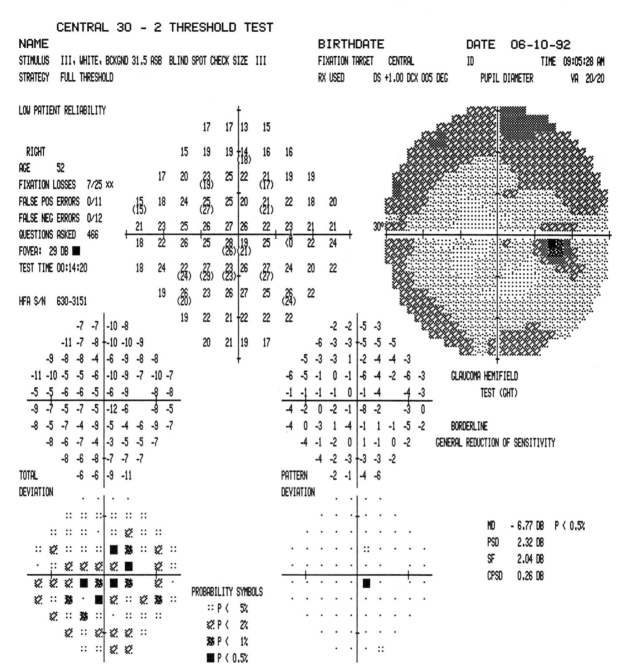

Figure 2-5. Edge artifact. Visual field of a patient with suspected glaucoma, which shows a superior arcuate defect and peripheral inferonasal defect on the graytone printout, central depression without peripheral depression on the total deviation plot, and normal pattern deviation plot. The abnormal graytone printout could be interpreted as nerve fiber layer field loss from optic nerve disease. However, the edge of the central field is subject to more variability than the center and sensitivity drops off as one moves away from the fovea, particularly superiorly,[2] and the edge artifact in the graytone printout shown above is not uncommon. Fortunately, the computer software accounts for the fact that sensitivity decreases away from the fovea[3, 4] and the edge points of this field are largely normalized in the total deviation plot and not at all abnormal in the pattern deviation plot. This field reinforces the importance of looking beyond the graytone printout to the total deviation and pattern deviation printouts when interpreting field abnormalities.

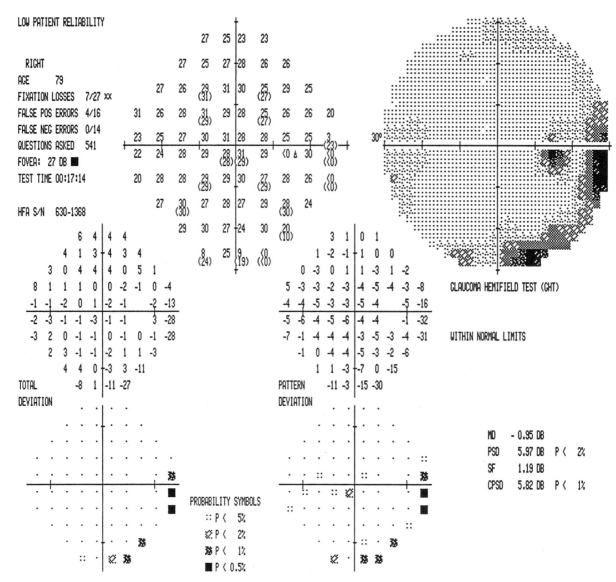

Figure 2-6. Edge artifact. Central 30° field with a defect along the inferotemporal edge on the graytone printout, total deviation, and pattern deviation plots. The defect disappeared on repeat testing. Fortunately, the peripheral inferotemporal quadrant is an unusual pattern of field loss (except perhaps in retinal disease or focal media opacity, both of which are easily seen with examination of the eye) so that this defect is easily recognized as artifact. Edge artifacts of this type are so common that the most peripheral ring of points on the 30-2 program are generally ignored when identifying glaucomatous visual field defects.[5] In addition, many perimetrists preferentially test the central 24° field because of the frequency of edge artifact when the visual field is tested to 30°.

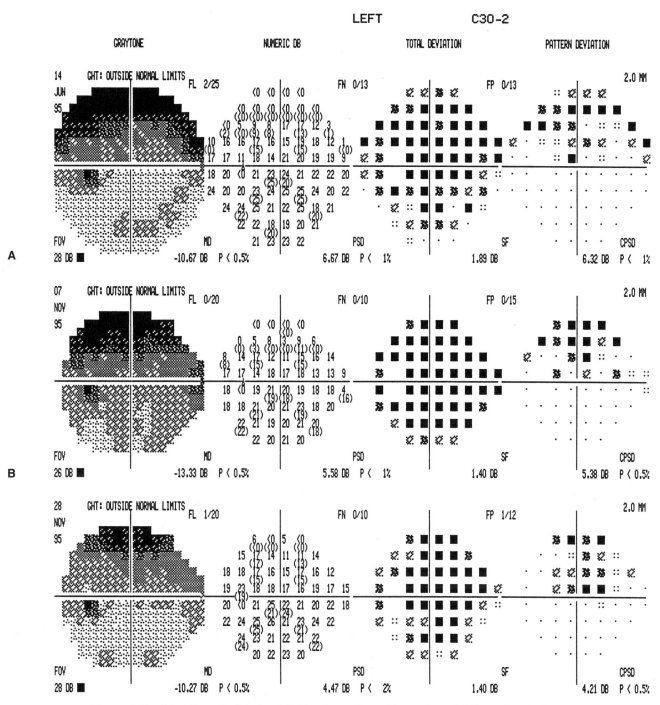

Figure 2-7. Lid artifact. Serial visual fields of a patient with ptosis and diffuse choroidal thickening of the left eye due to ocular lymphoma. Field **A** shows diffuse depression on the total deviation plot, which is worse superiorly on the graytone printout and total deviation plot. The left upper eyelid was taped open during this field test. Field **B**, performed 5 months later without the upper eyelid taped, showed worsening of the foveal threshold. The eyelid was not taped in the center field. The possibility of worsening was raised but the repeat field (*bottom*), performed with the upper eyelid taped, is more similar to the baseline field.

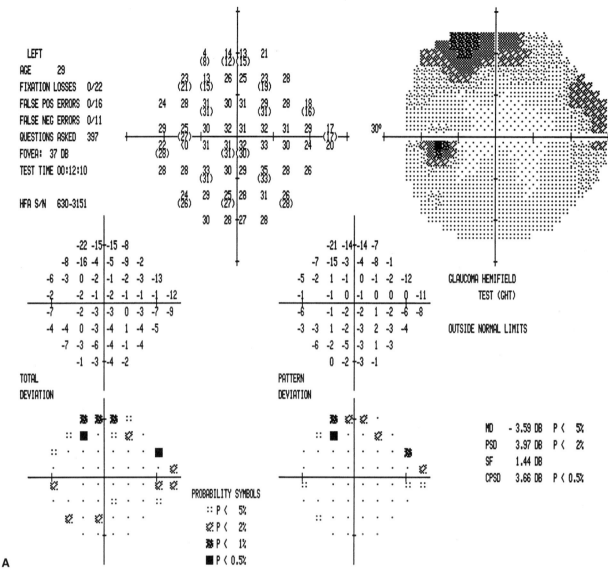

```
LEFT
AGE      29
FIXATION LOSSES   0/22
FALSE POS ERRORS  0/16
FALSE NEG ERRORS  0/11
QUESTIONS ASKED   397
FOVEA:  37 DB
TEST TIME 00:12:10

HFA S/N   630-3151
```

```
            4   14 13   21
           (8) (12)(15)
         23  13  26  25  23  28
        (21)(15)        (19)
      24  28  31  30 31  29  28  18
             (31)         (31)    (16)
    29  25  30  32 31  32  31  29  17
       (27)(0)                    (17)
       22      31  31 32  33  30  24  20
      (28)        (31)(30)
    28  28  33  30 29  35  28  26
           (31)        (33)
       24  29  25 28  31  26
      (26)    (27)        (28)
            30  28 27  28
```

30°

```
        -22 -15 -15 -8
      -8 -16 -4 -5 -9 -2
    -6 -3  0 -2 -1 -2 -3 -13
    -2   -2 -1 -2 -1 -1 -1 -12
    -7   -2 -3 -3  0 -3 -7 -9
    -4 -4  0 -3 -4  1 -4 -5
      -7 -3 -6 -4 -1 -4
        -1 -3 -4 -2
```

```
        -21 -14 -14 -7
      -7 -15 -3 -4 -8 -1
    -5 -2  1 -1  0 -1 -2 -12
    -1   -1  0 -1  0  0  0 -11
    -6   -1 -2 -2  1 -2 -6 -8
    -3 -3  1 -2 -3  2 -3 -4
      -6 -2 -5 -3  1 -3
         0 -2 -3 -1
```

GLAUCOMA HEMIFIELD
TEST (GHT)

OUTSIDE NORMAL LIMITS

TOTAL
DEVIATION

PATTERN
DEVIATION

```
MD    - 3.59 DB   P < 5%
PSD     3.97 DB   P < 2%
SF      1.44 DB
CPSD    3.66 DB   P < 0.5%
```

PROBABILITY SYMBOLS
```
:: P < 5%
▨ P < 2%
▩ P < 1%
■ P < 0.5%
```

A

Figure 2-8. Lid/brow artifact. Bilateral visual fields of a 29-year-old ophthalmology resident with a normal ocular examination. The graytone printout, total deviation plot, and pattern deviation plot show depression of the superior two rows of points. Ptosis or prominent superior orbital rims can cause the superior one or two rows of points to be depressed, as in this case. The superior orbital rim can obscure the superior visual field, especially if the head of the patient is inappropriately tilted forward during positioning.[6] Inexperience also caused a suspicious nasal defect in this case, which disappeared on repeat testing. The pattern standard deviation (PSD) is high in both eyes but the corrected pattern standard deviation (CPSD) is normal (0 dB) in the right eye **(A)** and markedly abnormal (3.66 dB) in the left eye **(B)**.

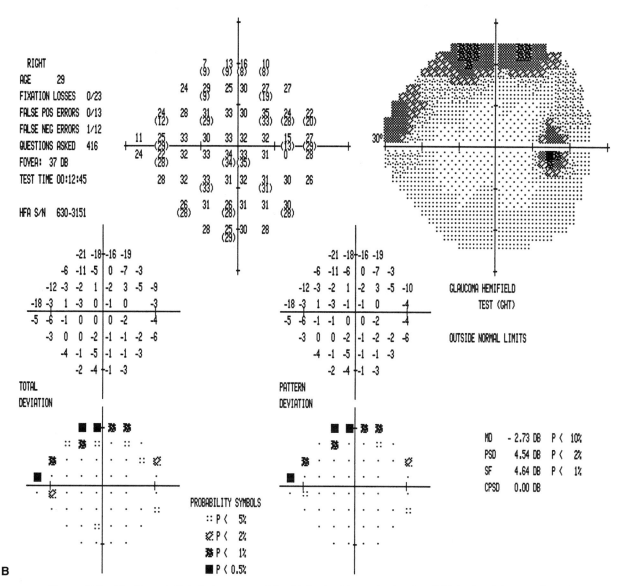

Figure 2-8. *Continued.* This is because of the high short-term fluctuation (SF) in the right eye. Recall that SF is subtracted from PSD to obtain the CPSD. The SF is high because of the variation in the two most superior points that are double determined as part of the calculation of short-term fluctuation, which happen to be at the edge of the scotoma caused by brow artifact and are physiologically highly variable. The remaining eight points used in the determination of SF are very reproducible. These fields reinforce the concept of obtaining a second baseline field, particularly when suspicious abnormalities are found on the first field or if the defects do not correspond to the clinical situation.

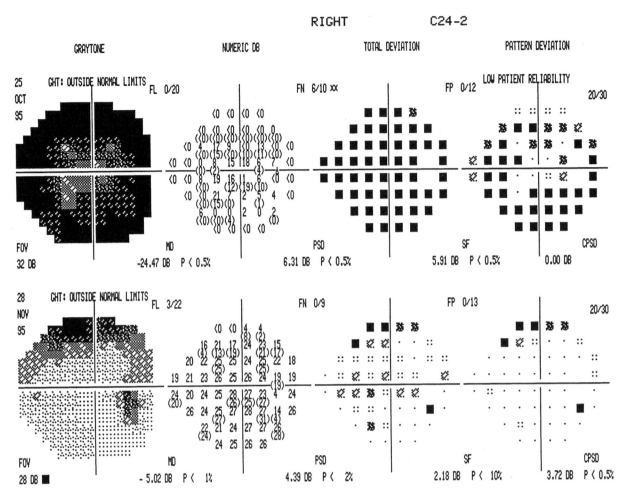

Figure 2-9. Learning effect. Patients undergoing automated perimetry for the first time often have an artificially poor field. Initial visual field (top) shows marked concentric contraction in the midperiphery with better sensitivity in the central and paracentral regions, a typical pattern for inexperienced fields[7]. Notice the high false negative rate that often accompanies artificially bad first fields.[7] The repeat field (*bottom*) shows mild superior depression, possibly due to lid artifact. Patients whose initial visual fields do not correlate with clinical findings should undergo repeat testing.[7] Completely normal visual fields usually do not need confirmation if the reliability parameters are normal.

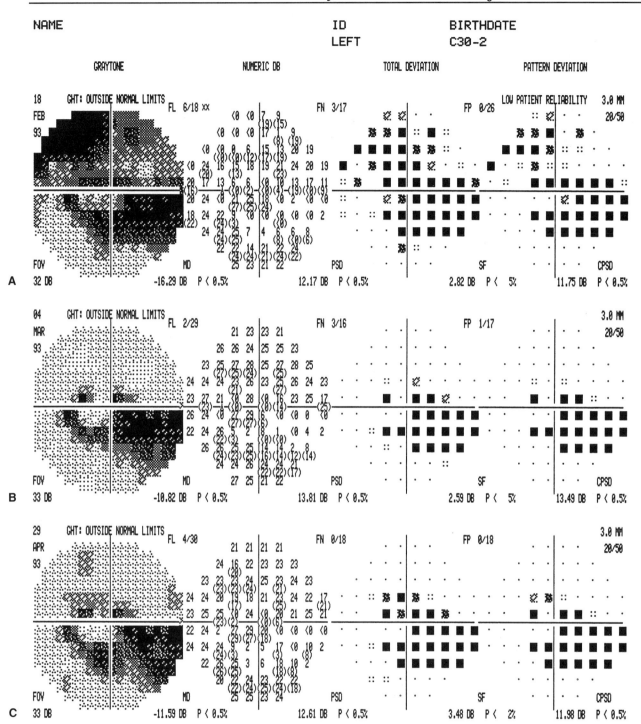

Figure 2-10. Learning effect. Visual fields of a glaucoma patient inexperienced in field taking. Field **A** shows a dense superotemporal defect and an inferior arcuate scotoma. Although the message "low patient reliability" is present, this is due to 30% fixation loss, which is considered particularly high by most perimetrists and may, in fact, be artifactually high due to incorrect determination of the blind spot (see Chapter 1). Field **B**, performed less than 1 month later, shows an inferior arcuate defect and superior paracentral defects but the dense superotemporal defect has disappeared. Field **C**, which is similar to field B, confirms that field A was artifactually poor. The perimetrist should consider obtaining a second baseline field on all patients for whom clinical decisions will be made based on comparison to a baseline field. If the two baseline fields are similar, these can be used for future comparison. If they differ, a third baseline field is advisable to determine which of the first two fields represents the patient's "true" visual field.

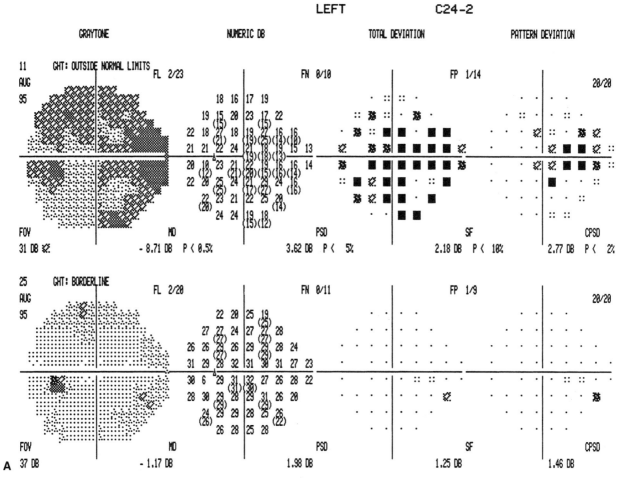

Figure 2-11. Learning effect OU. Initial and follow-up visual fields of a 68-year-old patient with elevated intraocular pressures and enlarged cup:disc ratio, **(A)** left, **(B)** right.

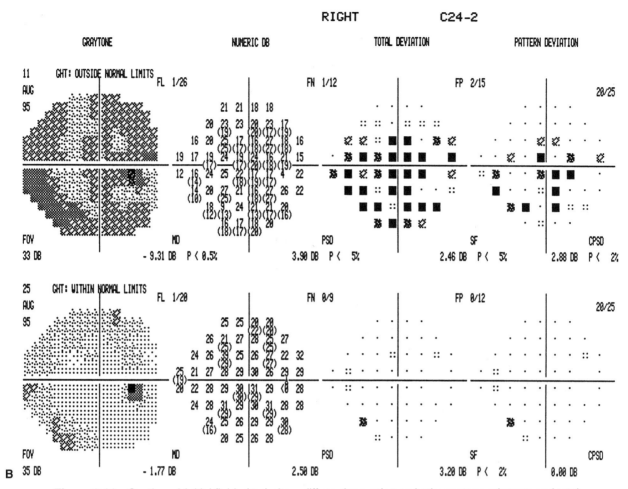

Figure 2-11. *Continued.* Initial fields (*top*) show diffuse depression on both graytone printouts and total deviation plots and superimposed localized defects, which could be consistent with early glaucoma. The glaucoma hemifield test, mean deviation, pattern standard deviation, and corrected pattern standard deviation are all abnormal at statistically significant levels. Note that the reliability parameters are excellent. However, follow-up baseline fields (*bottom*) were normal.

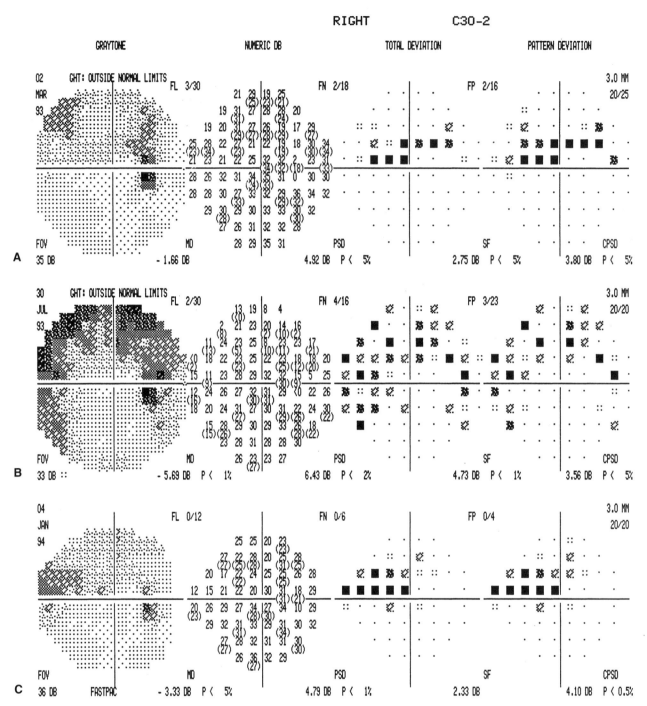

Figure 2-12. Long-term fluctuation. The concept of long-term fluctuation comes from the observation that, even after the patient has learned to perform automated perimetry and despite reliable test taking parameters, there is fluctuation in the results from session to session. This is evident in this series of fields obtained over several years on a glaucoma patient. Field **A** was the 11th automated field performed on the patient over a 3-year period and shows a superior arcuate defect that breaks into a nasal step, consistent with early glaucoma (see Tables 5-1 and 5-2). Field **B** shows worsening of the superior defect (see Table 5-5), a new inferonasal scotoma, and worsening of the mean deviation. The repeat field, **C**, performed to confirm the worsening in field B, is back to baseline.*

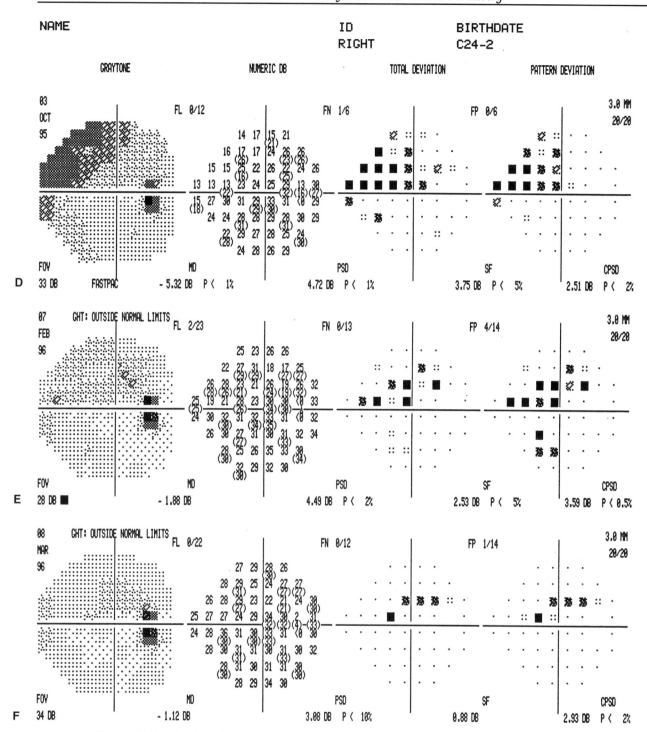

Figure 2-12. *Continued.* The field was stable until field **D** was performed, which shows enlargement of the superonasal step within the midperipheral superior nasal quadrant and worsening of the mean deviation. In field **E**, the superior defect is back to baseline (compare with A) but there is a new inferior paracentral scotoma that fits the criteria for minimal abnormality (Table 5-1). This disappears on the follow-up field (**F**). Note that the reliability parameters are normal in all of the fields. Long-term fluctuation is worse in moderately depressed fields due to fluctuation in and adjacent to relative scotomas. Long-term fluctuation must be suspected any time a field is worse, which is why any field that appears worse requires at least one, and possibly two,[8] confirmatory fields.

* Note that fields C and D were performed using the FASTPAC testing strategy, rather than full-threshold strategies used in fields A, B, E, and F. FASTPAC, as its name implies, reduces test taking time by 30% to 40% by altering the thresholding strategy without, according to some investigators,[9] compromising sensitivity to early glaucoma defects. The FASTPAC program, however, does not provide results of the glaucoma hemifield test, which is why this information is missing for fields C and D.

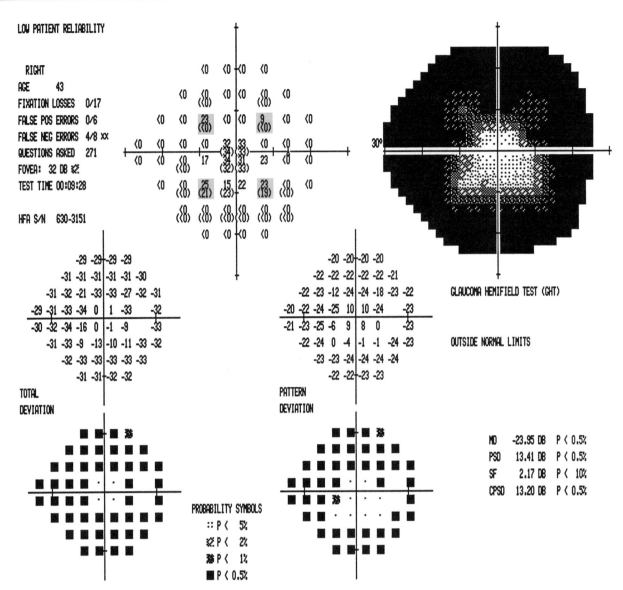

Figure 2-13. Fatigue effect. Visual field of a patient whose field is artifactually poor because of fatigue. The graytone printout shows the typical clover leaf pattern accompanying fatigue. Patients who fatigue will generally do well on the points tested early but lose concentration after these points are determined. The four primary points (*highlighted*) are checked first, and are double determined, which takes considerable time at the beginning of the test. Locations surrounding these points are then tested, followed by the midperipheral and peripheral field.

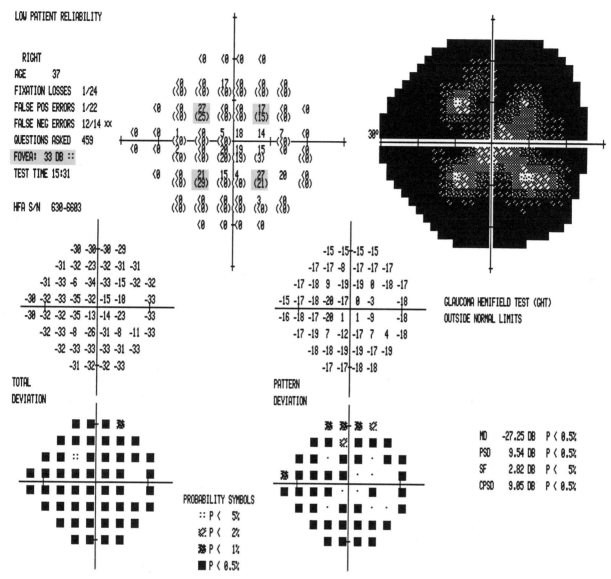

LOW PATIENT RELIABILITY

RIGHT
AGE 37
FIXATION LOSSES 1/24
FALSE POS ERRORS 1/22
FALSE NEG ERRORS 12/14 xx
QUESTIONS ASKED 459
FOVEA: 33 DB ::
TEST TIME 15:31

HFA S/N 630-6603

GLAUCOMA HEMIFIELD TEST (GHT)
OUTSIDE NORMAL LIMITS

```
TOTAL
DEVIATION
  -30 -30 -30 -29
-31 -32 -23 -32 -31 -31
-31 -33 -6 -34 -33 -15 -32 -32
-30 -32 -33 -35 -32 -15 -18    -33
-30 -32 -32 -35 -13 -14 -23    -33
-32 -33 -8 -26 -31 -8 -11 -33
  -32 -33 -33 -33 -31 -33
    -31 -32 -32 -33
```

```
PATTERN
DEVIATION
  -15 -15 -15 -15
-17 -17 -8 -17 -17 -17
-17 -18 9 -19 -19 0 -18 -17
-15 -17 -18 -20 -17 0 -3    -18
-16 -18 -17 -20 1 1 -9    -18
-17 -19 7 -12 -17 7 4 -18
  -18 -18 -19 -19 -17 -19
    -17 -17 -18 -18
```

PROBABILITY SYMBOLS
:: P < 5%
※ P < 2%
▓ P < 1%
■ P < 0.5%

MD -27.25 DB P < 0.5%
PSD 9.54 DB P < 0.5%
SF 2.82 DB P < 5%
CPSD 9.05 DB P < 0.5%

Figure 2-14. Fatigue effect. Another severely depressed visual field showing the characteristic clover-leaf pattern of fatigue effect. The foveal threshold and four cardinal points are near normal (*highlighted*), whereas the remainder of the field is severely depressed. The patient probably stopped responding after determination of the central field. Note the high false negative errors, which are determined by the computer presenting suprathreshold stimuli at locations in the field previously determined to be sensitive to dimmer stimuli. The false negative rate is elevated since the patient failed to respond to these suprathreshold stimuli. The fixation loss rate and false positive rate are normal because these require the patient to make an active response.

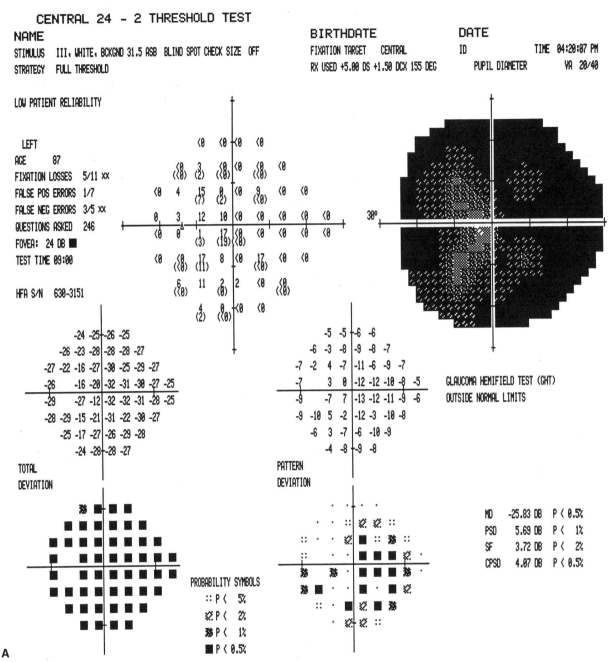

CENTRAL 24 - 2 THRESHOLD TEST

NAME

STIMULUS   III, WHITE, BCKGND 31.5 ASB   BLIND SPOT CHECK SIZE   OFF
STRATEGY   FULL THRESHOLD

BIRTHDATE   DATE
FIXATION TARGET   CENTRAL   ID   TIME 04:20:07 PM
RX USED +5.00 DS +1.50 DCX 155 DEG   PUPIL DIAMETER   VA 20/40

LOW PATIENT RELIABILITY

LEFT
AGE   87
FIXATION LOSSES   5/11 xx
FALSE POS ERRORS   1/7
FALSE NEG ERRORS   3/5 xx
QUESTIONS ASKED   246
FOVEA: 24 DB ■
TEST TIME 09:00

HFA S/N   630-3151

GLAUCOMA HEMIFIELD TEST (GHT)
OUTSIDE NORMAL LIMITS

TOTAL
DEVIATION

PATTERN
DEVIATION

PROBABILITY SYMBOLS
:: P < 5%
▨ P < 2%
▩ P < 1%
■ P < 0.5%

MD   -25.83 DB   P < 0.5%
PSD   5.69 DB   P < 1%
SF   3.72 DB   P < 2%
CPSD   4.07 DB   P < 0.5%

A

Figure 2-15. Fatigue effect. Bilateral visual fields in an elderly patient status post cerebrovascular accident with a right homonomous hemianopia. The right visual field, **(B)** which has poor reliability as evidenced by a high false negative rate, shows a complete right hemianopia and nonspecific constriction of the left hemifield. The left field is almost completely extinguished. The eye that is tested second, in this case the left eye, **(A)** will show a more pronounced fatigue effect in patients who tend to fatigue. Patients who fatigue during automated perimetry will generally show less reliability and decreased retinal sensitivity[10] as time elapses, so it can be helpful to know which eye was tested second and how long each eye took to be tested. The time the test was started is printed in the upper right-hand corner of the visual field printout and can be used to determine which eye was tested second. The time it took the patient to perform an individual field is printed underneath the reliability parameters and foveal threshold.

CENTRAL 24 - 2 THRESHOLD TEST

NAME

STIMULUS   III, WHITE, BCKGND 31.5 ASB   BLIND SPOT CHECK SIZE III
STRATEGY   FULL THRESHOLD

BIRTHDATE
FIXATION TARGET   CENTRAL
RX USED +4.75 DS +2.25 DCX 100 DEG

DATE   12-18-95
ID   TIME 04:08:28 PM
PUPIL DIAMETER   VA 20/30

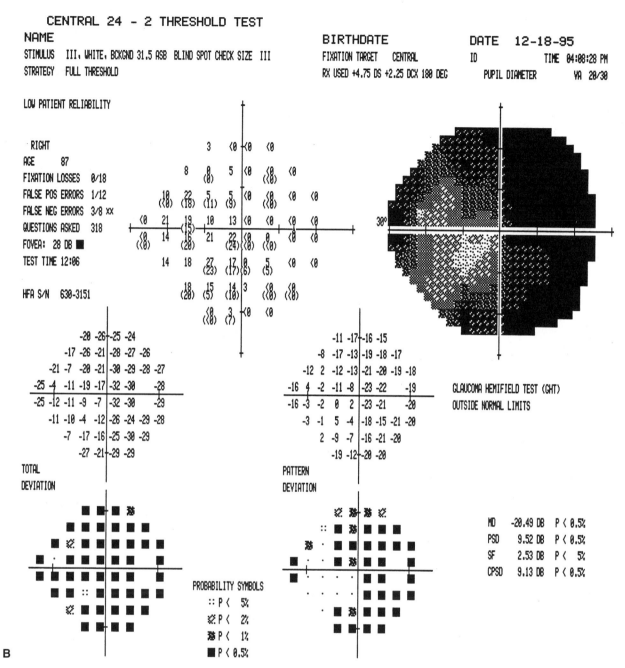

LOW PATIENT RELIABILITY

RIGHT
AGE   87
FIXATION LOSSES   0/18
FALSE POS ERRORS 1/12
FALSE NEG ERRORS 3/8 xx
QUESTIONS ASKED   318
FOVEA: 28 DB ■
TEST TIME 12:06

HFA S/N   630-3151

GLAUCOMA HEMIFIELD TEST (GHT)
OUTSIDE NORMAL LIMITS

TOTAL
DEVIATION

PATTERN
DEVIATION

MD	-20.49 DB	P < 0.5%
PSD	9.52 DB	P < 0.5%
SF	2.53 DB	P < 5%
CPSD	9.13 DB	P < 0.5%

PROBABILITY SYMBOLS

:: P < 5%
✼ P < 2%
▩ P < 1%
■ P < 0.5%

B

Figure 2-15. *Continued.*

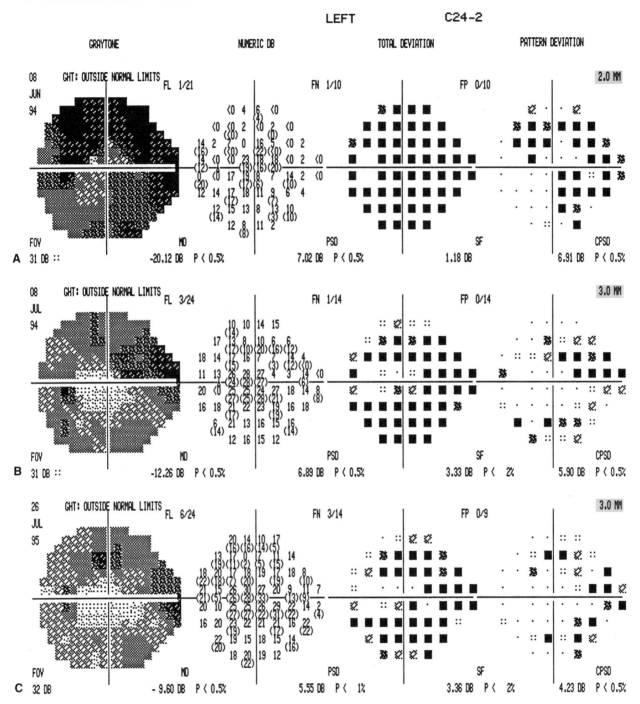

Figure 2-16. Effect of pupil size. Visual fields of a glaucoma patient on miotic therapy tested without pupillary dilation (Field **A**) and subsequently with pupillary dilation (Fields **B** and **C**). All three fields show a superior arcuate defect and inferonasal scotoma, but the first field is worse because of pupillary constriction. Patients receiving miotic therapy for glaucoma can have artifactually depressed fields owing to decreased retinal illumination through the small pupil.[11] Although a miotic pupil usually causes diffuse depression of sensitivity,[12] localized defects can be produced and pre-existing areas of decreased sensitivity may be affected more that normal areas.[13] When performing serial visual fields in patients on miotic therapy, the pupil should be either undilated or dilated for all examinations for the sake of accurate comparison. The problem comes in trying to compare fields on miotics and off miotics (or dilated fields). Careful attention should be paid to the pupil diameter message, which appears on the visual field printout (*highlighted*) if entered by the perimetrist at the start of the test.

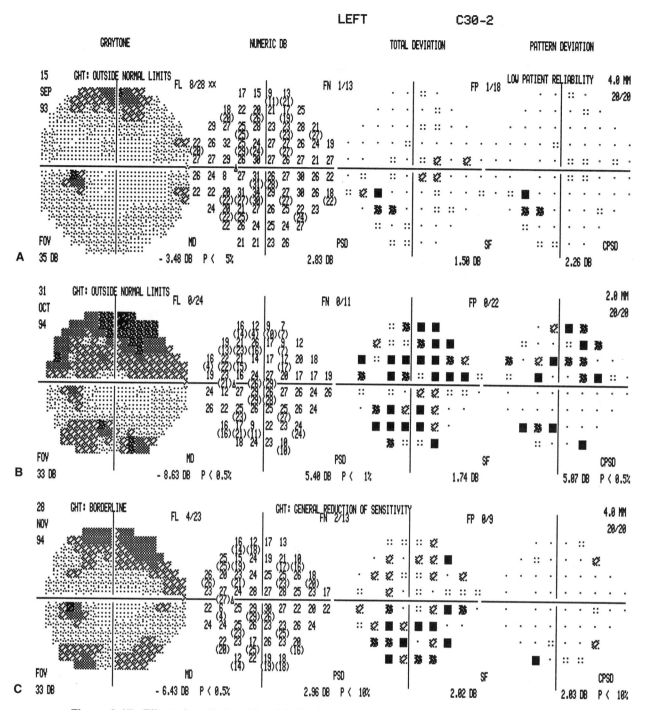

Figure 2-17. Effect of pupil size. Visual field of a glaucoma patient before pilocarpine therapy (Field **A**), on pilocarpine therapy (Field **B**), and after pupillary dilation (Field **C**). Field A shows an early inferior arcuate defect which emanates from the blind spot on the pattern deviation plot (see Table 5-1 for criteria). Field B shows diffuse depression on the total deviation plot and a new superior field defect on the pattern deviation plot, which could have resulted in the false conclusion that the patient's glaucoma was progressing. Field C, performed with pupillary dilation, does not contain any localized defects.

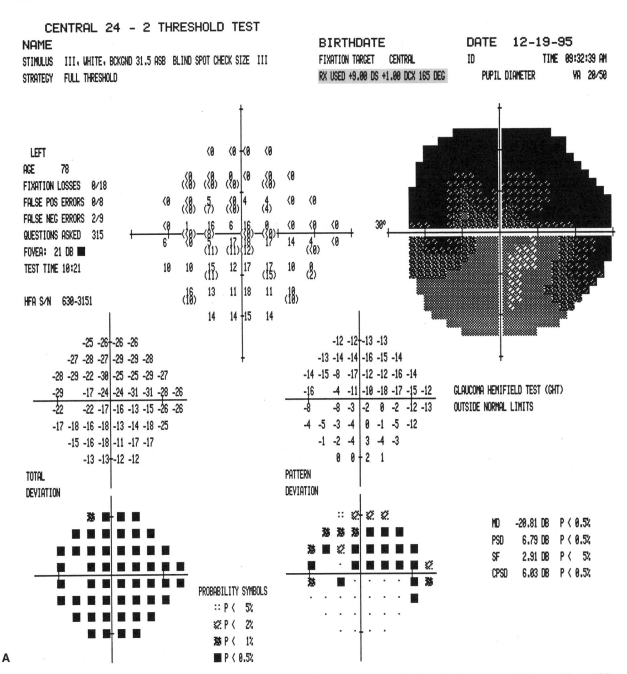

Figure 2-18. Incorrect refraction. The technician read the patient's refraction as +6.00 +1.00 × 165 in the first field (**A**) and added a +3.00 add for a total of +9.00 +1.00 × 165, in the trial frame. The correct refraction was −6.00 +1.00 × 165, and the correct trial frame was used in the second field (**B**). The 12 diopter error produced an increase in diffuse depression, best appreciated by comparing the graytone printouts. The pattern deviation plot was unchanged. The visual field should always be tested with the age appropriate add over the best refraction. Incorrect refraction of as little as 1 diopter can cause diffuse depression of the central field.[14,15]

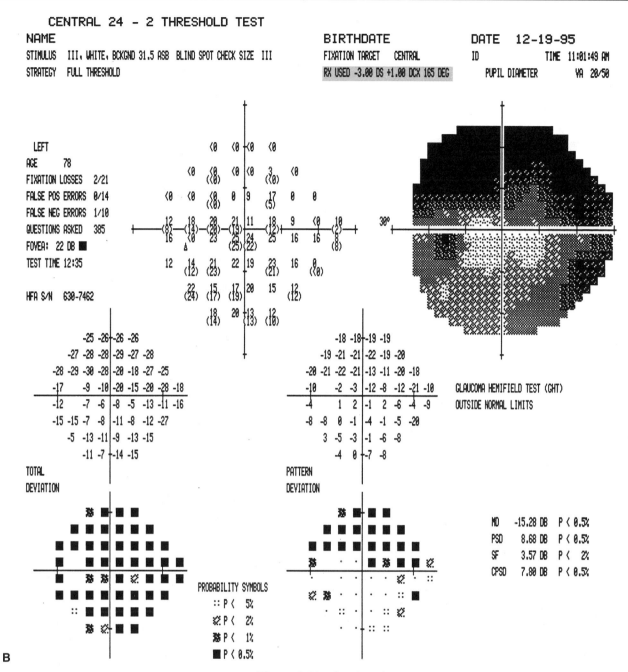

B

Figure 2-18. *Continued.*

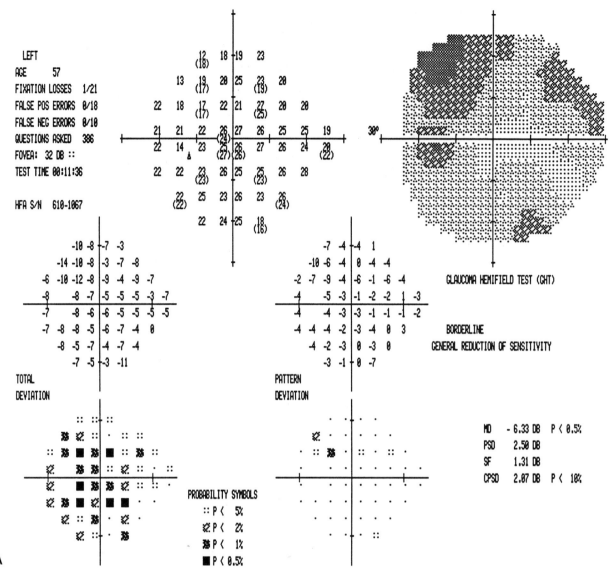

Figure 2-19. Refraction scotoma from staphyloma. Visual fields of a patient with suspected glaucoma who has an −18.00D refractive error and a posterior staphyloma from high myopia. Both graytone printouts show superior defects emanating from the blind spot, which is characteristic of this artifact.[16] These defects could have been interpreted as glaucomatous if the perimetrist was not aware of the artifact produced by the staphyloma.

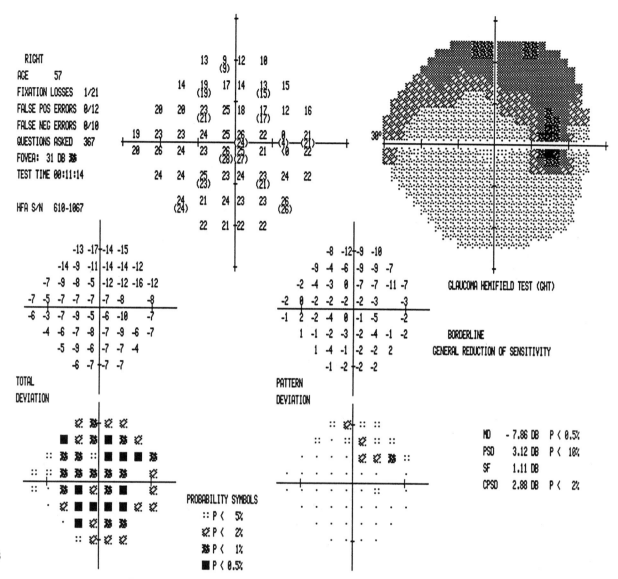

Figure 2-19. *Continued.*

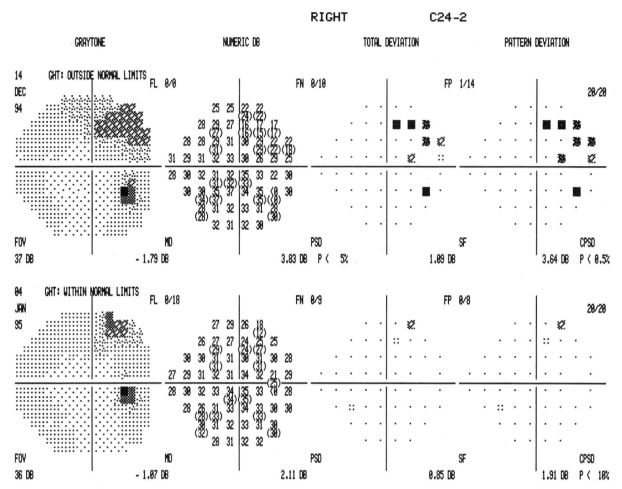

Figure 2-20. Incorrect fixation. The patient who performed the top visual field was fixating too low during the entire test, in the center of the diamond that is used in the initial stage of the test to determine foveal threshold. The blind spot is mapped lower than expected and an artifactual superior arcuate defect appears in the graytone printout, total deviation and pattern deviation plots. The reason these points are abnormal is because the portion of the retina being tested due to incorrect fixation is insensitive compared with the points that the analyzer uses for comparison. The follow-up field (*bottom*) was performed with the patient fixating correctly. (Courtesy of Robert Douville, M.D.)

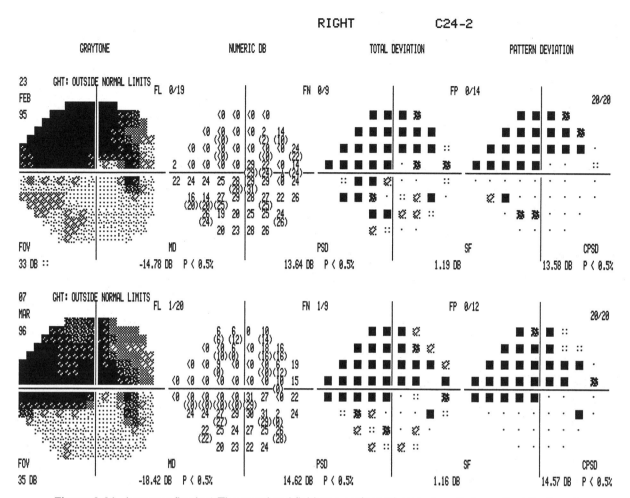

Figure 2-21. Incorrect fixation. The *top* visual field was performed properly, with the patient fixating at the central fixation light. This field shows a superior altitudinal defect that respects the horizontal meridian. The follow-up field (*bottom*) was performed with the patient fixating in the center of the diamond used in determination of the foveal threshold rather than at the central fixation light. The superior altitudinal defect, in this case secondary to glaucoma, crosses the horizontal meridian, which is physiologically impossible. The blind spot is also shifted inferiorly. Retesting showed a pattern similar to the top field.

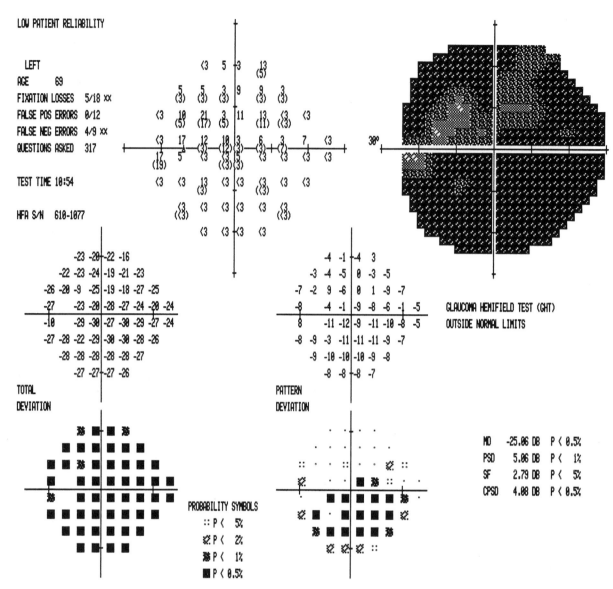

Figure 2-22. Dim projector bulb. The brightest stimulus generated by the Humphrey perimeter is the one with no attenuation and is designated 0 dB on the threshold plot. An absolute scotoma is composed of threshold values <0 dB on the threshold plot. However, if the projector bulb is dim, it may only generate a value of < 3 dB, as in this field. This indicates that the projector bulb is dim and should be replaced. (Courtesy of Ralph Lanciano, DO)

References

1. Zalta AH. Lens rim artifact in automated threshold perimetry. Ophthalmology 1989;96:1302.
2. Katz J, Sommer A. Asymmetry and variation in the normal hill of vision. Arch Ophthalmol 1986;104:65.
3. Åsman P, Heijl A. A clinical study of perimetric probability maps. Arch Ophthalmol 1989, 107:199.
4. Heijl A, Lindgren G, Ollson J, Åsman P. Visual field interpretation with empirical probability maps. Arch Ophthalmol 1989;107:204.
5. Anderson DR. Automated static perimetry. St. Louis: Mosby-Year Book, 1992:123.
6. Anderson DR. Automated static perimetry. St. Louis: Mosby-Year Book, 1992:274.
7. Heijl A, Lindgren G, Olsson J. The effect of perimetric experience in normal subjects. Arch Ophthalmol1989; 107:81.
8. Schulzer M. Errors in the diagnosis of visual field progression in normal-tension glaucoma. Ophthalmology 1994;101:1589.
9. Mills RP, Barnebey HS, Migliazzo CV, Li Y. Does saving time using FASTPAC or suprathreshold testing reduce quality of visual fields? Ophthalmology 1994;101:1596.
10. Johnson CA, Adams CW, Lewis RA. Fatigue effects in automated perimetry. Applied Optics 1988;27:1030.
11. Heuer DK, Anderson DR, Feuer WJ, Gressel MG. The influence of decreased retinal illumination on automated perimetric threshold measurements. Ophthalmology 1989;108:643.
12. Webster AR, Luff AJ, Canning CR, Elkington AR. The effect of pilocarpine on the glaucomatous visual field. Br J Ophthalmol 1993;77:721.
13. Rebolleda G, Muñoz F, Victorio JMF, Pellicer T, Castillo JM. Effects of pupillary dilation on automated perimetry in glaucoma patients receiving pilocarpine. Ophthalmology 1992;99:418.
14. Weinreb RN, Perlman JP. The effect of refractive correction on automated perimetric thresholds. Am J Ophthalmol 1986;101:706.
15. Heuer DK, Anderson DR, Feuer WJ, Gressel MG. The influence of refraction accuracy on automated perimetric threshold measurements. Ophthalmology 1987;94:1550.

3

Opacification of the Ocular Media

Donald L. Budenz

Diseases of the cornea, lens, pupillary space and vitreous generally cause diffuse depression of the visual field, although localized abnormalities are rarely seen.[1] Small pupil size from miotic use can also result in generalized depression of the visual field[2] from decreased retinal illumination.[3] Early glaucoma has been reported to cause generalized depression of the visual field[4–6] but was exceedingly rare in the absence of associated localized nerve fiber layer defects when a large number of patients were tested with automated perimetry.[7] Severe diffuse depression may be seen in the late stages of glaucoma but is preceded by widespread localized defects, which eventually coalesce to affect the entire visual field.

Figures 3.1–3.15 follow on pages 80–97.

References appear on page 98.

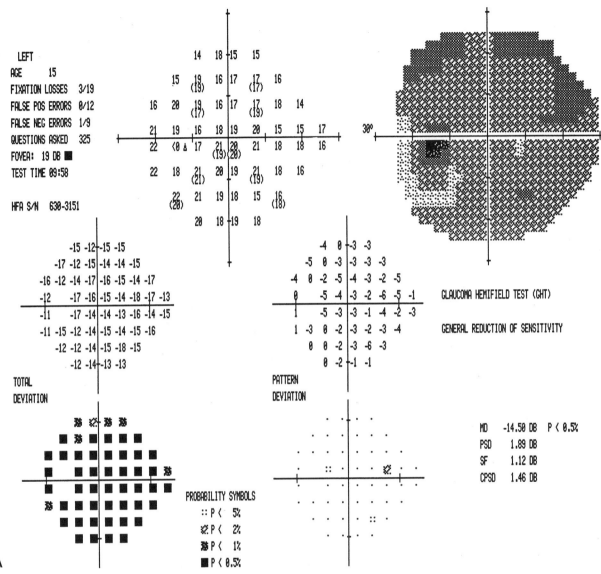

Figure 3-1. Posterior polymorphous dystrophy. Diffuse depression of visual fields in both eyes **(A)** left, **(B)** right, in a 15-year-old with reduced vision (20/50 OD and 20/80 OS) from posterior polymorphous dystrophy. Note the generalized depression of the graytone printout and total deviation plots with normal pattern deviation plots. This confirms that the depression is purely diffuse and there are no localized defects present. Diffuse depression from media opacification is also generally accompanied by reduced central visual acuity, reduced foveal threshold, reduced mean deviation, and the "general reduction of sensitivity" message on the glaucoma hemifield test (GHT). The intraocular pressures were elevated and there was mild cup:disc asymmetry in this patient, thus raising the question of a secondary glaucoma. However, no localized defects are noted on the visual field and treatment was not instituted.

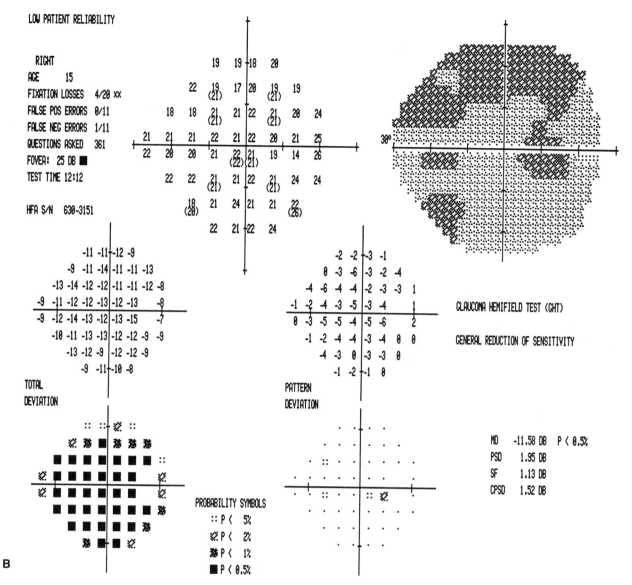

LOW PATIENT RELIABILITY

RIGHT
AGE   15
FIXATION LOSSES   4/20 xx
FALSE POS ERRORS 0/11
FALSE NEG ERRORS 1/11
QUESTIONS ASKED   361
FOVEA: 25 DB ■
TEST TIME 12:12

HFA S/N   630-3151

TOTAL
DEVIATION

PATTERN
DEVIATION

PROBABILITY SYMBOLS
:: P <   5%
⚏ P <   2%
⚏ P <   1%
■ P < 0.5%

GLAUCOMA HEMIFIELD TEST (GHT)

GENERAL REDUCTION OF SENSITIVITY

MD   -11.58 DB   P < 0.5%
PSD   1.95 DB
SF   1.13 DB
CPSD   1.52 DB

B

Figure 3-1. *Continued.*

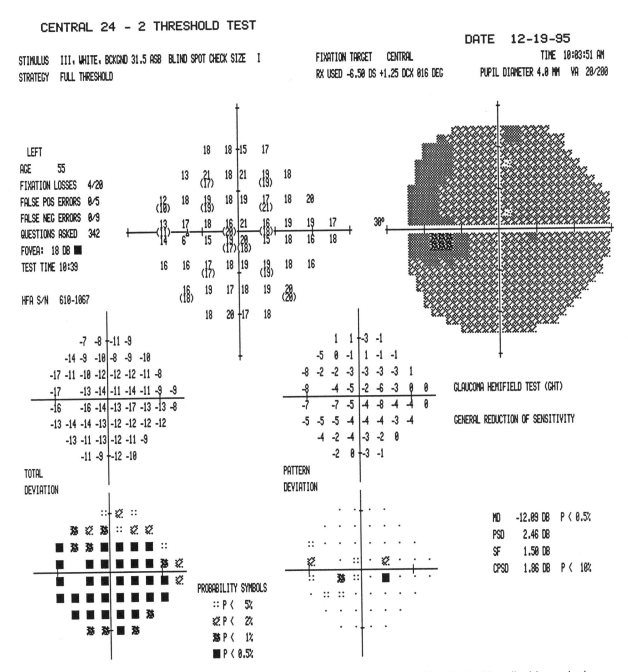

Figure 3-2. Pellucid marginal degeneration. Visual field of a 55-year-old patient with pellucid marginal degeneration of the cornea. The graytone printout and total deviation plots show diffuse depression of the visual field. The pattern deviation plot shows a few depressed points centrally, indicating that the central field is affected to a greater extent than the peripheral field. The foveal threshold and mean deviation are abnormal, as indicated by the presence of probability symbols adjacent to these values. The corrected pattern standard deviation (CPSD) is slightly abnormal, as a result of the mild predominance of central depression.

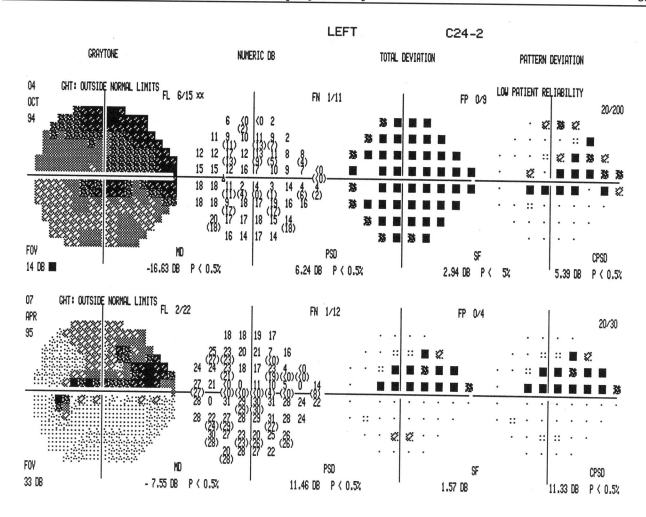

	GRAYTONE SYMBOLS					REV AK			
SYM									
ASB	.8 − .1	2.5 − 1	8 − 3.2	25 − 10	79 − 32	251 − 100	794 − 316	2512 − 1000	7943 − 3162	≥ 10000
DB	41 − 50	36 − 40	31 − 35	26 − 30	21 − 25	16 − 20	11 − 15	6 − 10	1 − 5	≤0

Figure 3-3. Corneal edema and glaucoma. Overview printout of the left eye of a patient who presented with corneal edema following cataract surgery and a history of glaucoma. In the top visual field, the graytone printout shows diffuse depression of the field with superimposed central and superior defects. The total deviation plot shows that all points are severely affected. The pattern deviation plot, which removes the affect from generalized depression, shows localized defects of the central and superior field. Unlike the previous two examples, the GHT is abnormal. In the bottom field, after resolution of the corneal edema, the localized defect persisted and was typical for glaucomatous visual field loss (*bottom*).

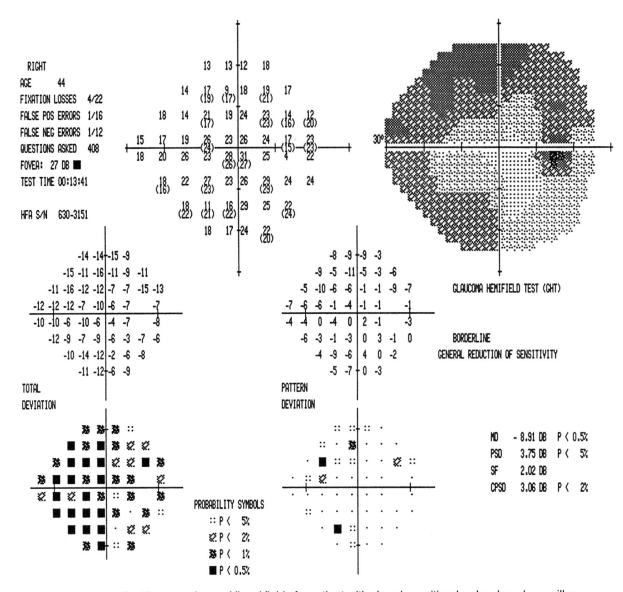

RIGHT

AGE   44

FIXATION LOSSES   4/22

FALSE POS ERRORS 1/16

FALSE NEG ERRORS 1/12

QUESTIONS ASKED   408

FOVEA: 27 DB ■

TEST TIME 00:13:41

HFA S/N   630-3151

TOTAL
DEVIATION

PATTERN
DEVIATION

GLAUCOMA HEMIFIELD TEST (GHT)

BORDERLINE
GENERAL REDUCTION OF SENSITIVITY

MD   - 8.91 DB   P < 0.5%

PSD   3.75 DB   P < 5%

SF   2.02 DB

CPSD   3.06 DB   P < 2%

PROBABILITY SYMBOLS

:: P < 5%

⌧ P < 2%

⅜ P < 1%

■ P < 0.5%

Figure 3-4. Pupillary membrane. Visual field of a patient with chronic uveitis who developed a pupillary membrane affecting the visual field in a diffuse fashion. The foveal threshold is reduced, the graytone printout and total deviation plot show diffuse depression of the field, and the pattern deviation plot shows a few scattered defects in a nonspecific pattern. The GHT reads "general reduction of sensitivity" and "borderline" owing to the cluster of abnormal points in the superonasal field, which were not thought to be clinically significant.

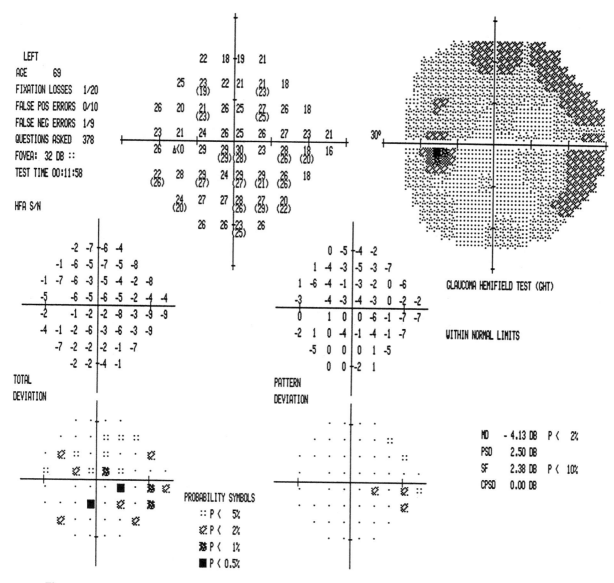

LEFT
AGE   69
FIXATION LOSSES   1/20
FALSE POS ERRORS 0/10
FALSE NEG ERRORS 1/9
QUESTIONS ASKED   378
FOVEA: 32 DB ::
TEST TIME 00:11:58

HFA S/N

		22	18	19	21	
	25	23 (19)	22	21	21 (23)	18
26	20	21 (23)	26	25	27 (25)	26	18
23	21	24	26	25	26	27	23	21
26	&<0	29	29 (29)	30 (28)	23	28 (26)	18 (20)	16
22 (26)	28	29 (27)	24	29 (27)	29 (21)	26 (26)	18
24 (20)	27	27	28 (26)	27 (29)	20 (22)
	26	26	23 (25)	26

30°

GLAUCOMA HEMIFIELD TEST (GHT)

WITHIN NORMAL LIMITS

TOTAL DEVIATION

```
          -2  -7 -6  -4
      -1  -6  -5 -7 -5 -8
  -1  -7  -6  -3 -5 -4 -2 -8
  -5   -6  -5 -6 -5 -2 -4 -4
  -2      -1  -2 -2 -8 -3 -9 -9
  -4  -1  -2  -6 -3 -6 -3 -9
     -7  -2  -2 -2 -1 -7
         -2  -2 -4 -1
```

PATTERN DEVIATION

```
           0  -5 -4 -2
       1  -4  -3 -5 -3 -7
   1  -6  -4  -1 -3 -2  0 -6
  -3      -4  -3 -4 -3  0 -2 -2
   0       1   0  0 -6 -1 -7 -7
  -2   1   0  -4 -1 -4 -1 -7
     -5   0   0  0  1 -5
          0   0 -2  1
```

PROBABILITY SYMBOLS
:: P < 5%
▨ P < 2%
▩ P < 1%
■ P < 0.5%

MD   - 4.13 DB   P < 2%
PSD   2.50 DB
SF   2.38 DB   P < 10%
CPSD   0.00 DB

Figure 3-5. Mild nuclear sclerotic cataract. The visual field of this patient with a 20/40 nuclear sclerotic cataract shows very mild scattered diffuse depression on the total deviation plot, which largely disappears on the pattern deviation plot. The foveal threshold and mean deviation are reduced but the GHT and CPSD do not show any evidence of localized loss, which is characteristic of the effect of cataracts on the visual field. Cataracts have been shown to effect all parts of the visual field uniformly.[8]

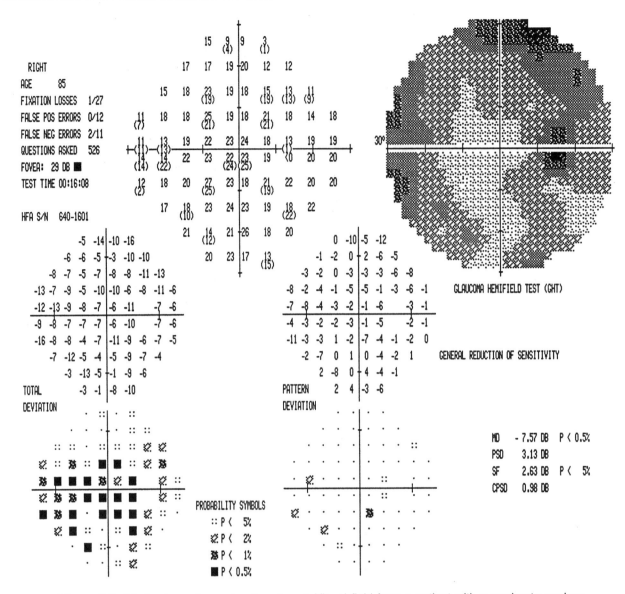

RIGHT

AGE   85

FIXATION LOSSES   1/27

FALSE POS ERRORS 0/12

FALSE NEG ERRORS 2/11

QUESTIONS ASKED   526

FOVEA: 29 DB ■

TEST TIME 00:16:08

HFA S/N   640-1601

GLAUCOMA HEMIFIELD TEST (GHT)

GENERAL REDUCTION OF SENSITIVITY

TOTAL DEVIATION

PATTERN DEVIATION

PROBABILITY SYMBOLS

:: P < 5%

▧ P < 2%

▨ P < 1%

■ P < 0.5%

MD   - 7.57 DB   P < 0.5%

PSD   3.13 DB

SF   2.63 DB   P < 5%

CPSD   0.98 DB

Figure 3-6. Moderate nuclear sclerotic cataract. Visual field from a patient with a moderate nuclear sclerotic cataract and 20/60 vision. The foveal threshold, mean deviation, total deviation plot, and GHT are all abnormal. The pattern deviation plot and CPSD are normal, confirming that the depression is diffuse and not localized. (Courtesy of Rick Davis, OD)

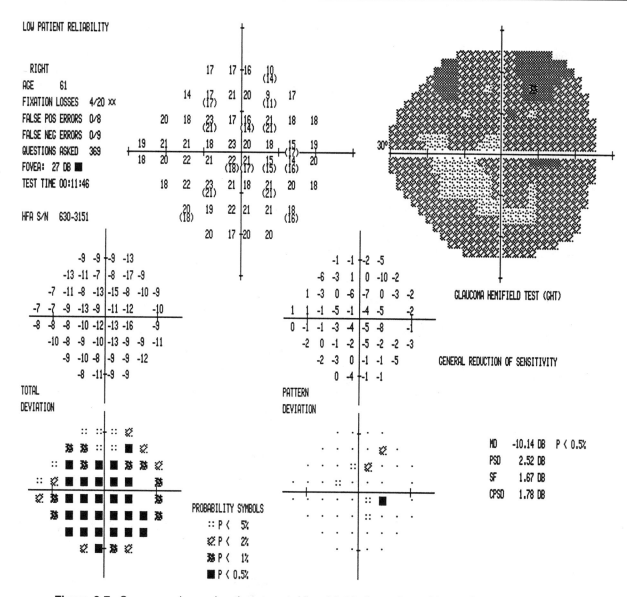

LOW PATIENT RELIABILITY

RIGHT

AGE   61
FIXATION LOSSES   4/20 xx
FALSE POS ERRORS   0/8
FALSE NEG ERRORS   0/9
QUESTIONS ASKED   369
FOVEA: 27 DB ■
TEST TIME 00:11:46

HFA S/N   630-3151

GLAUCOMA HEMIFIELD TEST (GHT)

GENERAL REDUCTION OF SENSITIVITY

TOTAL
DEVIATION

PATTERN
DEVIATION

PROBABILITY SYMBOLS
   :: P < 5%
   ▨ P < 2%
   ▩ P < 1%
   ■ P < 0.5%

MD   -10.14 DB   P < 0.5%
PSD   2.52 DB
SF   1.67 DB
CPSD   1.78 DB

Figure 3-7. Severe nuclear sclerotic cataract. Visual field of a patient with a 20/200 nuclear sclerotic cataract. The foveal threshold, total deviation plot, and mean deviation are markedly abnormal and the GHT reads "general reduction of sensitivity." The pattern deviation plot and CPSD are normal, supporting the interpretation that the abnormality is generalized and not localized.

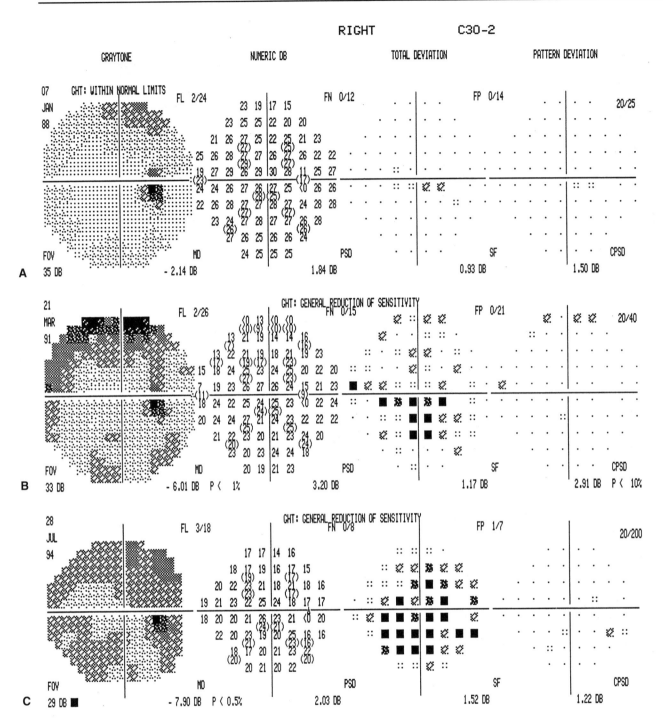

Figure 3-8. Progressive nuclear cataract and removal. Serial visual fields, presented in overview format, showing the effect of progressive nuclear sclerosis (Fields **A-C**) and effect of cataract extraction (Field **D**). Field A, performed when the visual acuity was 20/25, shows a mildly depressed (but not statistically abnormal) mean deviation, and minimally abnormal total deviation plot centrally. Field B, performed when the vision declined to 20/40, shows a depressed mean deviation, diffusely depressed total deviation plot, and "general reduction of sensitivity" on the GHT. Field C, performed when the vision had declined to 20/200, shows an abnormal foveal threshold and worsening of the mean deviation and total deviation plot. Note that the pattern deviation plot, pattern standard deviation, and CPSD remained normal as the cataract worsened. This provides evidence that no localized defects are developing, which was important in this patient, for whom glaucoma was also suspected.

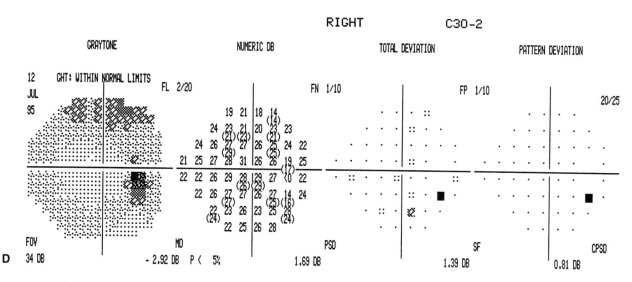

Figure 3-8. *Continued.* Field D was obtained after removal of the cataract. The abnormal parameters return to normal, and the field resembles the original field done before the development of the lens opacification. (*Figure continues on p. 90*)

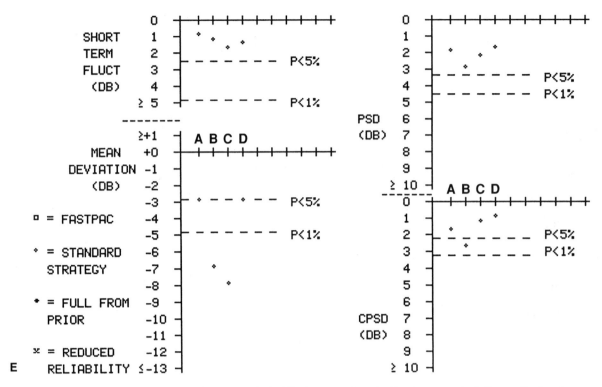

Figure 3-8. *Continued.* The change analysis (**E**) shows a slow decline in mean deviation until after the cataract is removed, after which the mean deviation returns to normal. Note that the CPSD plot over time is relatively stable.

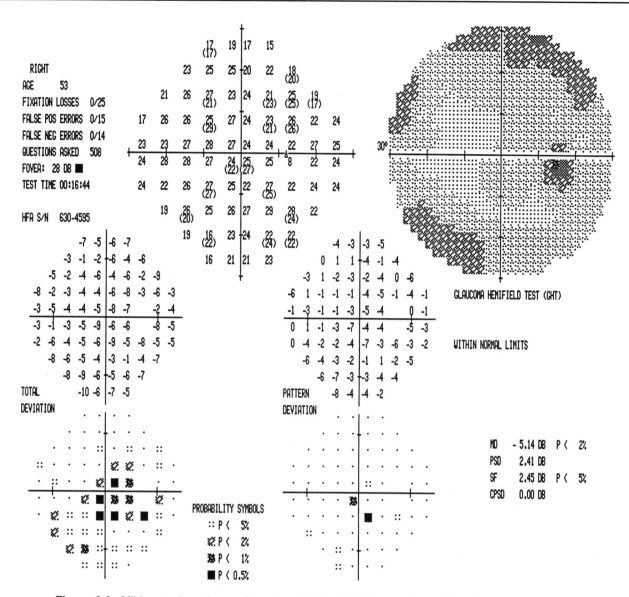

Figure 3-9. Mild posterior subcapsular cataract. Visual field of a patient with 20/20 visual acuity due to a posterior subcapsular cataract. Notice the abnormal foveal sensitivity, depressed mean deviation, and abnormal total deviation plot, which is worse centrally, as evidenced by the depressed central points on the pattern deviation plot. The GHT and CPSD are normal. Posterior subcapsular cataracts tend to be more focal and can effect the visual field more in some areas than others. (Courtesy of Rick Davis, OD)

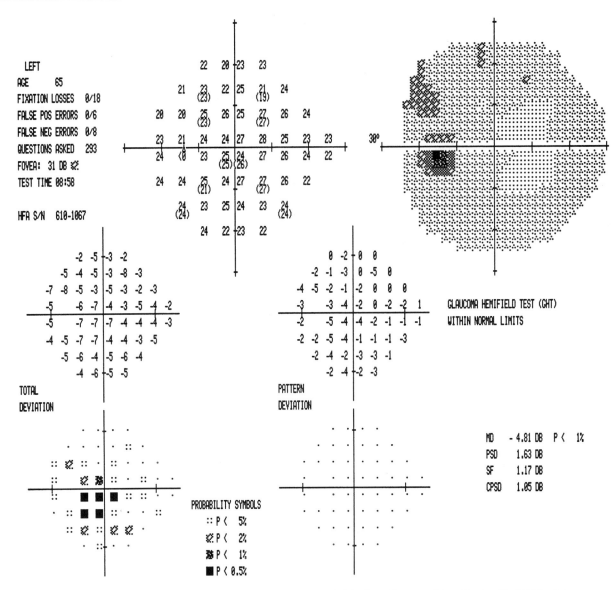

Figure 3-10. Posterior subcapsular cataract. Visual field of a 65-year-old patient with 20/40 vision secondary to a posterior subcapsular cataract. There is reduced foveal threshold and mean deviation, and the total deviation plot is abnormal. The pattern deviation plot, which subtracts the effect of generalized depression, is normal. Note similarity between this and the previous visual field.

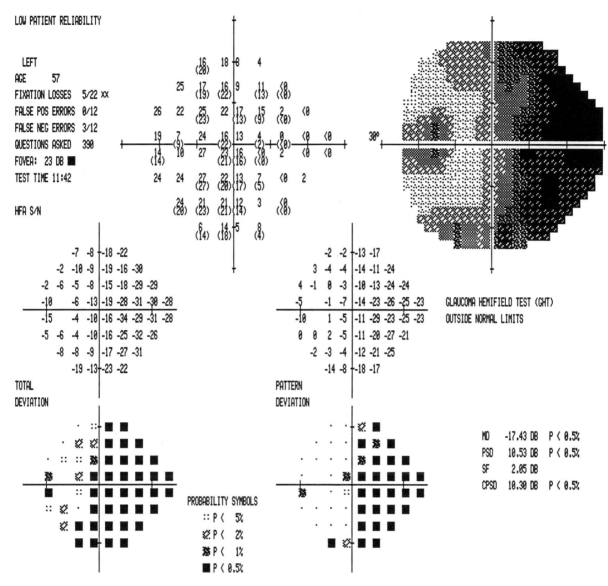

LOW PATIENT RELIABILITY

LEFT
AGE   57
FIXATION LOSSES   5/22 xx
FALSE POS ERRORS 0/12
FALSE NEG ERRORS 3/12
QUESTIONS ASKED   390
FOVEA: 23 DB ■
TEST TIME 11:42

HFA S/N

TOTAL
DEVIATION

PATTERN
DEVIATION

GLAUCOMA HEMIFIELD TEST (GHT)
OUTSIDE NORMAL LIMITS

PROBABILITY SYMBOLS
:: P < 5%
▨ P < 2%
▩ P < 1%
■ P < 0.5%

MD   -17.43 DB   P < 0.5%
PSD   10.53 DB   P < 0.5%
SF   2.05 DB
CPSD   10.30 DB   P < 0.5%

Figure 3-11. Localized field loss from posterior subcapsular cataract. Visual field of a 57-year-old woman who complained of progressive nasal field loss in the left eye. The visual acuity was 20/400. The visual field shows a right hemianopic defect which respects the vertical meridian on the graytone printout, total deviation, and pattern deviation plots. Although a central nervous system lesion might be suspected to cause such a defect, the visual field in the contralateral eye was completely normal. Optic nerve disease or a lesion compressing the lateral aspect of the optic chiasm can rarely cause a monocular nasal hemianopia but there was no abnormality of the optic nerve appearance or function (measured by the swinging flashlight test and color plates). The patient had a dense posterior subcapsular cataract, which was denser nasally. Removal of the cataract resulted in complete normalization of the visual field. Relatively focal media opacities of the posterior lens can cause localized abnormalities in the opposite visual field, whereas relatively focal media opacities of the cornea can cause a localized abnormality on the same side as the lesion.[1] (Courtesy of Carol Karp, M.D.)

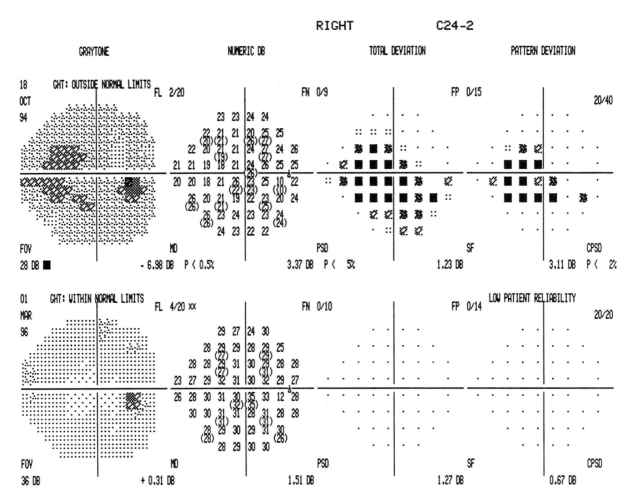

Figure 3-12. Effect of posterior subcapsular cataract removal. Visual fields performed before (*top*) and after (*bottom*) removal of a predominantly posterior subcapsular cataract. The top field shows reduced foveal threshold and mean deviation, diffuse depression which appears worse centrally on the total deviation and pattern deviation plots. The defect is worse inferiorly and the GHT is "outside normal limits." Removal of the cataract resulted in normalization of all parameters.

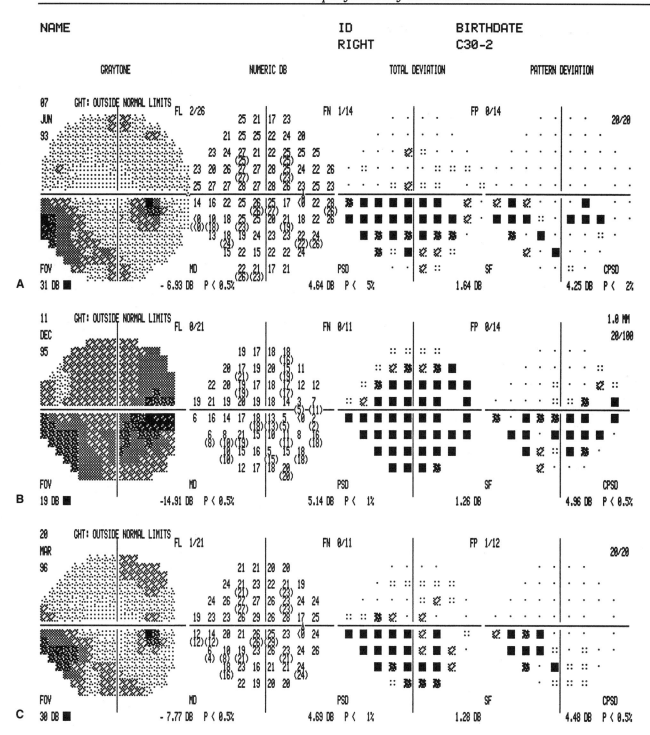

Figure 3-13. Effect of cataract on the glaucomatous visual field. Visual fields of a patient with glaucoma who developed a nuclear sclerotic cataract, which was subsequently removed. Field **A**, performed before the development of cataract, shows an inferior defect, worse nasally, which respects the horizontal meridian. This defect correlated with the patient's glaucomatous optic nerve damage and is typical of a moderate localized field defect from glaucoma (Table 5-3). The patient underwent glaucoma surgery but the visual acuity gradually worsened to 20/100 and the visual field (Field **B**) showed worsening of the foveal threshold, mean deviation, graytone printout, and total deviation plot. The superior hemifield, which was normal on the total deviation printout in field A, is markedly abnormal in field B. However, the pattern deviation plot and CPSD, which are measures of localized abnormality, are essentially unchanged between A and B. The intraocular pressure was controlled by glaucoma surgery during this interval. Cataract extraction resulted in return of the visual field (**C**) to baseline. Cataracts affect normal areas of the field the same amount as glaucomatous areas of the field,[9] and removal of cataracts in patients with glaucomatous visual fields results in significant improvement of global indices in all but the most severely depressed visual fields.[10]

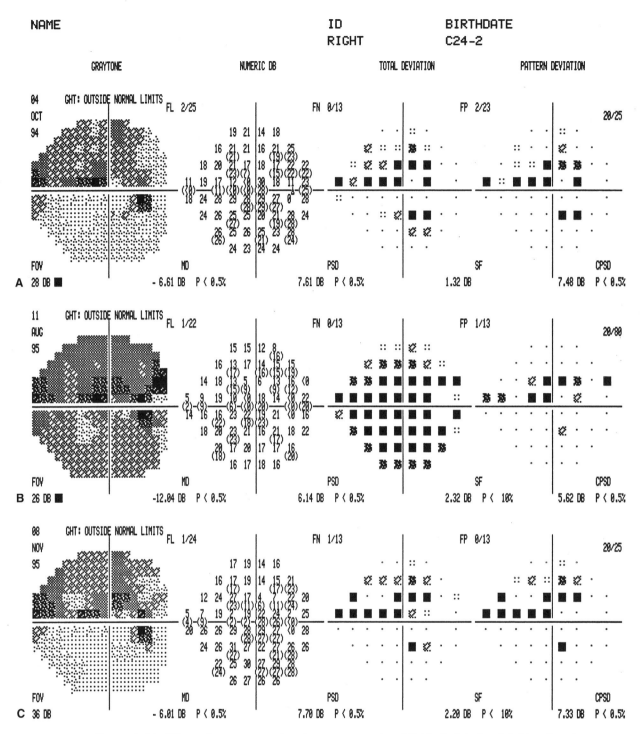

Figure 3-14. Effect of cataract on the glaucomatous visual field. Serial visual fields of a glaucoma patient who developed a cataract, and the visual field subsequent to cataract removal. Field **A** shows a severe superior arcuate defect (see Table 5-4) and an inferior paracentral scotoma that does not quite meet the criteria for early glaucomatous defect (Table 5-1), although it is probably real because of the reproducibility of the depression in this area over time (see Fields **B** and **C**). The patient developed a cataract, and field B shows the effect of diffuse depression over the entire graytone printout and total deviation plot. The mean deviation foreal and visual acuity worsened during this time. The pattern deviation plot is very similar between fields A and B. Note that the threshold, CPSD actually improves. This is due to the fact that, as diffuse depression worsens, the hill of vision becomes relatively smoother. After removal of the cataract, field C returns to baseline in all parameters.

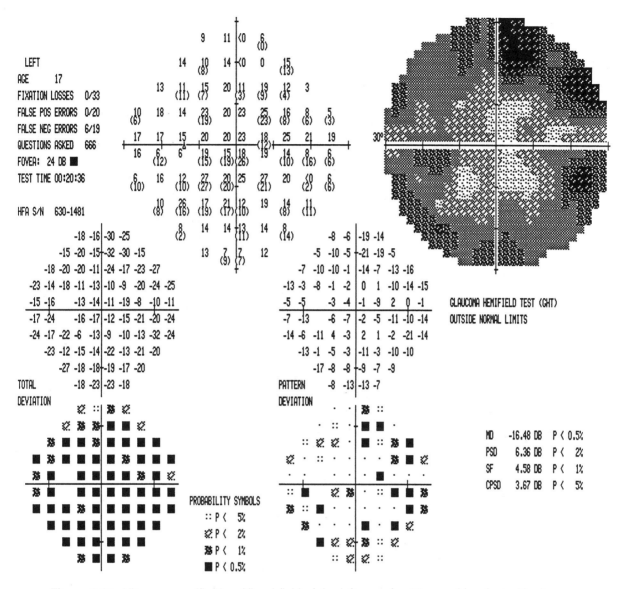

Figure 3-15. Vitreous opacification. Visual field of the left eye of a 17-year-old patient with vitreous cells secondary to pars planitis. Diffuse generalized depression is seen on the graytone printout and total deviation plot. Scattered areas of localized abnormality are seen superimposed on the generalized depression in the pattern deviation plot secondary to retinal scarring.

References

1. Lyne AJ, Phillips CI. Visual field defects due to opacities in the optical media. Br J Ophthalmol 1969;53: 119.
2. Webster AR, Luff AJ, Canning CR, Elkington AR. The effect of pilocarpine on the glaucomatous visual field. Br J Ophthalmol 1993;77:721.
3. Heuer DK, Anderson DR, Feuer WJ, Gressel MG. The influence of decreased retinal illumination on automated perimetric threshold measurements. Ophthalmology 1989;108:643.
4. Anctil J-L, Anderson DR. Early foveal involvement and generalized depression of the visual field in glaucoma. Arch Ophthalmol 1984;102:363.
5. Caprioli J, Sears M. Patterns of early visual field loss in open angle glaucoma. Doc Ophth Pro Ser 1987; 49:307.
6. Drance SM. Diffuse visual field loss in open-angle glaucoma. Ophthalmology 1991;98:1533.
7. Åsman P, Heijl A. Diffuse visual field loss and glaucoma. Acta Ophthal 1994;72:303.
8. Lam BL, Alward WLM, Kolder HE. Effect of cataract on automated perimetry. Ophthalmology 1991;98: 1066.
9. Budenz DL, Feuer W, Anderson DR. The effect of simulated cataract on the glaucomatous visual field. Ophthalmology 1993;100:511.
10. Chem PP, Budenz DL, The effect of cataract extract on the glaucomatous visual field. Submitted for publication.

4

Chorioretinal Disease

Donald L. Budenz

Chorioretinal diseases cause a wide variety of visual field defects. Although few generalizations can be made about the visual field defects caused by chorioretinal diseases as a whole, each class of disease causes characteristic visual field defects. For example, retinal vascular occlusive diseases typically produce dense scotomas in the hemifield opposite the occlusion, with sharp borders that often respect the horizontal meridian. Macular diseases, such as age-related macular degeneration and macular holes, produce central scotomas. Superotemporal lesions of the retina produce scotomas in the inferonasal visual fields. Fortunately, there tends to be close correspondence between the location and appearance of the disease ophthalmoscopically to the visual field appearance.

Figures 4.1–4.34 follow on pages 100–141.

References appear on page 142.

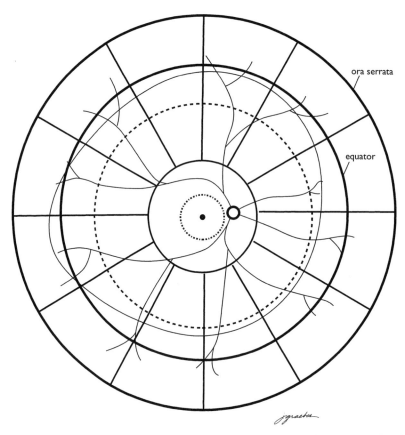

Figure 4-1. Appoximate anatomic relationship between retina and visual field tests. The V4e stimulus of the Goldmann perimeter is able to test the retina *(solid circle, second from rim).* This stimulus is useful for testing visual field loss in peripheral retinal disease, such as CMV retinitis, retinitis pigmentosa, retinal detachment, or retinoschisis. The full field test of the Humphrey perimeter tests the field 60° in each meridian *(broken-line circle, third from rim).* This suprathreshold test may be a useful alternative for following diseases of the periphereal retina because it takes only 6 to 8 minutes and does not require a Goldmann perimeter or a perimetrist skilled in performing manual perimetry. The central 30° field tests the macula and some of the nasal retina *(solid circle, fourth from rim).* This is the most commonly performed automated field test and is more useful for macular disease than peripheral retinal disease. The central 10 ° field tests the parafoveal region *(broken-line circle, fifth from rim).* This test is used to assess visual changes that accompany drug toxicity, such as chloroquine retinopathy.

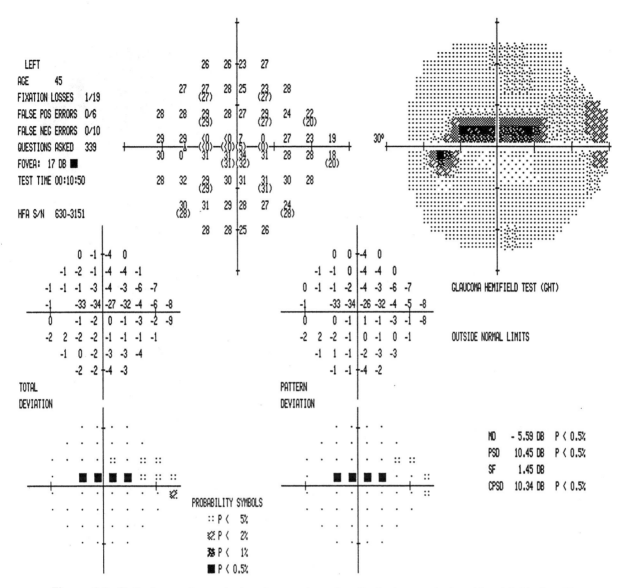

Figure 4-2. Retinal vascular occlusive disease: branch retinal artery occlusion. Visual field of a 45-year-old patient who presented with a Hollenhorst plaque at the first bifurcation of the inferotemporal branch of the central retinal artery. The visual field shows a small scotoma that is deep and has sharp margins in the opposite hemifield. Retinal vascular occlusions characteristically respect the horizontal meridian because the retinal vessels and the corresponding retina that they supply respect the horizontal raphe.

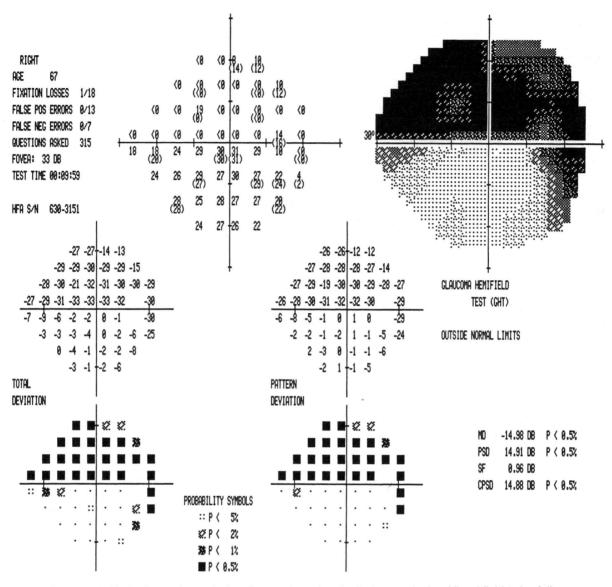

Figure 4-3. Retinal vascular occlusive disease: branch retinal artery occlusion. Visual field 1 day following acute visual loss from an occlusion of the inferotemporal branch of the central retinal artery in a 67-year-old man. Visual field demonstrates a superior altitudinal defect.

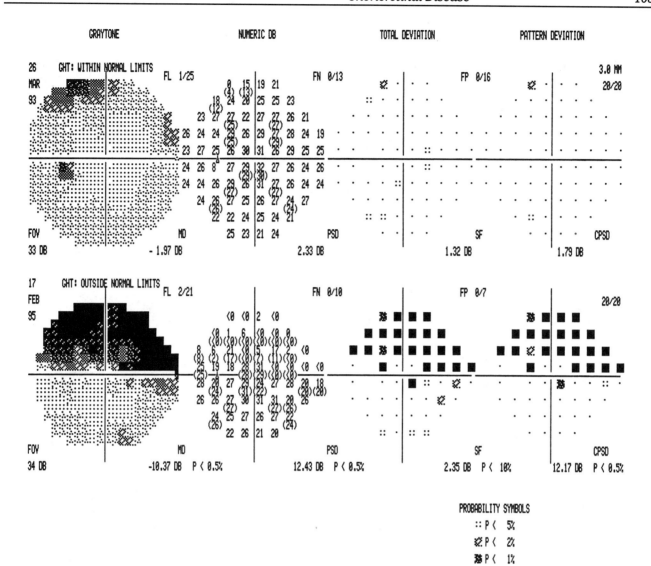

Figure 4-4. Retinal vascular occlusive disease: branch retinal artery occlusion. A 76-year-old patient with suspected glaucoma and a previously normal visual field *(top)* presented with a new, dense, superior arcuate defect that spares the fovea and respects the horizontal meridian *(bottom)*. Ophthalmoscopy revealed a cholesterol embolus at the first bifurcation of the inferior branch of the central retinal artery and ischemia in the distribution of the inferotemporal branch.

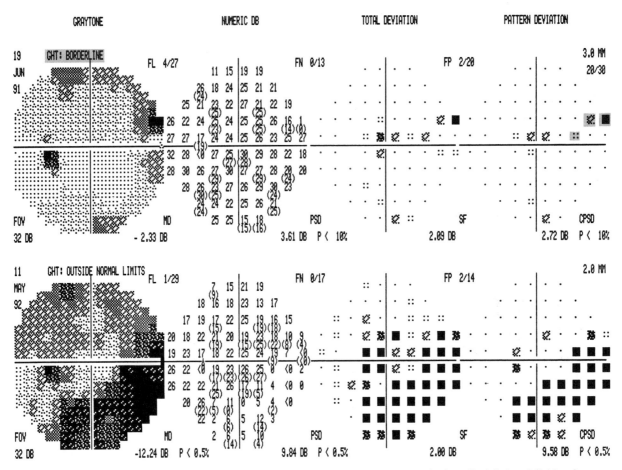

Figure 4-5. Retinal vascular occlusive disease: branch retinal artery occlusion. Serial visual fields of an 82-year-old patient who initially had an early superonasal defect from glaucoma *(top)*, with a borderline glaucoma hemifield test and three adjacent points in the pattern deviation plot that fit the minimal criteria (see Chapter 5, Table 5-1) for glaucomatous nerve fiber layer defect *(highlighted)*. The patient subsequently presented with a superior branch retinal artery occlusion. The field after the occlusion shows a larger, deeper superonasal glaucoma defect and a new dense inferior arcuate defect that respects the horizontal meridian *(bottom)*. This defect is similar in appearance to an arcuate defect from glaucoma. Ophthalmoscopy was necessary to distinguish between a new glaucomatous defect and retinal vascular occlusion in this patient. (Courtesy of Richard K. Parrish, M.D.)

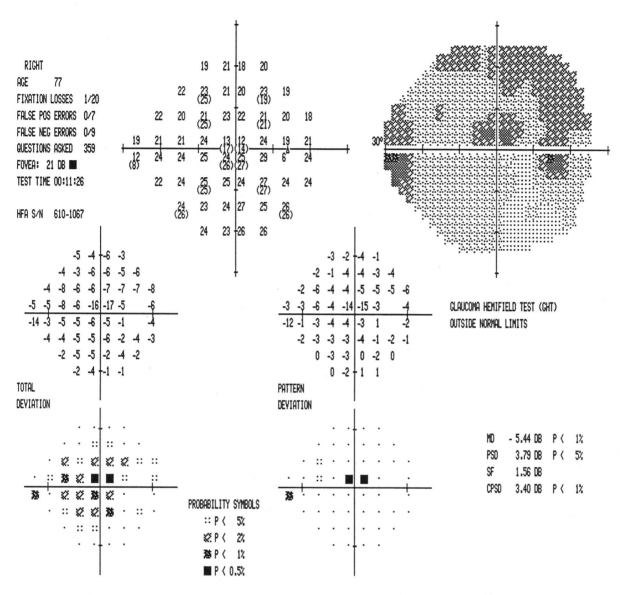

Figure 4-6. Retinal vascular occlusive disease: branch retinal vein occlusion. Visual field of a 77-year-old woman who presented with sudden visual loss to 20/400. A visual field was performed that shows central depression on the total deviation plot. The pattern deviation plot shows that the most depressed area is just above fixation. Ophthalmoscopy demonstrated moderate macular edema (causing reduced visual acuity, diffuse central depression on the total deviation plot, and poor foveal threshold) and an inferior branch retinal vein occlusion (causing severe depression just above fixation respecting the horizontal meridian).

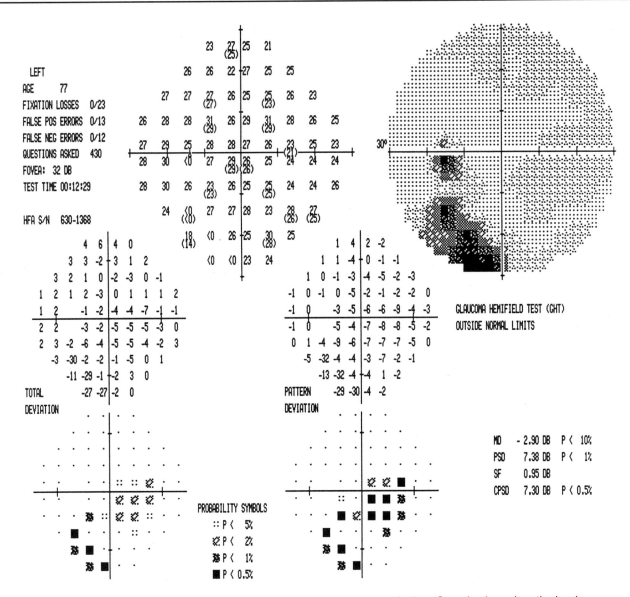

LEFT

AGE 77
FIXATION LOSSES 0/23
FALSE POS ERRORS 0/13
FALSE NEG ERRORS 0/12
QUESTIONS ASKED 430
FOVEA: 32 DB
TEST TIME 00:12:29

HFA S/N 630-1368

GLAUCOMA HEMIFIELD TEST (GHT)
OUTSIDE NORMAL LIMITS

TOTAL DEVIATION

PATTERN DEVIATION

PROBABILITY SYMBOLS
∷ P < 5%
▨ P < 2%
▩ P < 1%
■ P < 0.5%

MD   - 2.90 DB   P < 10%
PSD   7.38 DB   P < 1%
SF   0.95 DB
CPSD   7.30 DB   P < 0.5%

Figure 4-7. Vascular occlusive disease: branch retinal vein occlusion. Superior branch retinal vein occlusion causing peripheral inferior defect, seen on the graytone printout, total deviation plot, and pattern deviation plot. The pattern deviation plot also shows a central process in the temporal quadrant, which is not evident on the graytone printout. This second defect was due to an epiretinal membrane.

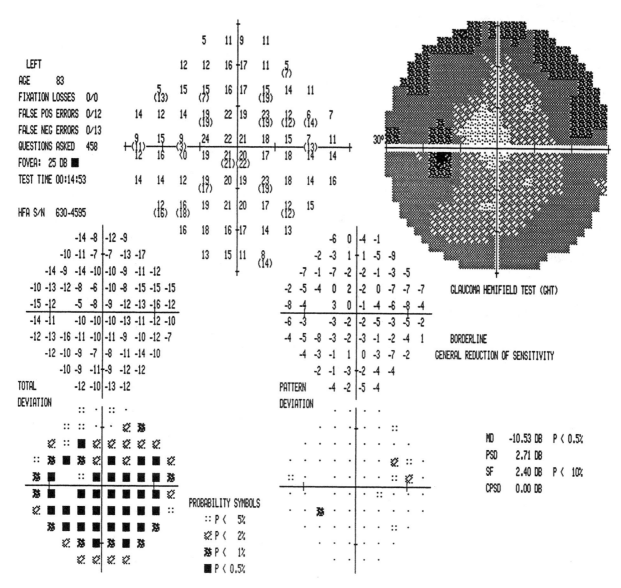

Figure 4-8. Vascular occlusive disease: central retinal vein occlusion. Visual field of an 83-year-old woman with a central retinal vein occlusion who also has suspected glaucoma, based on elevated intraocular pressure. Generalized depression secondary to the central retinal vein occlusion is noted on the graytone printout and total deviation plot. Diffuse retinal disease can cause generalized depression of the visual field. The visual field will be difficult to interpret for early glaucomatous changes. However, note that the pattern deviation plot and corrected pattern deviation (CPSD) are normal and the glaucoma hemifield test is not outside normal limits. A change in any of these three parameters in the future would suggest localized damage from glaucoma. Careful optic nerve analysis would also be important in follow-up of this patient for development of glaucoma.

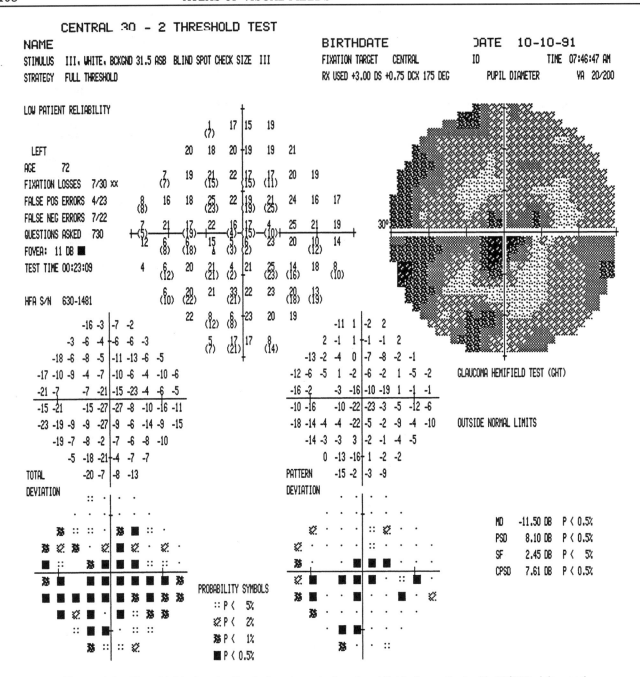

CENTRAL 30 - 2 THRESHOLD TEST

NAME

STIMULUS   III, WHITE, BCKGND 31.5 ASB BLIND SPOT CHECK SIZE III

STRATEGY   FULL THRESHOLD

BIRTHDATE

FIXATION TARGET   CENTRAL

RX USED +3.00 DS +0.75 DCX 175 DEG

DATE   10-10-91

ID   TIME 07:46:47 AM

PUPIL DIAMETER   VA 20/200

LOW PATIENT RELIABILITY

LEFT

AGE   72

FIXATION LOSSES   7/30 xx

FALSE POS ERRORS 4/23

FALSE NEG ERRORS 7/22

QUESTIONS ASKED   730

FOVEA: 11 DB ■

TEST TIME 00:23:09

HFA S/N   630-1481

GLAUCOMA HEMIFIELD TEST (GHT)

OUTSIDE NORMAL LIMITS

TOTAL DEVIATION

PATTERN DEVIATION

PROBABILITY SYMBOLS

:: P < 5%

⊠ P < 2%

▨ P < 1%

■ P < 0.5%

MD	-11.50 DB	P < 0.5%
PSD	8.10 DB	P < 0.5%
SF	2.45 DB	P < 5%
CPSD	7.61 DB	P < 0.5%

Figure 4-9. Choroidal ischemia. Central scotoma in the visual field of a patient with 20/200 vision and a normal retinal and optic nerve examination. Fluorescein angiography showed nonperfusion of the choroid in the peripapillary area on flourescein angiography. The scotoma does not respect the horizontal meridian as the blood supply of the choroid, unlike the blood supply of the retina, does not respect the horizontal raphe. An irregular central scotoma that is out of proportion to the appearance of the macula is characteristic of choroidal ischemia involving the fovea.[1] The fixation loss rate is high, typical of central scotomas, because patients have a difficult time fixating on the central fixation light. In this situation, redoing the test with the patient fixating in the center of the small or large diamond would reduce the fixation loss rate (Figure 1-9). The central scotoma on the pattern deviation plot does not respect the horizontal meridian since the chocoidal blood supply does not respect the horizontal raphe.

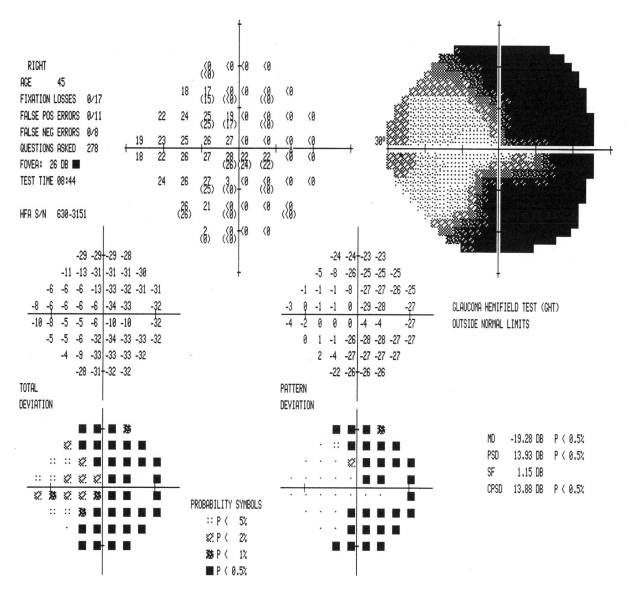

RIGHT

AGE 45

FIXATION LOSSES 0/17

FALSE POS ERRORS 0/11

FALSE NEG ERRORS 0/8

QUESTIONS ASKED 278

FOVEA: 26 DB ■

TEST TIME 08:44

HFA S/N 630-3151

GLAUCOMA HEMIFIELD TEST (GHT)
OUTSIDE NORMAL LIMITS

TOTAL DEVIATION

PATTERN DEVIATION

MD   -19.28 DB   P < 0.5%

PSD   13.93 DB   P < 0.5%

SF   1.15 DB

CPSD   13.88 DB   P < 0.5%

PROBABILITY SYMBOLS

:: P < 5%

▨ P < 2%

▩ P < 1%

■ P < 0.5%

Figure 4-10. Retinal detachment: rhegmatogenous. Central 30° field of a 45-year-old man, 20 years after a rhegmatogenous retinal detachment involving the nasal retina. The temporal field is mostly affected. Note that the defect has sharp borders, a typical feature of long-standing, but not recent, rhegmatogenous retinal detachments. Less chronic detachments tend to have sloping margins (ie, relative defect at the edge of the scotoma).[2]

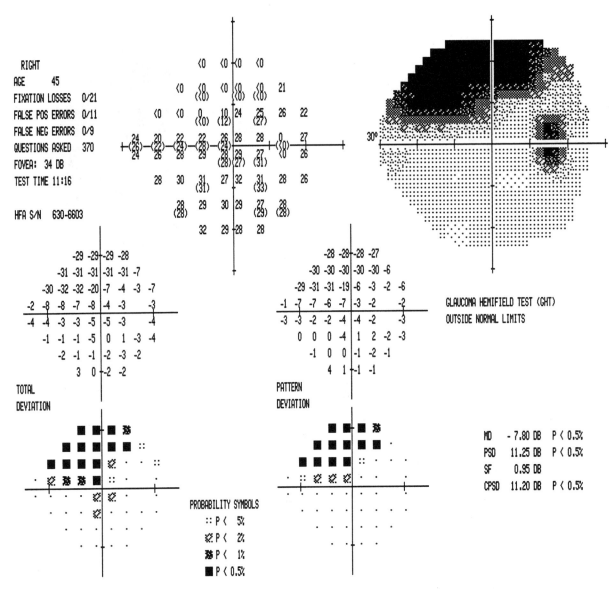

RIGHT

AGE 45

FIXATION LOSSES 0/21

FALSE POS ERRORS 0/11

FALSE NEG ERRORS 0/9

QUESTIONS ASKED 370

FOVEA: 34 DB

TEST TIME 11:16

HFA S/N 630-6603

```
                      <0   <0  <0   <0
                 <0   <0  <0  <0   <0   21
                           <0  (0)  (27)
            <0   <0   <0   10   24   25   26   22
                      (0) (12)       (27)
      24   20   22   22   26   28   28   0    27
     (26) (22) (24) (28) (24)          (0)  26
      24   26   28   28        28   27   27   26
                      (28)(27)(31)
           28   30   31   27  32   31   28   26
                     (31)         (33)
                28   29   30  29   27   28
               (28)              (29) (28)
                     32   29   28   28
```

```
TOTAL DEVIATION

      -29  -29  -29  -28
   -31  -31  -31  -31  -31  -7
 -30  -32  -32  -20  -7  -4  -3  -7
-2  -8  -8  -7  -8  -4  -3       -3
-4  -4  -3  -3  -5  -5  -3       -4
  -1  -1  -1  -5  0   1  -3  -4
    -2  -1  -1  -2  -3  -2
        3   0  -2  -2
```

```
PATTERN DEVIATION

      -28  -28  -28  -27
   -30  -30  -30  -30  -30  -6
 -29  -31  -31  -19  -6  -3  -2  -6
-1  -7  -7  -6  -7  -3  -2       -2
-3  -3  -2  -2  -4  -4  -2       -3
   0   0   0  -4   1   2  -2  -3
    -1   0   0  -1  -2  -1
        4   1  -1  -1
```

GLAUCOMA HEMIFIELD TEST (GHT)

OUTSIDE NORMAL LIMITS

PROBABILITY SYMBOLS

:: P < 5%

▨ P < 2%

▩ P < 1%

■ P < 0.5%

MD -7.80 DB   P < 0.5%

PSD 11.25 DB   P < 0.5%

SF 0.95 DB

CPSD 11.20 DB   P < 0.5%

Figure 4-11. Retinal detachment: rhegmatogenous. Visual field of a patient referred for glaucoma evaluation secondary to the above visual field defect. The visual field shows a dense superior nasal step with sharp borders. The defect has an arcuate component but does not emanate from the blind spot. Ophthalmoscopy revealed a healthy optic nerve but also evidence of an old inferior retinal detachment, which had resolved spontaneously although retinal function was lost in the area of the detachment. Visual field function may or may not return after reattachment of the retina, depending on the chronicity of the detachment.[2]

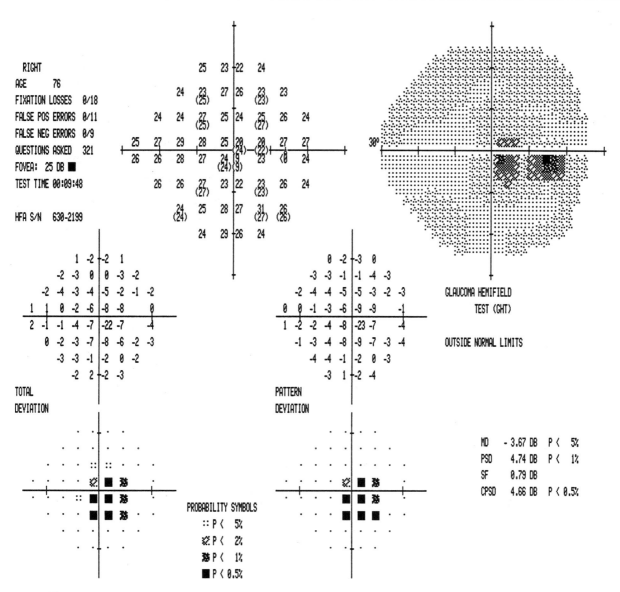

Figure 4-12. Retinal detachment: exudative. A 76-year-old woman with an exudative neurosensory retinal detachment involving the center of the macula, causing central scotoma and reduced visual acuity (20/200). Fluorescein angiography did not show a choroidal neovascular membrane or pigment epithelial detachment. The isolated neurosensory detachment was felt to be related to macular degeneration in this case because of the patient's age. The relative scotoma is evident on the graytone printout, total deviation plot, and pattern deviation plot. The foveal threshold is also reduced.

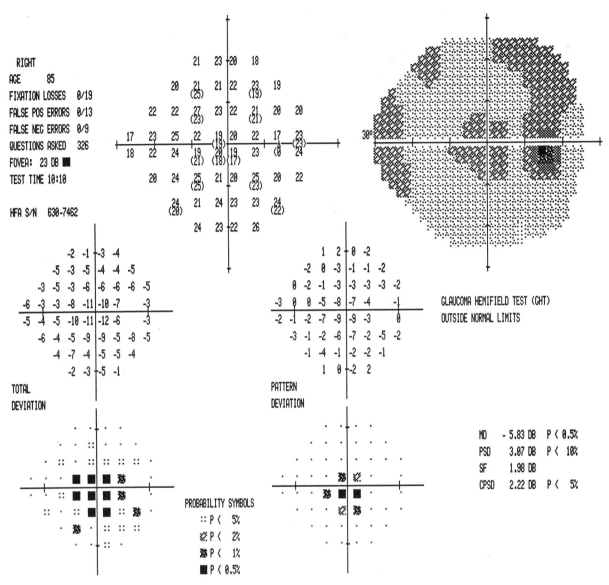

RIGHT

AGE 85

FIXATION LOSSES 0/19

FALSE POS ERRORS 0/13

FALSE NEG ERRORS 0/9

QUESTIONS ASKED 326

FOVEA: 23 DB ■

TEST TIME 10:10

HFA S/N 630-7462

```
                    21   23  20   18
               20   21   21  22   23   19
                   (25)          (19)
          22   22   27   23  22   21   20   20
                   (23)          (21)
     17   23   25   22   19  20   22   17   23
                        (18)              (23)
     18   22   24   19   20  19   23   0    24
                   (21)  (18)(17)
          20   24   25   21  20   25   20   22
                   (25)          (23)
               24   21   24  23   23   24
              (20)                   (22)
                    24   23  22   26
```

```
                -2  -1  -3  -4
             -5 -3 -5 -4 -4 -5
          -3 -5 -3 -6 -6 -6 -6 -5
       -6 -3 -3 -8 -11 -10 -7    -3
       -5 -4 -5 -10 -11 -12 -6   -3
          -6 -4 -5 -9 -9 -5 -8 -5
             -4 -7 -4 -5 -5 -4
                -2 -3 -5 -1
```

TOTAL
DEVIATION

```
                 1   2   0  -2
              -2  0  -3 -1 -1 -2
           0  -2 -1 -3 -3 -3 -3 -2
       -3  0  0 -5 -8 -7 -4    -1
       -2 -1 -2 -7 -9 -9 -3     0
          -3 -1 -2 -6 -7 -2 -5 -2
             -1 -4 -1 -2 -2 -1
                 1  0 -2  2
```

PATTERN
DEVIATION

GLAUCOMA HEMIFIELD TEST (GHT)

OUTSIDE NORMAL LIMITS

PROBABILITY SYMBOLS

:: P < 5%

▨ P < 2%

▩ P < 1%

■ P < 0.5%

MD   - 5.83 DB   P < 0.5%

PSD   3.07 DB   P < 10%

SF   1.98 DB

CPSD   2.22 DB   P < 5%

Figure 4-13. Macular degeneration: RPE atrophy. Visual field of an 85-year-old woman with 20/60 vision and atrophic age related macular degeneration OD in the center of the macula. A choroidal neovascular membrane was absent on flourescein angiography. The visual field demonstrates a central scotoma on the graytone printout, total deviation, and pattern deviation plots. RPE atrophy from age-related macular degeneration is more likely to cause visual field disturbance than drusen, which do not typically cause visual field dysfunction.[2]

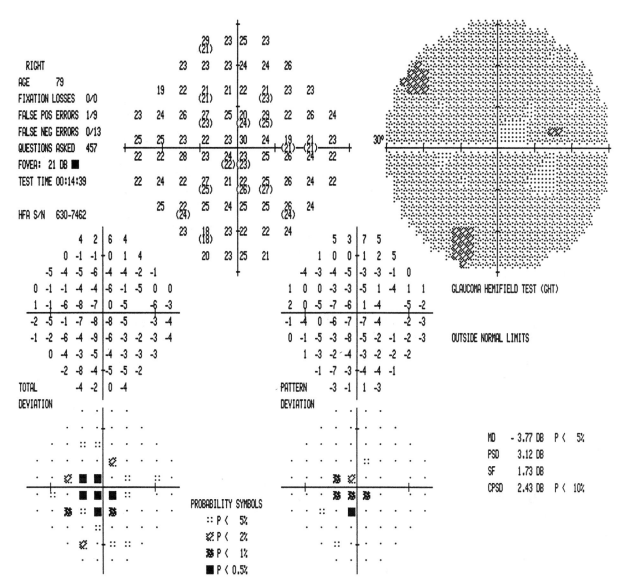

Figure 4-14. Macular degeneration: choroidal neovascular membrane. Visual field of a 79-year-old woman with atrophic age-related macular degeneration. The graytone printout is normal but the total deviation and pattern deviation plots show central depression secondary to neovascular membrane, diagnosed by intravenous flourescein angiography. The foveal threshold is markedly abnormal. The patient's central scotoma prohibited reliable central fixation, so the blind spot check function for evaluating fixation losses was turned off, accounting for the 0/0 fixation losses.

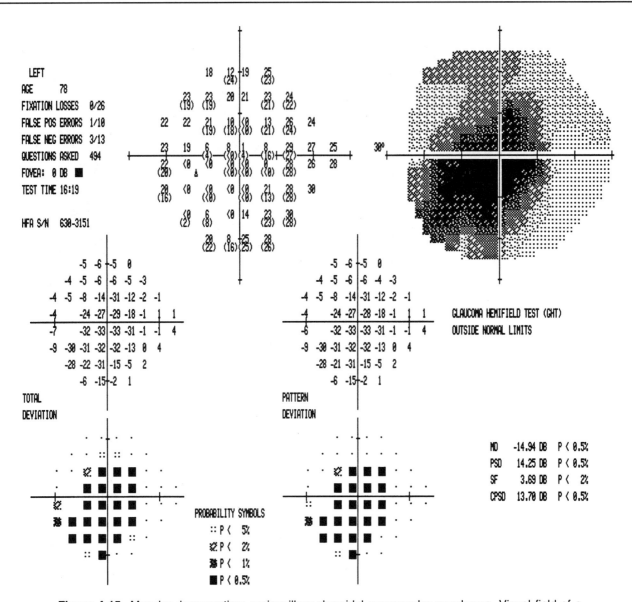

Figure 4-15. Macular degeneration: peripapillary choroidal neovascular membrane. Visual field of a 78-year-old man with a peripapillary choroidal neovascular membrane, which had been treated with laser in the left eye. A large, dense cecocentral scotoma is noted on the graytone printout, total deviation, and pattern deviation plots. The visual acuity was 20/400, and the foveal threshold was 0 dB. Subretinal neovascular membranes typically cause dense, irregular-shaped, central scotomas with sharp margins.[1]

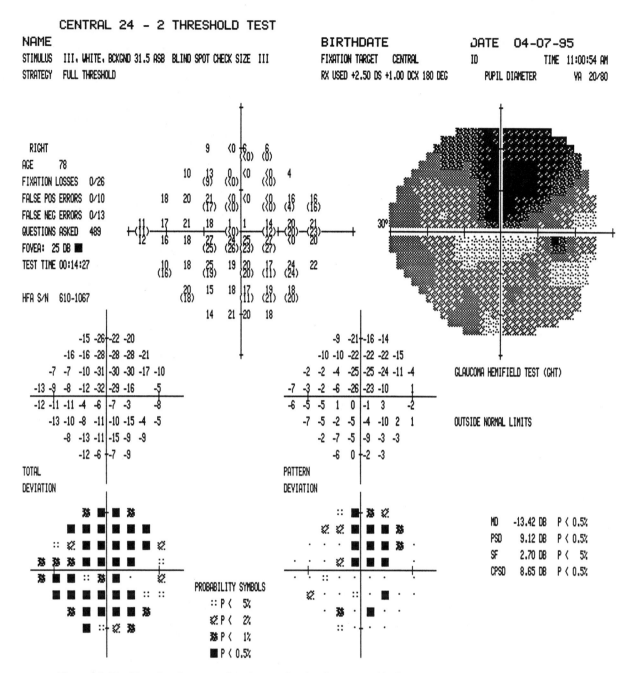

Figure 4-16. Macular degeneration: hemorrhagic pigment epithelial detachment. Visual field of a 78-year-old man who presented with visual acuity of 20/80 OD, elevated intraocular pressure and cup:disc of 0.8. Retinal examination revealed a hemorrhagic pigment epithelial detachment inferior to the fovea. The visual field shows diffuse depression on the graytone printout and total deviation plots from macular degeneration but a denser superior paracentral visual field defect on the pattern deviation plot that corresponded to the location of the hemorrhagic pigment epithelial detachment.

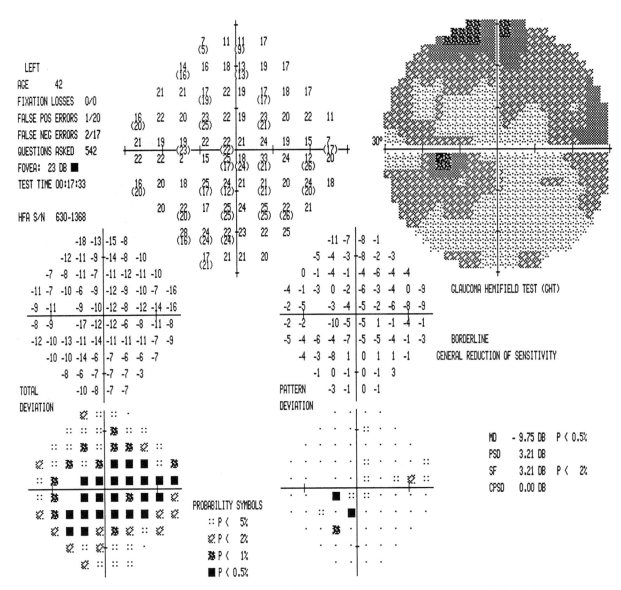

Figure 4-17. Diabetic retinopathy: macular edema. Visual field of a 42-year-old diabetic patient with clinically significant macular edema. The visual acuity was 20/200, and the visual field shows reduced foveal threshold, high mean deviation, and diffuse depression on the total deviation plot. The pattern deviation plot does not show any significant localized defects. The glaucoma hemifield test reads "borderline" (owing to the small cluster of abnormal points inferiorly on the pattern deviation plot) as well as generalized reduction of sensitivity. The CPSD is normal, further evidence that the field is diffusely depressed. Central visual field abnormalities have been demonstrated in 100% of patients with ophthalmoscopically visible diabetic retinopathy and 39.4% of diabetics without visible retinopathy.[3]

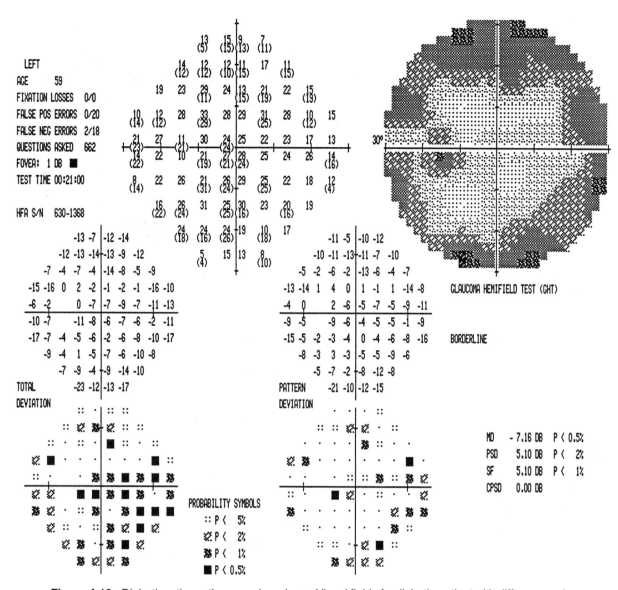

Figure 4-18. Diabetic retinopathy: macular edema. Visual field of a diabetic patient with diffuse macular edema before photocoagulation. The entire central field is affected diffusely, best seen in the total deviation plot. The pattern deviation plot shows scattered areas of depression over the entire central 30°. The glaucoma hemifield test reads "borderline." Although the pattern standard deviation is high, the high short-term fluctuation cancels this out, resulting in a corrected pattern standard deviation of 0 dB.

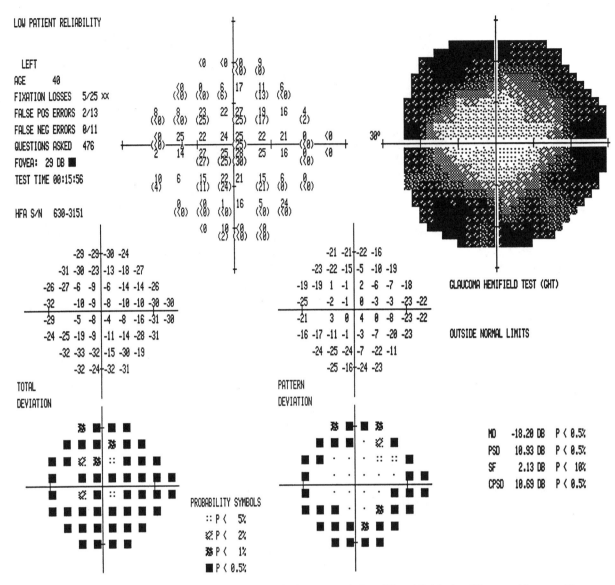

Figure 4-19. Diabetic retinopathy: panretinal photocoagulation. Visual field of a 40-year-old man with proliferative diabetic retinopathy who underwent heavy panretinal photocoagulation. The total deviation plot shows diffuse depression and the visual acuity (20/50) and foveal threshold are depressed from retinal disease. The graytone printout and pattern deviation plot show the effects of panretinal photocoagulation, which has resulted in dense peripheral field constriction sparing the central 15°. Panretinal photocoagulation for proliferative diabetic retinopathy produces dense constriction of the peripheral visual field, whereas focal laser treatment for macular edema has been shown to produce small localized scotomas in the central region of the field.[4] The patient whose fields are shown above is also a glaucoma suspect with ocular hypertension and normal optic nerves. Because nerve fiber defects from glaucoma are most likely to appear between 20° and 30° from fixation, following the visual field for glaucomatous change will be difficult in this patient. In cases such as this, careful optic disc observation is important.

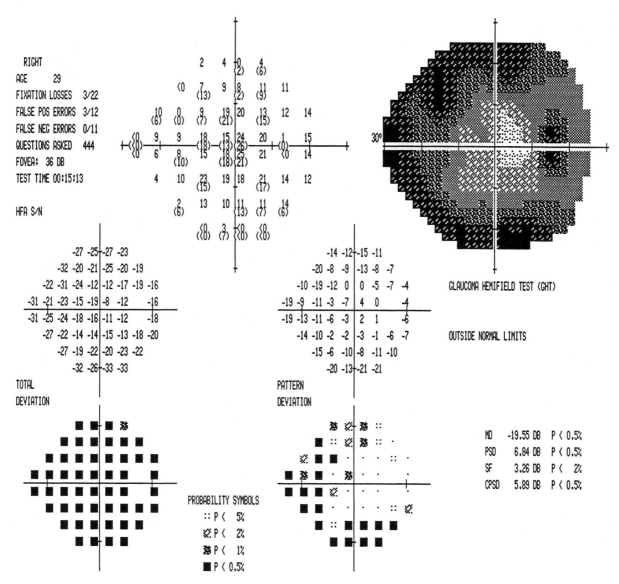

Figure 4-20. Retinitis pigmentosa (RP). Visual field of the right eye of a 29-year-old patient with 20/30 vision and RP with simplex inheritance pattern. The field is diffusely depressed on the total deviation plot but the depression is more severe peripherally. Note how the nasal constriction is contiguous across the horizontal meridian, which is typical of diffuse retinal disease. This is in contrast to retinal vascular disease and optic nerve diseases (such as glaucoma or optic neuropathies), which do not usually cross the horizontal meridian. RP affects rod function before cone function preferentially, thereby causing peripheral field loss. The field defects in typical RP start as isolated scotomas in the midperiphery of the visual field. These coalesce over time, and a ring scotoma is produced, usually in both eyes symmetrically.[1] The contralateral eye in this patient was so severely affected that there were no normal areas in the central 30°, even with a size V stimulus. Early central involvement is rare but may be seen in certain early-onset subtypes of RP and in cases with secondary causes of visual loss (eg, cystoid macular edema).[5]

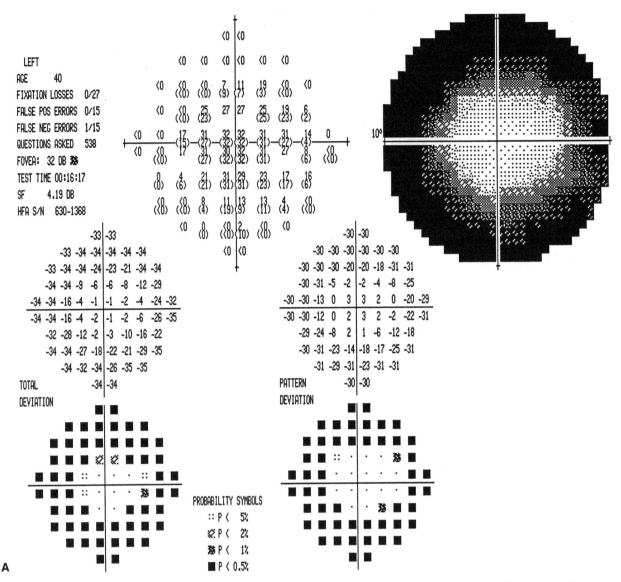

Figure 4-21. Severe retinitis pigmentosa (RP). Bilateral 10° visual fields of a 39-year-old patient with RP, **(A)** left eye, **(B)** right eye. Graytone, total deviation plot, and pattern deviation plot all show symmetric constriction to within the central 10° with central sparing. The patient's visual acuity was 20/30 in both eyes. Automated perimetry may be performed in the light- and dark-adapted states to help define the subtypes of RP.[6]

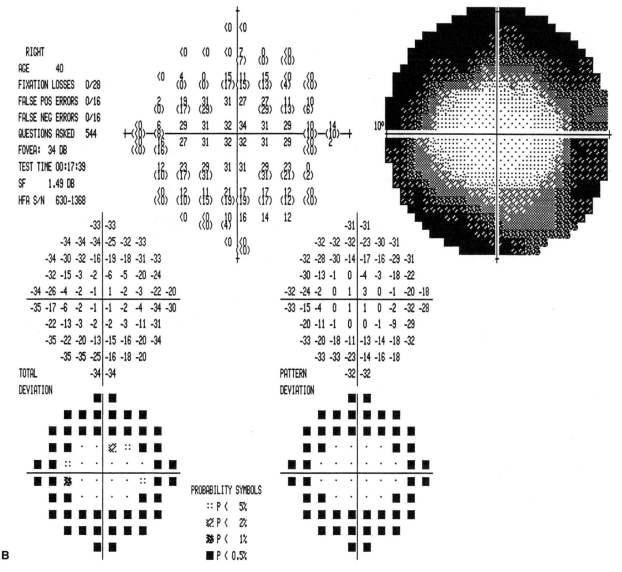

RIGHT

AGE   40

FIXATION LOSSES   0/28

FALSE POS ERRORS   0/16

FALSE NEG ERRORS   0/16

QUESTIONS ASKED   544

FOVEA: 34 DB

TEST TIME 00:17:39

SF   1.49 DB

HFA S/N   630-1368

TOTAL   -34 -34
DEVIATION

PATTERN   -32 -32
DEVIATION

PROBABILITY SYMBOLS

:: P < 5%

▨ P < 2%

▩ P < 1%

■ P < 0.5%

B

Figure 4-21. *Continued.*

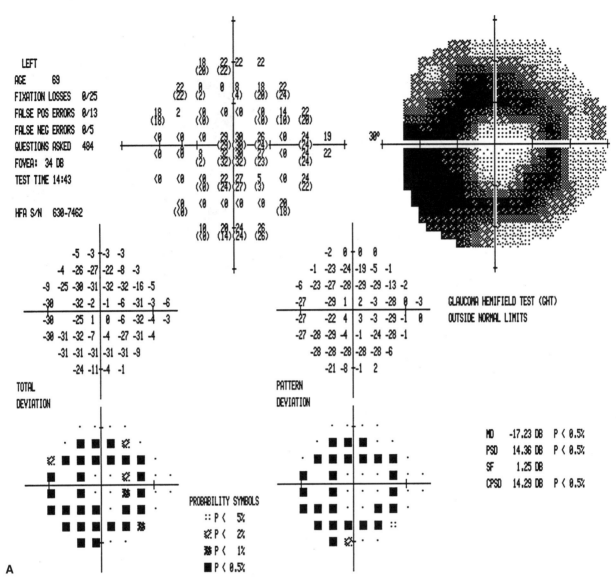

LEFT

AGE   69

FIXATION LOSSES   0/25

FALSE POS ERRORS   0/13

FALSE NEG ERRORS   0/5

QUESTIONS ASKED   484

FOVEA: 34 DB

TEST TIME 14:43

HFA S/N   630-7462

TOTAL
DEVIATION

PATTERN
DEVIATION

GLAUCOMA HEMIFIELD TEST (GHT)

OUTSIDE NORMAL LIMITS

PROBABILITY SYMBOLS

:: P < 5%

▨ P < 2%

▩ P < 1%

■ P < 0.5%

MD   -17.23 DB   P < 0.5%

PSD   14.36 DB   P < 0.5%

SF   1.25 DB

CPSD   14.29 DB   P < 0.5%

A

Figure 4-22. Inherited disorders of night blindness: atypical retinitis pigmentosa OU. Visual fields of a 69-year-old woman with pigmentary changes causing a ring scotoma in the paracentral (10° to 20°) region, **(A)** left eye, **(B)** right eye. This atypical location is more characteristic of later onset retinitis pigmentosa, which is more slowly progressive and less likely to affect fixation. The typical location for ring scotomas on the visual field in retinitis pigmentosa is 20° to 30°.[1] Note that the ring scotoma is contiguous across the horizontal meridian, distinguishing this from nerve fiber layer defects form optic nerve disorders.

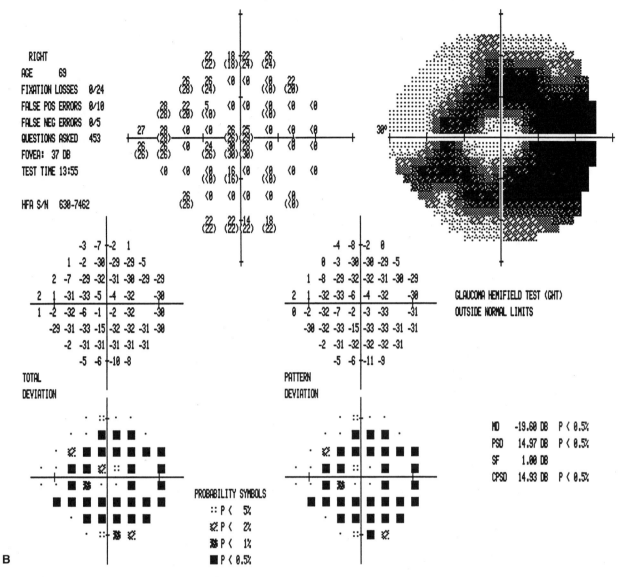

RIGHT

AGE   69
FIXATION LOSSES   0/24
FALSE POS ERRORS   0/10
FALSE NEG ERRORS   0/5
QUESTIONS ASKED   453
FOVEA: 37 DB
TEST TIME 13:55

HFA S/N   630-7462

TOTAL
DEVIATION

PATTERN
DEVIATION

GLAUCOMA HEMIFIELD TEST (GHT)
OUTSIDE NORMAL LIMITS

PROBABILITY SYMBOLS
:: P < 5%
P < 2%
P < 1%
P < 0.5%

MD   -19.60 DB   P < 0.5%
PSD   14.97 DB   P < 0.5%
SF   1.00 DB
CPSD   14.93 DB   P < 0.5%

B

Figure 4-22. *Continued.*

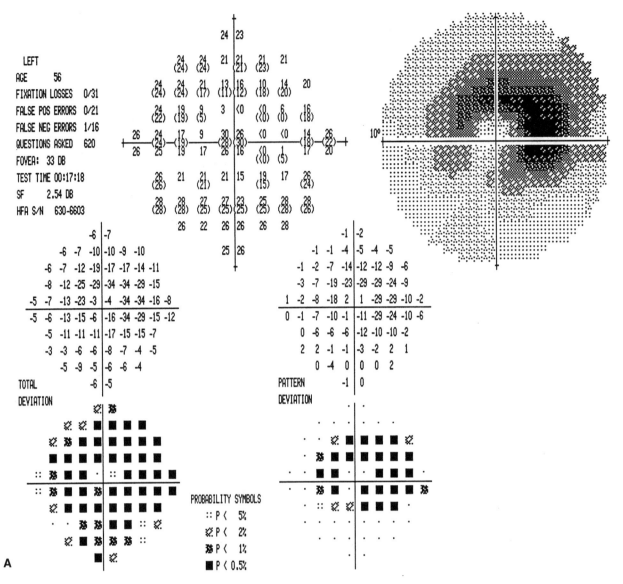

Figure 4-23. Drug toxicity: hydroxychloroquine and chloroquine. Visual fields of a 56-year-old woman receiving therapy with hydroxychloroquine and chloroquine for subacute cutaneous lupus erythomatosus who presented with vague visual complaints and 20/20 visual acuity, **(A)** left eye, **(B)** right eye. Central 10° visual field performed with a white test object revealed bilateral central ring scotomas. A central 10-2 field is recommended before the institution of therapy and every 6 months while on treatment. Defects are typically within the central 10° and are most prominent in the superior field near the vertical meridian.[7] (Courtesy of John Clarkson, MD)

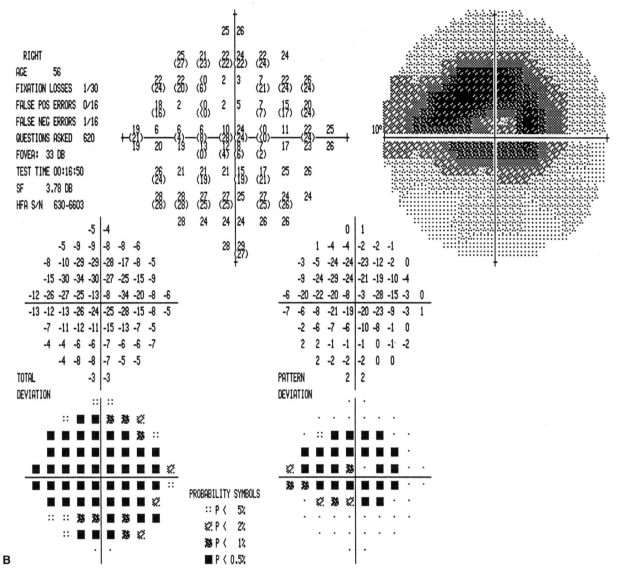

Figure 4-23. *Continued.*

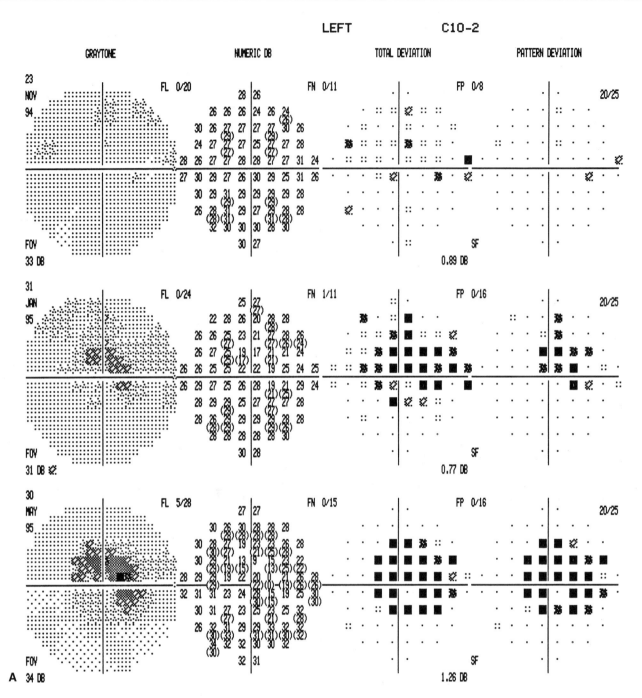

Figure 4-24. Drug toxicity: hydroxychloroquine. Visual fields of a 64-year-old woman **(A)** left eye, **(B)** right eye, who was under treatment with hydroxychloroquine for 2 1/2 years before the *top* 10° visual fields, which showed nonspecific abnormalities in both eyes. The *middle field*, performed 2 months later, shows a central scotoma in the left eye and an early ring scotoma in the right eye, which prompted discontinuation of the medication. Despite discontinuing the medication, the field progressed over the next 3 months to complete ring scotomas OU (*bottom fields*). Repeated testing with a red Amsler grid was normal throughout this period, and no pigmentary changes were noted in the macula. This case underscores the need for frequent visual field testing with automated perimetry using threshold test strategy within the central 10°, which is more sensitive to early visual complications than other measures of visual function or ophthalmoscopy.[7,8] The visual field defects, which are usually accompanied by subtle macular pigmentary abnormalities, do not resolve and may even progress after discontinuation of the medications due to prolonged systemic retention of the drug.[7,8] (Courtesy of Lori Ventura, MD)

RIGHT   C10-2

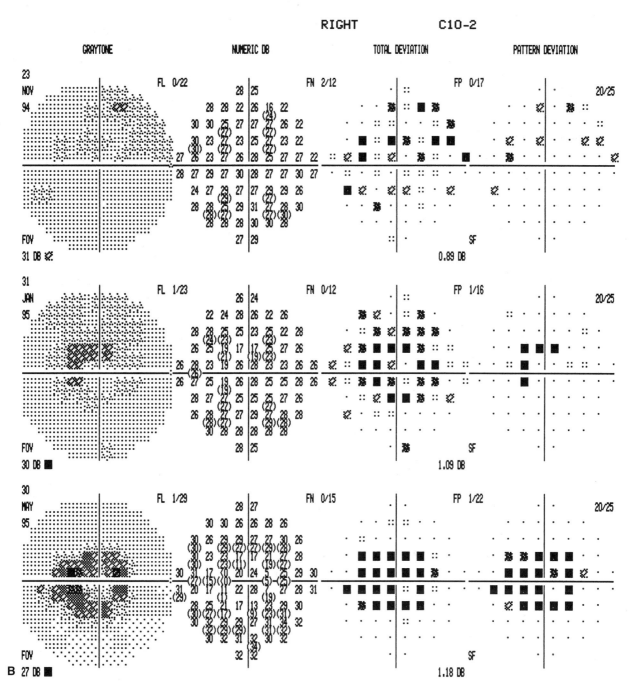

Figure 4-24. *Continued.*

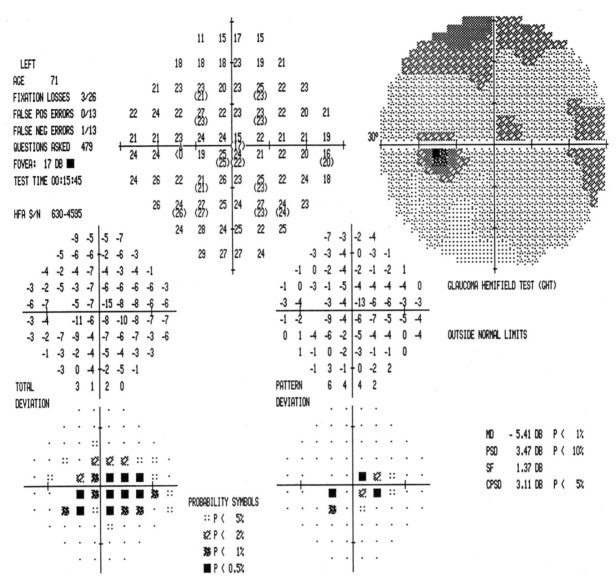

Figure 4-25. Macular hole. Central 30° visual field of a 71-year-old-patient with a macular hole and 20/60 visual acuity. Note markedly depressed foveal threshold and central scotoma on the graytone printout, total deviation, and pattern deviation plots. Other macular or optic nerve processes can cause a central scotoma. Diagnosis is made ophthalmoscopically. (Courtesy of Rick Davis, OD)

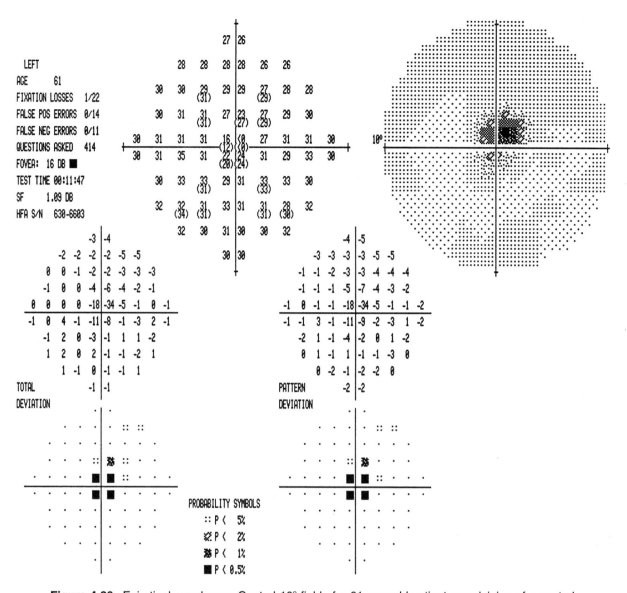

Figure 4-26. Epiretinal membrane. Central 10° field of a 61-year-old patient complaining of a central scotoma OS. An epiretinal membrane was noted ophthalmoscopically. The vision was 20/25, the foveal threshold was reduced, and the graytone printout, total deviation, and pattern deviation plots all showed a central scotoma. A central 10° field is an excellent way to diagnose and document subtle central scotomas. Another example of visual field defect from an epiretinal membrane may be found in figure 4-7. (Courtesy of Rick Davis, OD)

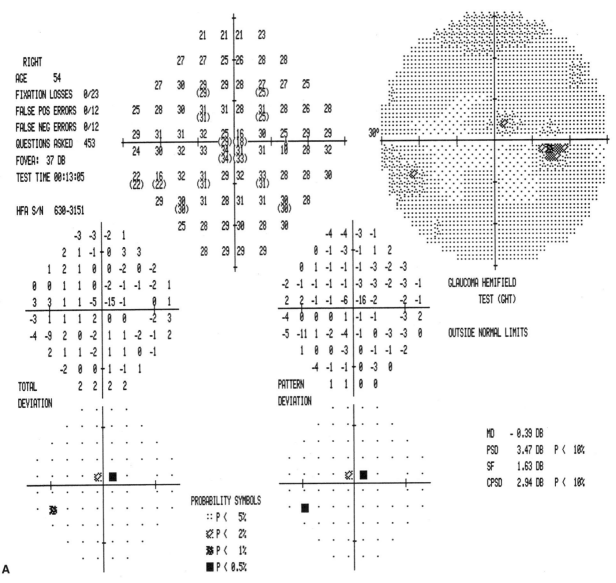

Figure 4-27. Parafoveal retinal pigment epithelium abnormality. Central 30° field (**A**) of a patient with only one functioning eye and 20/20 vision who was sent for glaucoma evaluation secondary to elevated intraocular pressure and the visual field defect seen here. Two abnormal points just above fixation on the 30° field prompted retesting with a central 10° field (**B**), which provides more detail of the scotoma. Ophthalmoscopy revealed a small cup in the optic nerve and an area of retinal pigment epithelial abnormality just inferior to the foveal, which appeared as a window defect on intravenous fluorescein angiography. The etiology of the retinal abnormality was unclear, although the patient had a history of blunt ocular trauma. Small lesions within the center of the macula are best characterized and followed for progression using a central 10° or central 5° field because these tests provide more points for analysis in the area of interest.

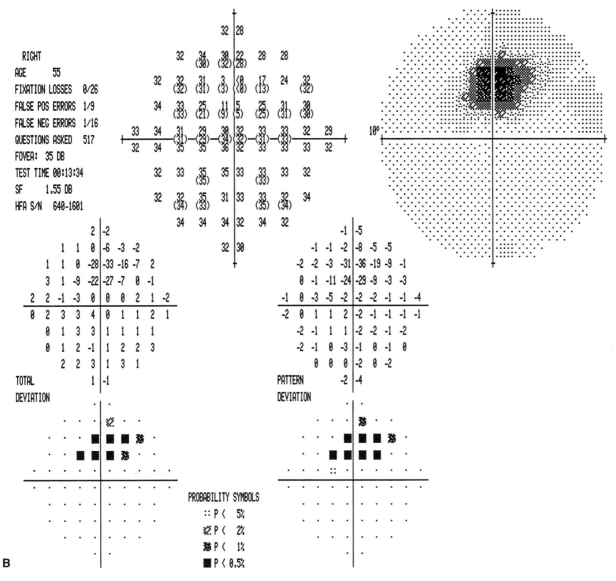

PROBABILITY SYMBOLS

∷ P < 5%
▨ P < 2%
▩ P < 1%
■ P < 0.5%

Figure 4-27. *Continued.*

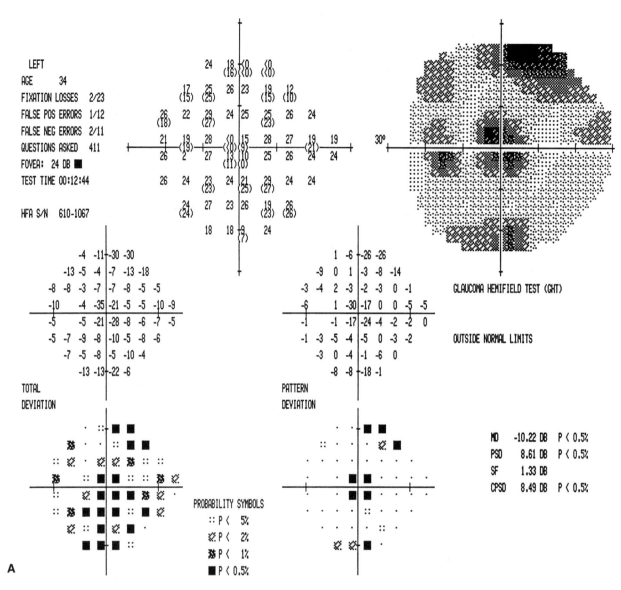

Figure 4-28. Acute zonal occult outer retinopathy. Visual fields of a 34-year-old patient complaining of an enlarging dark cloud in the center of his vision in the left eye. Visual acuity was 20/15. Acute zonal occult outer retinopathy, a disorder of the photoreceptor layer of the retina, was diagnosed. The central 24° field (**A**) shows a central scotoma on the pattern deviation plot. This field also shows a superonasal scotoma that corresponded to an area of retinal atrophy inferiorly from old CMV retinitis. The 10° field (**B**) shows the scotoma in more detail. Acute zonal occult outer retinopathy characteristically presents as rapidly enlarging visual field defects, which may or may not correspond to a region of depigmentation of the retinal pigment epithelium.[9]

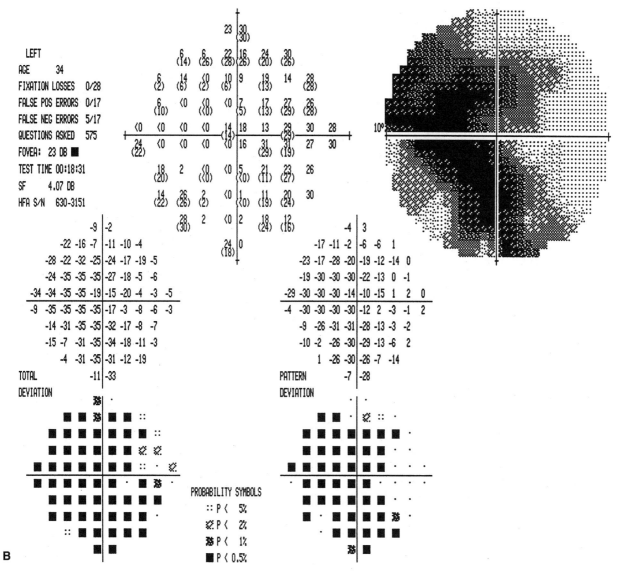

B

Figure 4-28. *Continued.*

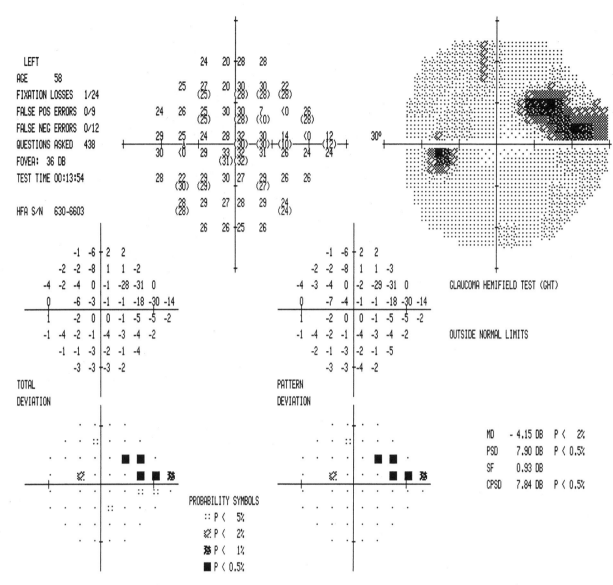

Figure 4-29. Toxoplasmosis chorioretinal scar. Left visual field of a 58-year-old man referred for glaucoma consultation. A superonasal defect which respected the horizontal meridian is seen on the above visual field. Ophthalmoscopy revealed a normal optic nerve but a 1-disc diameter chorioretinal scar inferotemporal to the fovea but not adjacent to the horizontal raphe. Toxoplasmosis affects the inner retinal layers, including the nerve fiber layer, which courses through the lesion. Therefore, the visual field may show a nerve fiber layer defect beginning at the site of the lesion and extending to the horizontal meridian. Even small toxoplasmosis lesions, if located close to the optic disc, can produce large arcuate nerve fiber layer defects, unlike choroiditis (such as histoplasmosis), which characteristically spares the nerve fiber layer intact and only causes focal defects in the visual field.[10]

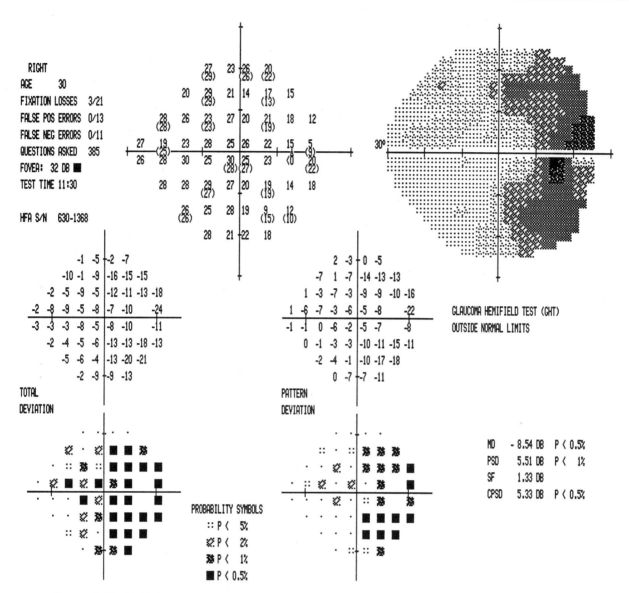

Figure 4-30. Multiple evanescent white dot syndrome. Visual field of a 30-year-old woman who presented with a complaint of a shadow in the temporal portion of the right visual field. The visual acuity was 20/100. Ophthalmoscopy revealed mild optic disc swelling and multiple discrete white dots in the macular and midperipheral retina. Visual field shows diffuse depression on the total deviation plot and extensive enlargement of the blind spot. All of the ophthalmoscopic findings resolved within 5 weeks, and the visual field returned to normal. Disc swelling and an enlarged blind spot on the visual field may accompany the multiple evanescent white dot syndrome.[11,12]

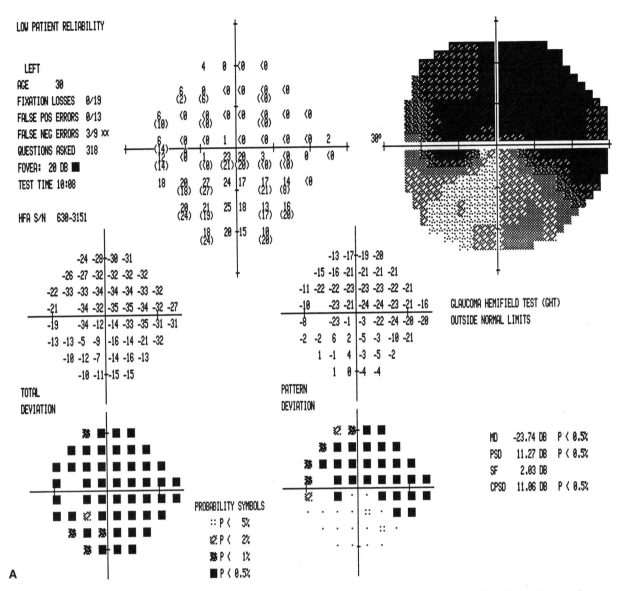

Figure 4-31. Serpiginous choroiditis (geographic helicoid peripapillary choroidopathy). Visual fields of a 30-year-old patient with an 18-year history of recurrent uveitis and charcoal-gray colored scars in the peripapillary region as well as elsewhere in the choroid, presumed secondary to sirpiginous choroiditis, **(A)** left eye, **(B)** right eye. Notice the absolute nature of the scotomas and the pattern of visual field defects in the central 24° fields, which respect neither the horizontal nor vertical meridian. Because large areas of the choroid may be affected, suprathreshold testing of the full field (60° in each meridian) may be more useful. This is true of all inflammatory diseases that affect the retina or choroid diffusely. Serial visual fields are helpful in following the outcome of therapy in these patients.[13]

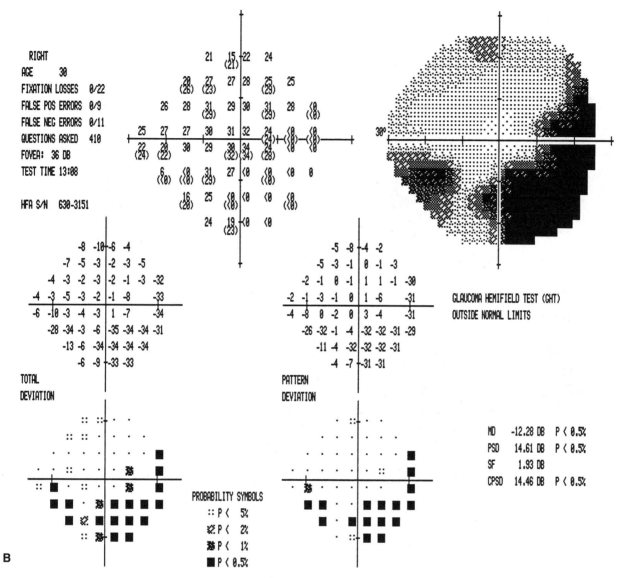

RIGHT

AGE   30

FIXATION LOSSES   0/22

FALSE POS ERRORS   0/9

FALSE NEG ERRORS   0/11

QUESTIONS ASKED   410

FOVEA: 36 DB

TEST TIME 13:08

HFA S/N   630-3151

```
                        21  15  22   24
                           (21)
                    20  27      27  28   25   25
                   (26)(23)                 (29)
               26  28  31   29  30   31   28   (0)
                      (29)            (29)      (0)
        25  27  27  30  31  32   24   (0   (0
                                   (24)  (0   (0
        22  20  30  29   30  34   24   (0   (0
       (24)(22)        (32)(34)  (28)
            6   0   31  27   0   (0   (0   0
          (0)  (0)  (29)       (0)
               16  25   0   (0   0   (0
              (20)      (0)           (0)
                   24  19  (0   (0
                      (23)
```

```
            -8  -10  -6  -4
        -7  -5  -3  -2  -3  -5
    -4  -3  -2  -3  -2  -1  -3  -32
-4  -3  -5  -3  -2  -1  -8      -33
-6  -10 -3  -4  -3   1  -7      -34
   -28 -34 -3  -6  -35 -34 -34 -31
      -13 -6  -34 -34 -34 -34
          -6  -9  -33 -33
```

TOTAL
DEVIATION

```
            -5  -8  -4  -2
        -5  -3  -1   0  -1  -3
    -2  -1   0  -1   1   1  -1  -30
-2  -1  -3  -1   0   1  -6      -31
-4  -8   0  -2   0   3  -4      -31
   -26 -32 -1  -4  -32 -32 -31 -29
      -11 -4  -32 -32 -32 -31
          -4  -7  -31 -31
```

PATTERN
DEVIATION

GLAUCOMA HEMIFIELD TEST (GHT)

OUTSIDE NORMAL LIMITS

MD	-12.28 DB	P < 0.5%
PSD	14.61 DB	P < 0.5%
SF	1.93 DB	
CPSD	14.46 DB	P < 0.5%

PROBABILITY SYMBOLS

:: P < 5%

⚄ P < 2%

▨ P < 1%

■ P < 0.5%

B

Figure 4-31. *Continued.*

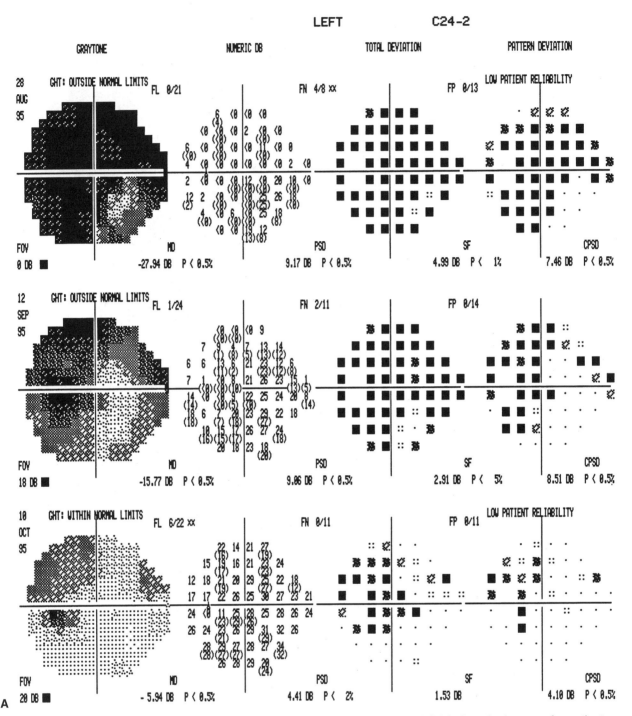

Figure 4-32. Cat scratch disease associated neuroretinitis. Visual fields from both eyes of a patient with bilateral neuroretinitis from cat scratch disease. The left eye **(A)** had a swollen disc and a complete macular star figure. The left field shows diffuse depression, which improved on therapy but shows residual enlargement of the blind spot, reduced central visual acuity, and depressed foveal threshold. The right eye **(B)** had a swollen disc and a partial macular lipid star figure. The initial field shows diffuse depression on the total deviation plot. On the pattern deviation plot, an enlarged blind spot and nasal defect are noted. The right field normalized on therapy.

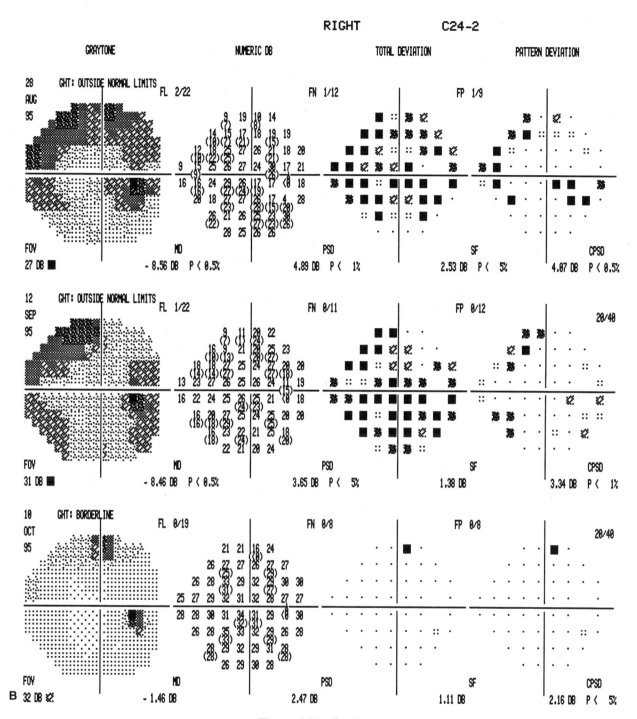

Figure 4-32. *Continued.*

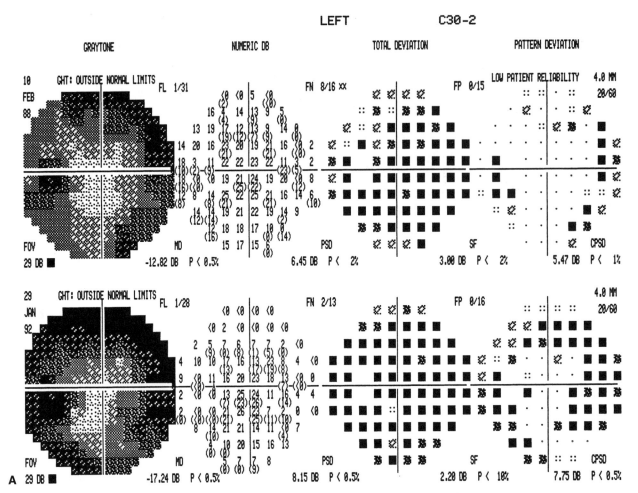

Figure 4-33. Progressive myopic degeneration. Visual fields of an elderly woman with worsening visual field secondary to myopic degeneration. In 1988, the field in the left eye **(A)** showed diffuse depression on the total deviation plot, worse in the area around the blind spot and nasally on the pattern deviation plot. The field in the left eye became progressively constricted over the ensuing 4 years, and the mean deviation worsened from −12.82 dB to −17.24 dB. The field in the right eye **(B)** showed diffuse depression, which was worse inferiorly and in the area of the blind spot. The field in the right eye also became progressively constricted over the ensuing 4 years and the mean worsened from -7.86 dB to −11.76 dB. This patient also had elevated intraocular pressures, raising the question of whether the progressive visual field changes were due to glaucoma or myopic degeneration. However, serial optic disc photographs had not changed in this patient. Because patients with high axial myopia may have anomalous discs, following patients with degenerative myopia for glaucomatous progression can be difficult because the visual field findings may be similar.

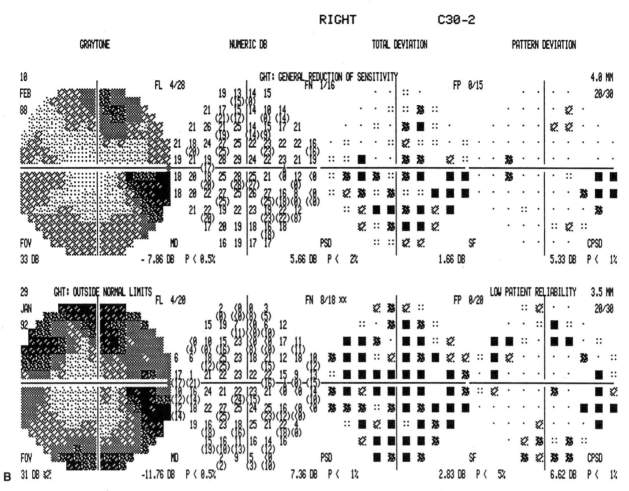

Figure 4-33. *Continued.*

References

1. Harrington DO. Visual field defects in retinal disease. In Straatsma BR, Hall MO, Allan RA, Crescitelli F, eds. The retina: morphology, function, and clinical characteristics. Berkeley: University of California Press, 1969:485.
2. Feldon SE. Visual fields in retinal disease. In Ryan SJ, ed. Retina 2nd ed, St. Louis: Mosby, 1994:167.
3. Roth JA. Central visual field in diabetes. Br J Ophthalmol 1969;53:16.
4. Zingirian M, Pisano E, Gandolfo E. Visual field damage after photocoagulative treatment for diabetic retinopathy. Doc Ophthalmologica Proc Ser 1977;14:265.
5. Weleber RG. Retinitis pigmentosa and allied disorders. In Ryan SJ, ed. Retina. 2nd ed. St Louis: Mosby, 1994:335.
6. Jacobson SG, Voigt WJ, Parel J-M, et al. Automated light- and dark-adapted perimetry for evaluating retinitis pigmentosa. Ophthalmology 1986;93:1604.
7. Hart WM Jr, Burde RM, Johnston GP, Drews RC. Static perimetry in chloroquine retinopathy: perifoveal patterns of visual field depression. Arch Ophthalmol 1984;102:377.
8. Swartz, M. Other diseases: drug toxicity and metabolic and nutritional conditions. In Ryan SJ, ed. Retina. 2nd ed. St Louis: Mosby, 1994:1760.
9. Gass JDM. Acute zonal occult outer retinopathy. J Clin Neuro-ophth 1993;13:79.
10. Martin WG, Brown GC, Parrish RK, Kimball R, Naidoff MA, Benson WE. Ocular toxoplasmosis and visual field defects. Am J Ophthalmol 1980;90:25.
11. Dodwell DG, Jampol LM, Rosenberg M, Berman A, Zaret CR. Optic nerve involvement associated with the multipleevanescent white-dot syndrome. Ophthalmology 1990;97:862.
12. Singh K, de Frank MP, Shults WT, Watzke RC. Acute idiopathic blind spot enlargement. A spectrum of disease. Ophthalmology 1991;98:497.
13. Schatz H, McDonald HR, Johnson RN. Geographic helicoid peripapillary choroidopathy (serpiginous choroiditis). In: Ryan SJ. Retina. 2nd ed. St. Louis: Mosby, 1994:1721.

5

Glaucomatous Visual Field Loss

Donald L. Budenz

Automated static perimetry is most often used in the diagnosis and follow-up of glaucoma. For this reason, considerable attention is given to these topics in this chapter.

The hallmark of the glaucomatous visual field is the nerve fiber bundle defect. (Figure 5-1) These defects respect the horizontal meridian (with the exception of the temporal wedge defect) and almost always are detectable within the central 30°.[1] Because the initial optic nerve damage caused by glaucoma most commonly occurs at the superior and inferior poles, the earliest visual field defects are found in an arcuate pattern in the superior and inferior hemifields and nasally along the horizontal meridian within 30° of fixation. The papillomacular bundle and nasal nerve fibers are typically spared until very late in the disease. Therefore, the very center of the visual field and the peripheral temporal field are usually spared until late in the disease. An exception is in the presence of axial myopia, in which the macular region may be severely affected at an earlier stage of the disease process.

For the purpose of setting treatment goals, our glaucoma service recommends classifying visual field defects as early, moderate, or severe. These divisions are arbitrary but very useful in managing patients.

EARLY GLAUCOMATOUS VISUAL FIELD DEFECTS

There are several characteristic patterns to the early visual field defects in glaucoma. Nearly always, some groups of nerve fibers are affected before others, so that characteristic field abnormalities include the paracentral scotoma, the arcuate scotoma (emanating from the blind spot in an arched fashion around fixation), the nasal step, and the temporal wedge defect.[2-4] Mild diffuse depression without localized defect is a rare early finding in glaucoma.[5,6] An increase in the short-term fluctuation without localized field loss may precede development of a detectable visual field defect.[7]

The goal of visual field testing in the patient with suspected glaucoma is to detect the earliest possible lesion so that treatment can be initiated. To reduce false positive findings, which would result in treating patients unnecessarily, it is very important that any suspi-

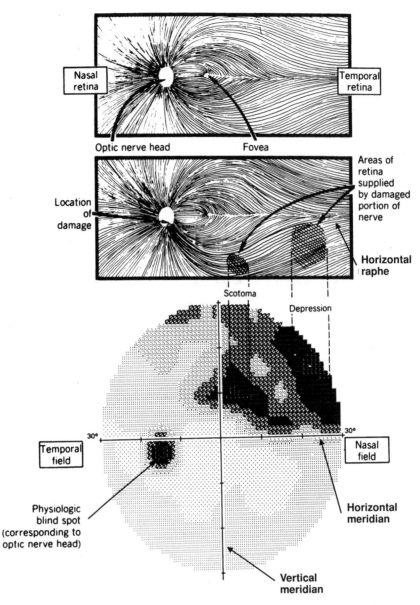

Figure 5-1. Anatomic basis of the nerve fiber defect in glaucoma. Glaucomatous damage most often first occurs to optic nerve fibers that enter the optic nerve at the superior and inferior poles. These ganglion cells originate from the retina temporal to the optic disc excluding the papillomaculary bundle. Ganglion cells in a particular hemifield respect the horizontal raphe of that hemifield and travel in an arcuate fashion around the papillomaculary bundle. Visual field defects in early glaucoma, therefore, take the form of paracentral scotomas, which respect the horizontal meridian and are most commonly found nasal to the blind spot. (Used with permission from Anderson DR. Automated static perimetry. St. Louis: Mosby–Year Book 1992:45).

Table 5-1. *Criteria for Minimal Abnormality in Glaucoma*

Three or more adjacent points in an expected location of the central 24° field* that have P < 5% on the pattern deviation plot, one of which must have P < 1%
Glaucoma hemifield test "outside normal limits"
Corrected pattern standard deviation with P < 5%

---

* Must be nonedge points in central 30° field.
Adapted from Anderson DR. Automated Static Perimetry. St. Louis: Mosby–Year Book, 1992.

cious defect be confirmed on a second test. There are no proven criteria for diagnosing an early nerve fiber layer defect, but Anderson has developed a rational arbitrary set of criteria that I have found extremely helpful and which is summarized in Table 5-1. If any of the three criteria for minimal abnormality are met, the defect is considered significant if reproducible. All three criteria need not be present to meet the criteria for minimal abnormality.

In using these criteria, Anderson points out several important caveats. First, a positive finding in any single criteria is not absolutely specific or sensitive. It is critical to evaluate fields that meet these criteria in light of the clinical situation. Second, the glaucoma hemifield test may be the most accurate of the criteria. And third, suspicious or early defects should be confirmed on a second test.

Table 5-2 outlines three arbitrary criteria, developed by Elizabeth Hodapp, MD, that may be used for defining a glaucomatous field defect as early. In general, a defect is early if it is neither extensive nor near fixation.

Table 5-2. *Criteria for Early Defect in Glaucoma*

Mean deviation no worse than −6 dB
On pattern deviation plot, fewer than 25% of points depressed below the 5% level and fewer than 15% of points depressed below 1% level
No point within central 5° with sensitivity less than 15 dB

Adapted from Hodapp E, Parrish RK, Anderson DR. Clinical decisions in glaucoma. St. Louis: Mosby, 1993:53.

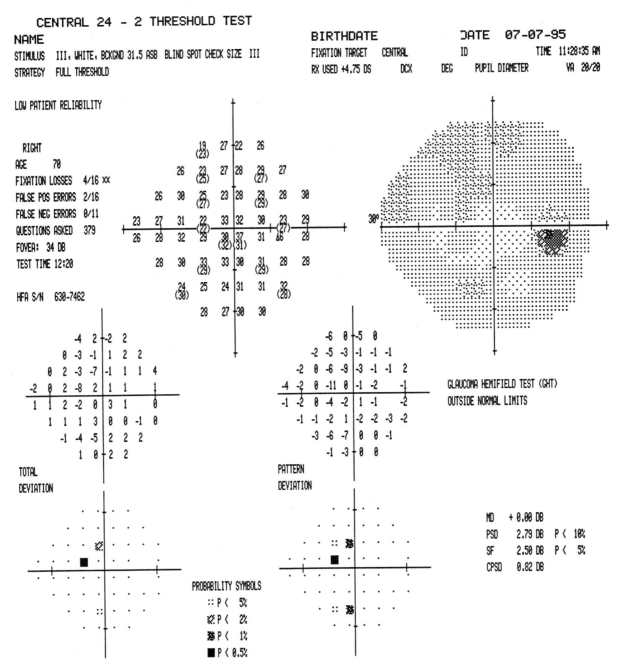

CENTRAL 24 - 2 THRESHOLD TEST

NAME   BIRTHDATE   DATE   07-07-95
STIMULUS   III, WHITE, BCKGND 31.5 ASB BLIND SPOT CHECK SIZE III   FIXATION TARGET   CENTRAL   ID   TIME 11:28:35 AM
STRATEGY   FULL THRESHOLD   RX USED +4.75 DS   DCX   DEG   PUPIL DIAMETER   VA 20/20

LOW PATIENT RELIABILITY

RIGHT

AGE   70
FIXATION LOSSES   4/16 xx
FALSE POS ERRORS   2/16
FALSE NEG ERRORS   0/11
QUESTIONS ASKED   379
FOVEA: 34 DB
TEST TIME 12:20

HFA S/N   630-7462

TOTAL
DEVIATION

PATTERN
DEVIATION

GLAUCOMA HEMIFIELD TEST (GHT)
OUTSIDE NORMAL LIMITS

PROBABILITY SYMBOLS
:: P < 5%
⊠ P < 2%
▦ P < 1%
■ P < 0.5%

MD   + 0.00 DB
PSD   2.79 DB   P < 10%
SF   2.50 DB   P <   5%
CPSD   0.82 DB

Figure 5-2. Early paracentral defect from glaucoma. Visual field of the right eye, with three adjacent points on the pattern deviation plot in the superior hemifield in the paracentral region, that meet Anderson's criteria for minimal abnormality. The 3 points have P values that are < 5%, at least one of which has a P value < 1%. The glaucoma hemifield test is also abnormal. The corrected pattern standard deviation (CPSD) is normal. There is a high number of fixation losses, and the short-term fluctuation is abnormal, but this defect was reproducible on subsequent fields. The two abnormal points in the inferior hemifield do not meet Anderson's criteria and were not reproducible on subsequent testing.

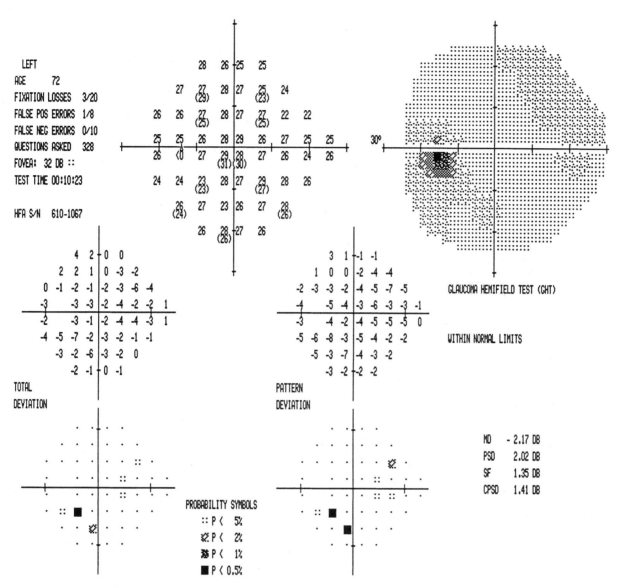

Figure 5-3. Early arcuate defect from glaucoma. Visual field of the left eye of a 72-year-old woman with early glaucoma. The pattern deviation plot contains three adjacent points just below the blind spot that are depressed at the $P < 5\%$ level, two at the $P < 0.5\%$ level, meeting Anderson's criterion for minimal abnormality. The glaucoma hemifield test and CPSD are normal. There are four adjacent points in the nasal field that are depressed but they straddle the horizontal meridian (uncharacteristic of glaucomatous nerve fiber layer defects except for temporal wedge defects) and are not sufficiently depressed to meet the criteria. The first defect described was reproducible, but the second disappeared on subsequent testing.

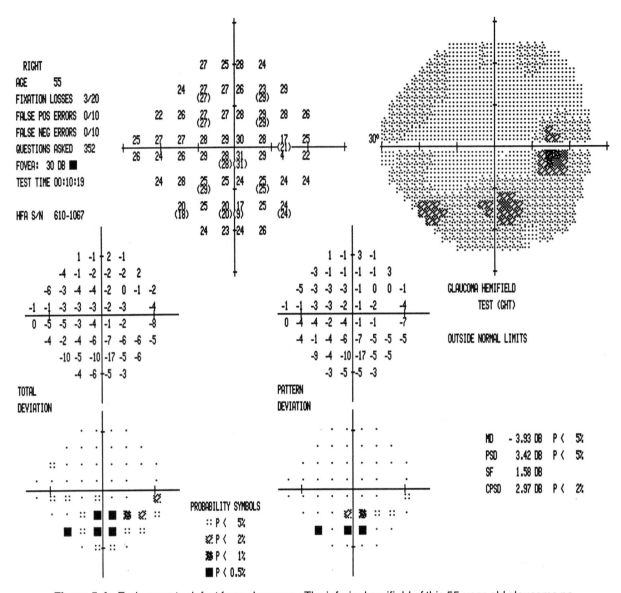

Figure 5-4. Early arcuate defect from glaucoma. The inferior hemifield of this 55-year-old glaucoma patient has an early arcuate defect. There are six adjacent points in the inferior hemifield that are depressed at least at the $P < 5\%$ level, one at the $P < 1\%$ level and two at the $P < 0.5\%$ level. The glaucoma hemifield test is outside normal limits. The CPSD is abnormal at the $P < 2\%$ level. The defect is early since the mean deviation is not worse than -6 dB, there are relatively few depressed points, and none of the points within 5° of fixation is less than 15 dB (see Table 5-2). Note how the defect widens as it gets further away from the blind spot, a frequent characteristic of an arcuate glaucomatous defect.

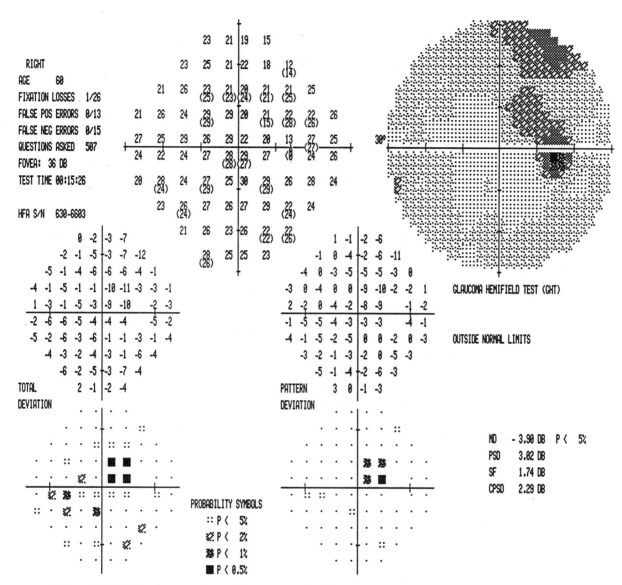

RIGHT

AGE 60

FIXATION LOSSES 1/26

FALSE POS ERRORS 0/13

FALSE NEG ERRORS 0/15

QUESTIONS ASKED 507

FOVEA: 36 DB

TEST TIME 00:15:26

HFA S/N 630-6603

GLAUCOMA HEMIFIELD TEST (GHT)

OUTSIDE NORMAL LIMITS

MD −3.90 DB P < 5%

PSD 3.02 DB

SF 1.74 DB

CPSD 2.29 DB

PROBABILITY SYMBOLS

∷ P < 5%

▨ P < 2%

▩ P < 1%

■ P < 0.5%

TOTAL DEVIATION

PATTERN DEVIATION

Figure 5-5. Early glaucomatous defect emanating from blind spot. The graytone printout of this 60-year-old patient with suspected glaucoma shows a typical early arcuate scotoma emanating from the blind spot on the graytone printout. Looking at the pattern deviation plot, there are three or more adjacent points in an expected location of the field, two of which are abnormal at the $P < 1\%$ level and one or more at the $P < 0.5\%$ level. The glaucoma hemifield test is abnormal, although the CPSD is not statistically abnormal. The defect is considered early since the mean deviation is not worse than −6 dB, fewer than 25% of points are depressed at the $P < 5\%$ level and fewer than 15% at the $P < 1\%$ level on the pattern deviation plot, and there is no point within 5° of fixation with a sensitivity of < 15 dB.

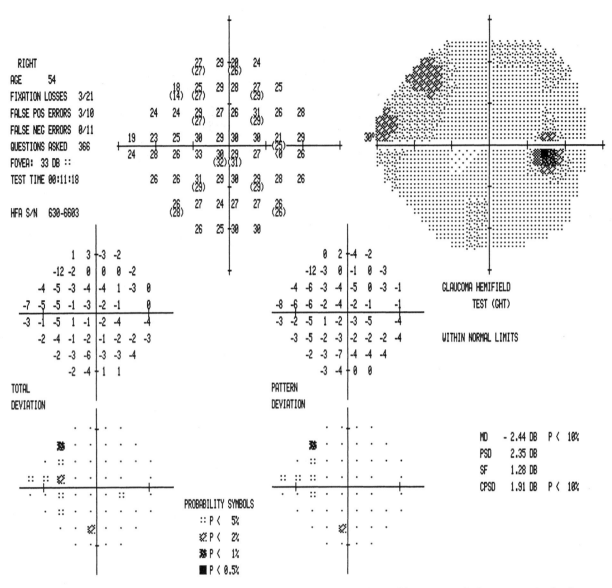

RIGHT

AGE   54

FIXATION LOSSES   3/21

FALSE POS ERRORS 3/10

FALSE NEG ERRORS 0/11

QUESTIONS ASKED   366

FOVEA: 33 DB ::

TEST TIME 00:11:18

HFA S/N   630-6603

```
                    27   29  28   24
                   (27)      (26)
               18   25   29  28   27   25
              (14) (27)           (29)
          24   24   29   27  26   31   26   28
                   (27)           (29)
     19   23   25   30   29  30   30   21   29
                                     (25)
     24   28   26   33   30  29   27   0    26
                       (32)(31)
          26   26   31   29  30   28   28   26
                   (29)           (29)
               26   27   24  27   27   26
              (28)                (26)
                    26   25  30   30
```

```
          1   3 -3  -2
     -12  -2  0  0   0  -2
      -4  -5 -3 -4  -4   1  -3   0
  -7  -5  -5 -1 -3  -2  -1       0
  -3  -1  -5  1 -1  -2  -4      -4
     -2  -4 -1 -2  -1  -2  -2  -3
         -2 -3 -6  -3  -3  -4
            -2 -4  1   1
```

TOTAL
DEVIATION

```
               0   2 -4  -2
     -12  -3  0 -1   0  -3
      -4  -6 -3 -4  -5   0  -3  -1
  -8  -6  -6 -2 -4  -2  -1      -1
  -3  -2  -5  1 -2  -3  -5      -4
     -3  -5 -2 -3  -2  -2  -2  -4
         -2 -3 -7  -4  -4  -4
            -3 -4  0   0
```

PATTERN
DEVIATION

GLAUCOMA HEMIFIELD

TEST (GHT)

WITHIN NORMAL LIMITS

MD   - 2.44 DB   P < 10%
PSD   2.35 DB
SF   1.28 DB
CPSD   1.91 DB   P < 10%

PROBABILITY SYMBOLS

:: P < 5%

※ P < 2%

▒ P < 1%

■ P < 0.5%

Figure 5-6. Early nasal step. Visual field of a 54-year-old patient with suspected glaucoma who had been followed-up for 2 years with normal visual fields. An early nasal step (defect that comes up to, but does not cross, the horizontal meridian in the nasal quadrant) appeared and was confirmed on subsequent testing. On the pattern deviation plot, five adjacent points are noted in the superonasal quadrant that are depressed at the $P < 5\%$ level, 1 at the $P < 1\%$ level. The pattern deviation plot is the only criterion for minimal abnormality that is met since the glaucoma hemifield test is normal and the CPSD is only depressed at the $P < 10\%$ level.

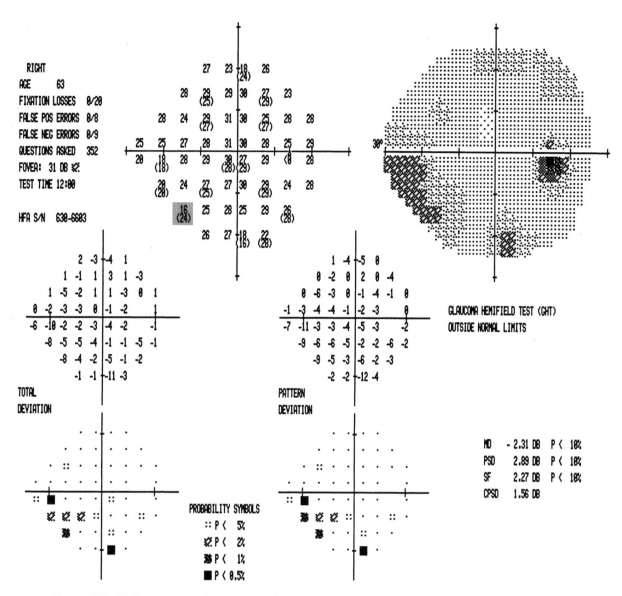

Figure 5-7. Early nasal step. Visual field of a 63-year-old glaucoma patient that shows an inferonasal step. There are a number of adjacent points in the inferonasal quadrant on the pattern deviation plot that are depressed at least at the *P* < 5% level, and three are depressed to the *P* < 1% level or worse. The glaucoma hemifield test is outside normal limits. The CPSD is normal. Note that the short-term fluctuation (SF) is somewhat abnormal because of a single variable point within the relative scotoma (highlighted) that was double determined as part of the short-term fluctuation calculation.

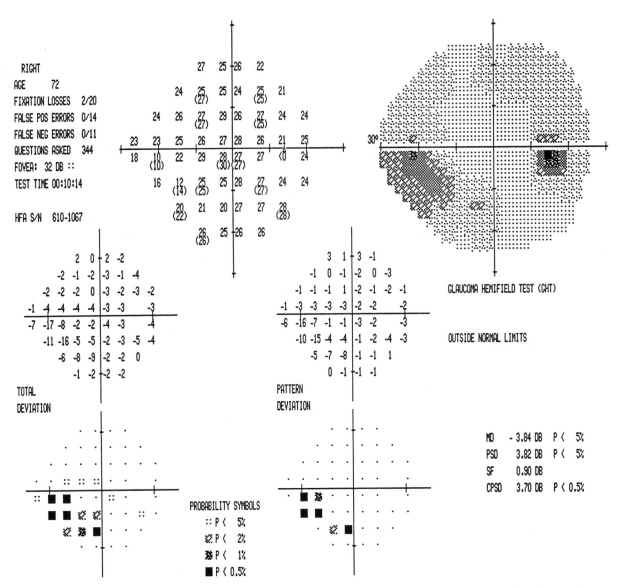

RIGHT
AGE 72
FIXATION LOSSES 2/20
FALSE POS ERRORS 0/14
FALSE NEG ERRORS 0/11
QUESTIONS ASKED 344
FOVEA: 32 DB ::
TEST TIME 00:10:14

HFA S/N 610-1067

TOTAL DEVIATION

PATTERN DEVIATION

GLAUCOMA HEMIFIELD TEST (GHT)

OUTSIDE NORMAL LIMITS

MD - 3.84 DB P < 5%
PSD 3.82 DB P < 5%
SF 0.90 DB
CPSD 3.70 DB P < 0.5%

PROBABILITY SYMBOLS
:: P < 5%
P < 2%
P < 1%
■ P < 0.5%

Figure 5-8. Early nasal step. Visual field of a 72-year-old patient with glaucoma (contralateral eye of visual field shown in figure 5-3) showing an early inferonasal step. The defect fits the pattern deviation plot criteria requiring at least three depressed points depressed at the *P* < 5% level and at least one point at the *P* < 1% level. The glaucoma hemifield test (GHT) is outside normal limits and the CPSD is abnormal at the *P* < 0.5% level, thus fitting all three of Anderson's criteria for minimal abnormality. The defect is still early since it meets the criteria found in Table 5-2.

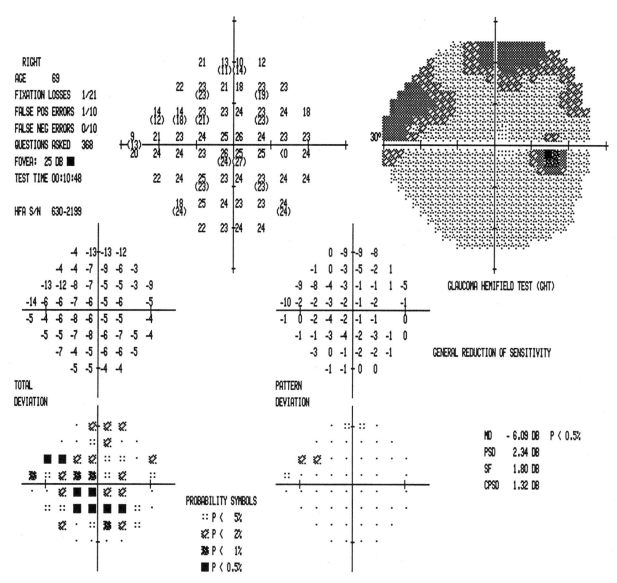

HFA S/N 630-2199

Figure 5-9. Early nasal step superimposed on generalized depression. The visual field of a patient with early glaucoma and a mild cataract demonstrates the usefulness of the pattern deviation plot. The total deviation plot shows diffuse depression, but the pattern deviation plot shows a localized defect consistent with an early nasal step. This defect does not quite fit Anderson's criteria for the presence of minimally detectable abnormality (the two worse points are only abnormal at the *P* < 2% level, the GHT reads only general reduction of sensi-tivity, and the CPSD is normal). The defect was reproducible and in keeping with other clinical findings, so was considered glaucomatous even without meeting any of the criteria, which are not 100% sensitive. The mean deviation is higher than that allowed for an early defect according to Table 5-2 but the majority of the abnormality is from diffuse depression rather than localized loss, and the glaucomatous portion of the field loss is early.

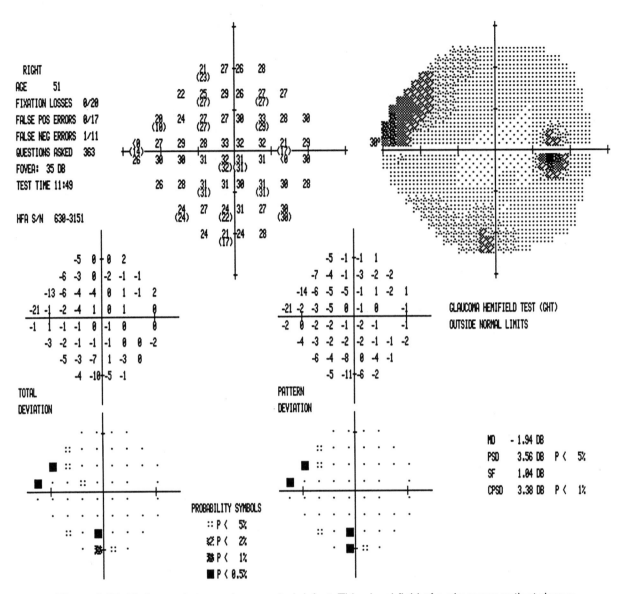

RIGHT

AGE   51

FIXATION LOSSES   0/20

FALSE POS ERRORS   0/17

FALSE NEG ERRORS   1/11

QUESTIONS ASKED   363

FOVEA: 35 DB

TEST TIME 11:49

HFA S/N   630-3151

TOTAL
DEVIATION

PATTERN
DEVIATION

GLAUCOMA HEMIFIELD TEST (GHT)

OUTSIDE NORMAL LIMITS

MD   - 1.94 DB

PSD   3.56 DB   P <   5%

SF   1.04 DB

CPSD   3.38 DB   P <   1%

PROBABILITY SYMBOLS

:: P <   5%

P <   2%

P <   1%

■ P < 0.5%

Figure 5-10. Early nasal step and paracentral defect. This visual field of a glaucoma patient demonstrates an early superonasal step and an inferior paracentral scotoma, both of which satisfy the criteria for minimal abnormality according to Anderson (Table 5-1). The intial field finding of a paracentral defect and nasal step together is common, although the two typically occur within the same hemifield. However, the superior and inferior hemifield can become involved almost at the same time.[2]

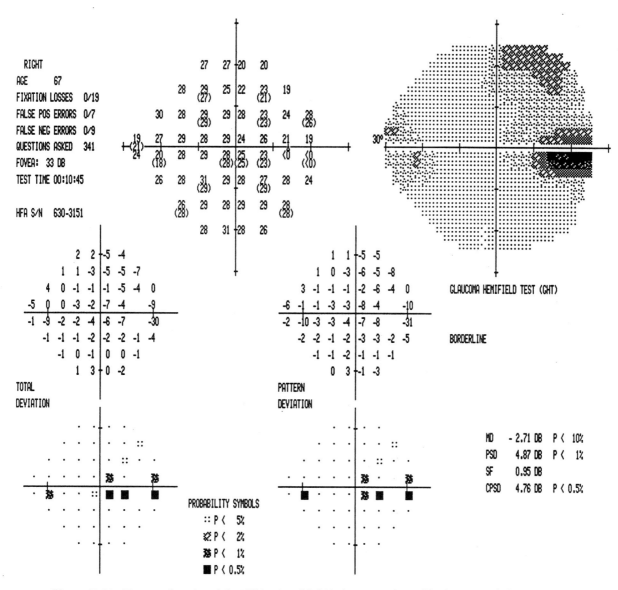

Figure 5-11. Temporal wedge defect This visual field is from a patient with glaucoma and an epiretinal membrane in the center of the macula. A temporal wedge defect is present, extending temporally from the blind spot. The defect between the blind spot and fixation is secondary to the epiretinal membrane. Temporal wedge defects are infrequent in glaucoma, representing fewer than 5% of defects.[2,3] Diagnosis of a temporal wedge defect is difficult using a central 24° field because only two points are tested temporal to the blind spot in this test. If a temporal wedge defect is suspected, a follow-up field testing the central 30° may provide confirmatory information.

MODERATE GLAUCOMATOUS VISUAL FIELD DEFECTS

As glaucoma progresses, paracentral defects coalesce and become continuous with the blind spot. A defect that seems to emanate from the blind spot is a characteristic of a well established glaucomatous field defect. In contrast, neurologic field defects are either central or "point toward fixation." Glaucomatous defects that encroach on fixation are quite worrisome. Specific arbitrary criteria that our service uses for diagnosing moderate glaucomatous field defects, developed by Elizabeth Hodapp, MD, are found in Table 5-3. In general, moderate visual field defects should not have profound central field loss or involve both upper and lower hemifields to a significant degree.

Table 5-3. *Criteria for Moderate Defect in Glaucoma*

Mean deviation worse than -6 dB but no worse than -12 dB
On pattern deviation plot, fewer than 50% of points depressed below the 5% level and fewer than 25% of points depressed below 1% level
No point within central 5° with sensitivity less than or equal to 0 dB
Only 1 hemifield containing a point with sensitivity less than 15 dB within 5° of fixation

Adapted from Hodapp E, Parrish RK, Anderson DR. Clinical decisions in glaucoma. St. Louis: Mosby, 1993:56.

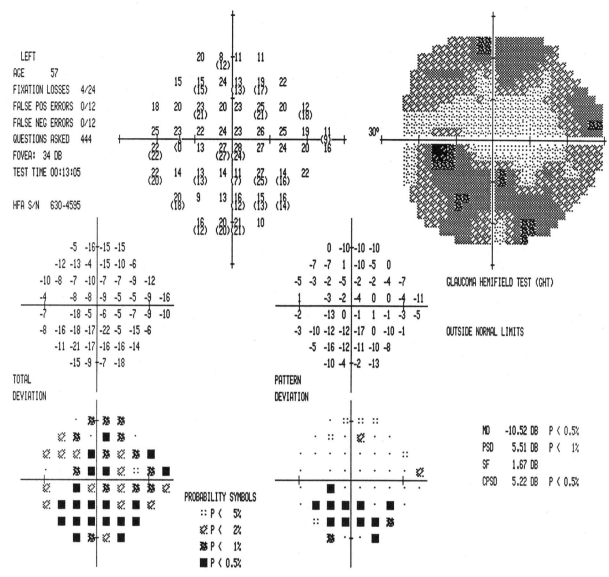

Figure 5-12. Moderate inferior arcuate scotoma. Visual field of the left eye of a patient with moderately advanced glaucoma. Note how the defect emanates from the blind spot inferiorly and expands nasally. The widening of the arcuate defect as it passes nasally is characteristic of a nerve fiber layer defect and is a feature that may help distinguish this defect from lens rim artifact, for instance. The mean deviation (MD) is worse than −6 dB but not worse than −12 dB, and there are no points within the central 5° with a sensitivity of < 15 dB. Exactly 25% of points on the pattern deviation plot are depressed at the *P* < 1% level but less than 50% of points are depressed at the *P* < 5% level on the pattern deviation plot. The defect, therefore, would be classified as moderate to severe.

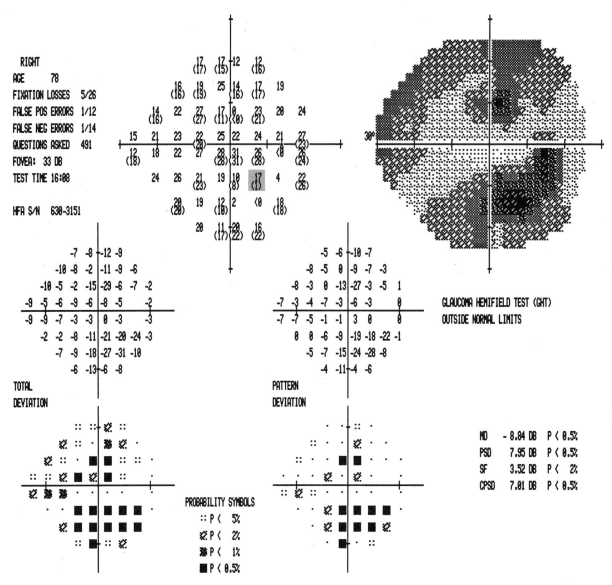

RIGHT
AGE   78
FIXATION LOSSES   5/26
FALSE POS ERRORS 1/12
FALSE NEG ERRORS 1/14
QUESTIONS ASKED   491
FOVEA: 33 DB
TEST TIME 16:08

HFA S/N   630-3151

TOTAL
DEVIATION

PATTERN
DEVIATION

GLAUCOMA HEMIFIELD TEST (GHT)
OUTSIDE NORMAL LIMITS

MD   - 8.84 DB   P < 0.5%
PSD   7.95 DB   P < 0.5%
SF   3.52 DB   P < 2%
CPSD   7.01 DB   P < 0.5%

PROBABILITY SYMBOLS
:: P < 5%
� P < 2%
✖ P < 1%
■ P < 0.5%

Figure 5-13. Moderate glaucomatous field loss involving both hemispheres. The inferior hemisphere contains an arcuate defect emanating from the blind spot, and there is a cluster of points on the pattern deviation plot superior to fixation that meets the criterion for minimal abnormality (Table 5-1). The mean deviation is between − 6 and − 12 dB, more than 25% but fewer than 50% of the points are depressed at the P < 5% level and more than 15% but less than 25% are depressed at the P < 1% level. There are no points within the central 5° with a sensitivity less than 15 dB. Note that the short-term fluctuation is high, not because of poor reliability but because one of the 10 points that is double-determined to assess short term fluctuation is within the inferior arcuate scotoma.

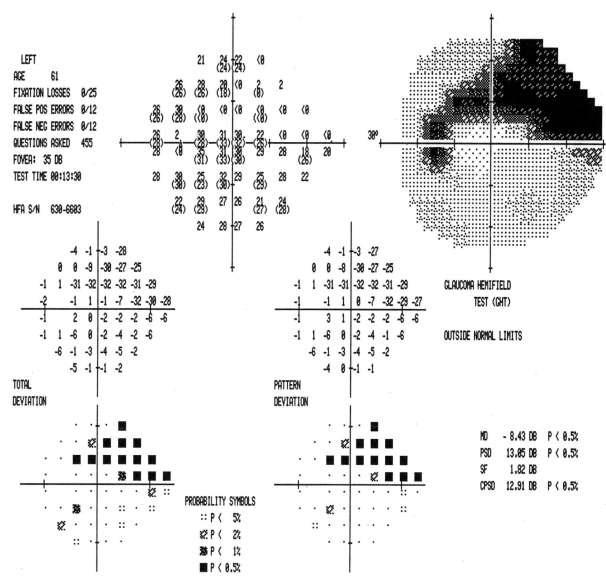

```
LEFT                                    21   24 22  <0
AGE       61                                (24)(24)
FIXATION LOSSES   0/25              26   28   20  <0    2    2
                                   (26) (26) (18)    (0)
FALSE POS ERRORS  0/12        26   30  <0    <0   <0  <0    <0   <0
                             (26) (28) (<0)         (<0)
FALSE NEG ERRORS  0/12        26   2   30   31  30   22  <0    <0   <0
QUESTIONS ASKED   455    ----(28)--A-(28)-(33)(32)-(25)--<0----<0----<0---
                             28   <0   35   31 30   29   28   18   20
FOVEA:  35 DB                          (31) (33)(30)              (26)
TEST TIME  00:13:30      28   30   25  32  29   25   28   22
                             (30) (23) (30)   (29)
HFA S/N   630-6603            22   20  27  26   21   24
                             (24) (29)          (27) (28)
                              24   28  27  26
```

```
     -4  -1 -3  -28                        -4  -1 -3  -27
  0   0  -9 -30 -27 -25                  0   0  -8 -30 -27 -25
-1  1 -31 -32 -32 -32 -31 -29          -1  1 -31 -31 -32 -32 -31 -29    GLAUCOMA HEMIFIELD
-2    -1  1 -1  -7 -32 -30 -28         -1    -1  1  0  -7 -32 -29 -27       TEST (GHT)
-1    2  0 -2 -2 -2 -6 -6             -1    3  1 -2 -2 -2 -6 -6
-1  1 -6  0 -2 -4 -2 -6               -1  1 -6  0 -2 -4 -1 -6          OUTSIDE NORMAL LIMITS
  -6  -1 -3 -4 -5 -2                    -6  -1 -3 -4 -5 -2
     -5  -1 -1 -2                          -4   0 -1 -1

TOTAL                                  PATTERN
DEVIATION                              DEVIATION
```

Probability symbols plots (Total Deviation and Pattern Deviation)

```
PROBABILITY SYMBOLS
   :: P < 5%
   ▨ P < 2%
   ▩ P < 1%
   ■ P < 0.5%
```

```
MD    - 8.43 DB   P < 0.5%
PSD    13.05 DB   P < 0.5%
SF      1.82 DB
CPSD   12.91 DB   P < 0.5%
```

Figure 5-14. Dense superior defect breaking into nasal step. As glaucoma progresses, isolated paracentral scotomas and nasal steps coalesce into arcuate defects, which often spare fixation, as in this moderately depressed visual field. The defect is moderate because the field has a mean deviation between −6 and −12 dB, more than 25% but fewer than 50% of points in the pattern deviation plot are depressed at the P < 5% level, more than 15% but fewer than 25% of points in the pattern deviation plot are depressed at the P < 1% level, and there is no point within 5° of fixation with a sensitivity less than 10 dB.

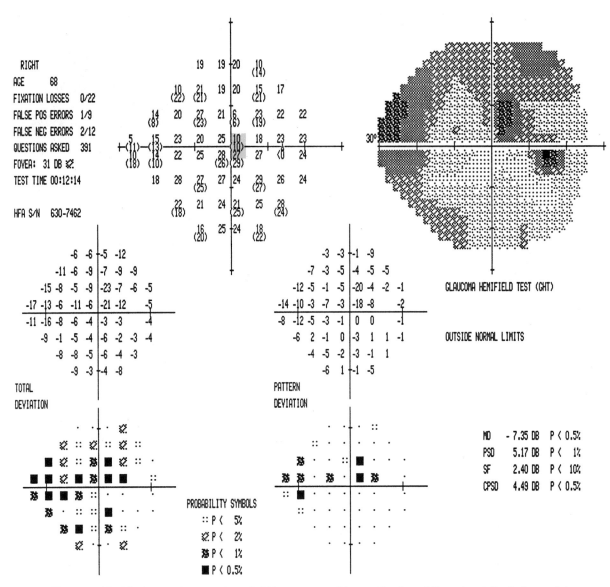

RIGHT

AGE   68

FIXATION LOSSES   0/22

FALSE POS ERRORS 1/9

FALSE NEG ERRORS 2/12

QUESTIONS ASKED   391

FOVEA: 31 DB

TEST TIME 00:12:14

HFA S/N   630-7462

TOTAL
DEVIATION

PATTERN
DEVIATION

GLAUCOMA HEMIFIELD TEST (GHT)

OUTSIDE NORMAL LIMITS

MD   - 7.35 DB   P < 0.5%
PSD   5.17 DB   P < 1%
SF   2.40 DB   P < 10%
CPSD   4.49 DB   P < 0.5%

PROBABILITY SYMBOLS

:: P < 5%
⚡ P < 2%
▩ P < 1%
■ P < 0.5%

Figure 5-15. Moderate glaucomatous field loss encroaching on fixation. Although relatively few points are statistically abnormal on the pattern deviation plot and the mean deviation is worse than −6 dB and one of the points within 5° of fixation has a sensitivity < 15 dB (*highlighted*). Although glaucoma typically does not affect fixation until late in the disease, it is not uncommon to see a mild depression of foveal threshold accompanying a localized defect near fixation,[8] as in this patient with 20/20 visual acuity.

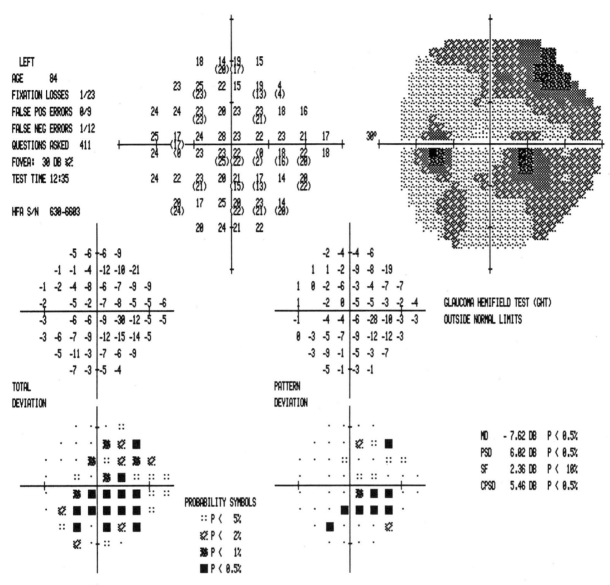

LEFT
AGE 84
FIXATION LOSSES 1/23
FALSE POS ERRORS 0/9
FALSE NEG ERRORS 1/12
QUESTIONS ASKED 411
FOVEA: 30 DB
TEST TIME 12:35

HFA S/N 630-6683

Figure 5-16. Moderate glaucomatous visual field defect close to fixation in normal tension glaucoma. This inferior arcuate defect comes quite close to fixation, which is more commonly recognized in patients with normal tension glaucoma than high tension glaucoma early in the disease,[9] with the exception of high tension glaucoma patients with high axial myopia. The field is classified as moderately depressed because the mean deviation is worse than −6 dB but not worse than 12 dB, there more than 25% but fewer than 50% of points in the pattern deviation plot are depressed at the $P < 5\%$ level, and more than 15% but fewer than 25% of points in the pattern deviation plot are depressed at the $P < 1\%$ level.

SEVERE GLAUCOMATOUS VISUAL FIELD DEFECTS

As glaucoma progresses further, it can involve almost the entire visual field, typically sparing fixation and the temporal portion of the field, outside the central 30°. A defect that splits fixation is considered severe because it threatens the center of vision.

The hallmarks of the severely affected visual field are widespread dense field loss and encroachment on, or loss of, fixation. Arbitrary criteria for defining severe glaucomatous field loss, developed by Elizabeth Hodapp, MD, are provided in Table 5-4.

Table 5-4. *Criteria for Severe Defect in Glaucoma*

Mean deviation worse than −12 dB

On pattern deviation plot, more than 50% of points depressed below the 5% level and more than 25% of points depressed below 1% level

Any point within central 5° with sensitivity less than or equal to 0 dB

Both hemifields containing a point(s) with sensitivity less than 15 dB wthin 5° of fixation

Adapted from Hodapp E, Parrish RK, Anderson DR. Clinical decisions in glaucoma. St. Louis: Mosby, 1993:59.

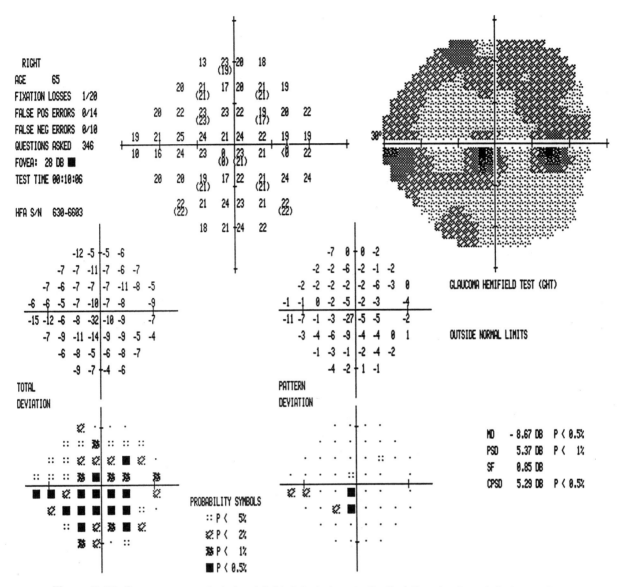

RIGHT

AGE   65

FIXATION LOSSES   1/20

FALSE POS ERRORS 0/14

FALSE NEG ERRORS 0/10

QUESTIONS ASKED   346

FOVEA: 28 DB ■

TEST TIME 00:10:06

HFA S/N   630-6603

```
            13  23 +20  18
               (19)
         20  21   17 |20  21   19
            (21)        (21)
      20  22  23  23 |22  19   20  22
            (23)         (17)
   19  21  25 |24  21 |24  22  19  19
   10  16  24  23   0 |23  21  (0  22
                    (0)|(21)
         20  20  19  17 |22  21  24  24
               (21)        (21)
            22  21  24 |23  21  22
           (22)              (22)
            18  21 +24  22
```

```
      -12 -5 +-5  -6
      -7  -7 -11|-7  -6  -7
   -7  -6  -7  -7 |-7 -11 -8  -5
-6 -6  -5 -7 -10|-7 -8      -9
-15 -12 -6  -8 -32|-10 -9       -7
   -7  -9 -11 -14|-9  -9  -5  -4
      -6  -8  -5 |-6  -8  -7
         -9  -7 +-4  -6
```

TOTAL
DEVIATION

```
         -7  0 + 0  -2
      -2 -2  -6 |-2  -1  -2
   -2  -2  -2  -2 |-2  -6  -3   0
-1 -1   0 -2  -5 |-2 -3      -4
-11 -7  -1  -3 -27|-5  -5      -2
   -3 -4  -6  -9 |-4  -4   0   1
      -1  -3  -1 |-2 -4  -2
         -4  -2 + 1  -1
```

PATTERN
DEVIATION

GLAUCOMA HEMIFIELD TEST (GHT)

OUTSIDE NORMAL LIMITS

PROBABILITY SYMBOLS

:: P < 5%

⊠ P < 2%

▧ P < 1%

■ P < 0.5%

MD   - 8.67 DB   P < 0.5%

PSD   5.37 DB   P < 1%

SF   0.85 DB

CPSD   5.29 DB   P < 0.5%

Figure 5-17. Severe paracentral visual field defect close to fixation. Despite the relatively small size of the paracentral defect on the pattern deviation plot, this dense scotoma is adjacent to fixation and contains a point that has 0 dB sensitivity, qualifying it as a severe visual field defect. None of the other criteria from Table 5-4 are met.

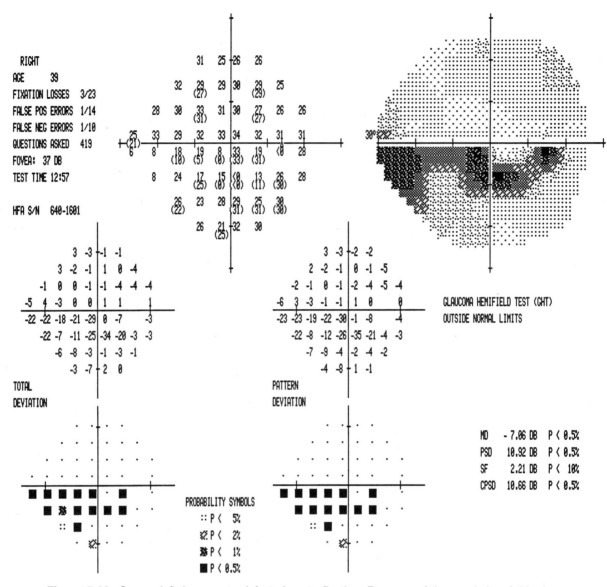

```
RIGHT                                          31   25  26   26

AGE      39                                 32   29   29  30   28    25
                                                (27)           (23)
FIXATION LOSSES  3/23
                                         28  30   33   31 30   27    26   26
FALSE POS ERRORS  1/14                           (31)         (27)

FALSE NEG ERRORS  1/10
                                             25  33   29   32  33 34  32  31   31
QUESTIONS ASKED   419                       -(21)
                                             6    8   18   19   8  33  19   0   28
FOVEA:  37 DB                                    (10) (5)  (0)(33)(31)

TEST TIME 12:57                              8   24   17   15  0  13   26   28
                                                    (25) (0)(0)(11)  (30)

HFA S/N   640-1601                              26   23   28  29  25   30
                                               (22)          (31)(31)(30)

                                                26   21  32   30
                                                   (25)
```

```
           3  -3  -1  -1                                3  -3  -2  -2
        3  -2  -1   1   0  -4                        2  -2  -1   0  -1  -5
     -1   0   0  -1  -1  -4  -4  -4                -2  -1   0  -1  -2  -4  -5  -4
   -5   4  -3   0   0   1   1      1             -6   3  -3  -1  -1   1   0      0
   -22 -22 -18 -21 -29  0  -7     -3             -23 -23 -19 -22 -30 -1  -8     -4
   -22  -7 -11 -25 -34 -20 -3 -3                 -22  -8 -12 -26 -35 -21 -4 -3
      -6  -8  -3 -1  -3  -1                          -7  -9  -4 -2  -4  -2
         -3  -7   2   0                                -4  -8   1  -1
```

TOTAL   PATTERN
DEVIATION   DEVIATION

GLAUCOMA HEMIFIELD TEST (GHT)
OUTSIDE NORMAL LIMITS

PROBABILITY SYMBOLS

:: P < 5%

▨ P < 2%

▩ P < 1%

■ P < 0.5%

MD   - 7.06 DB   P < 0.5%

PSD   10.92 DB   P < 0.5%

SF   2.21 DB   P < 10%

CPSD   10.66 DB   P < 0.5%

Figure 5-18. Severe inferior arcuate defect close to fixation. Because of the proximity of this dense defect to fixation, this inferior arcuate scotoma, which breaks into a nasal step, would be considered severe. None of the other criteria for a severe glaucomatous defect are met. Although the involved point adjacent to fixation had a sensitivity of 8 dB the first time it was checked, the number in parentheses (the value obtained when the threshold was determined a second time) indicates 0 dB sensitivity.

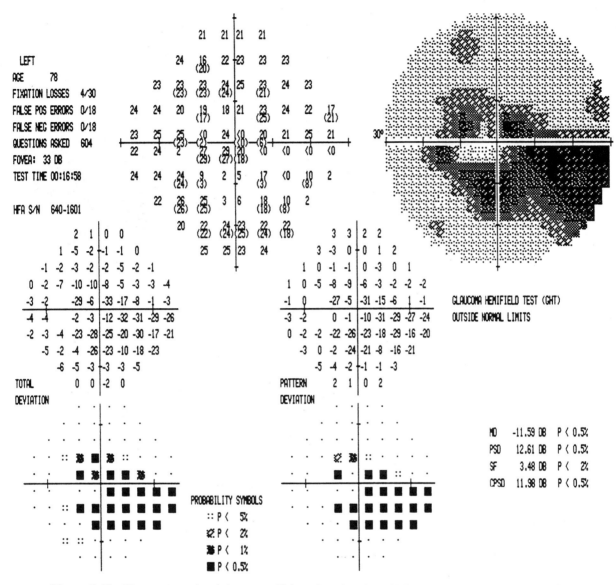

LEFT

AGE 78
FIXATION LOSSES 4/30
FALSE POS ERRORS 0/18
FALSE NEG ERRORS 0/18
QUESTIONS ASKED 604
FOVEA: 33 DB
TEST TIME 00:16:58

HFA S/N 640-1601

GLAUCOMA HEMIFIELD TEST (GHT)
OUTSIDE NORMAL LIMITS

PROBABILITY SYMBOLS
:: P < 5%
▧ P < 2%
▨ P < 1%
■ P < 0.5%

MD	-11.59 DB	P < 0.5%
PSD	12.61 DB	P < 0.5%
SF	3.48 DB	P < 2%
CPSD	11.98 DB	P < 0.5%

Figure 5-19. Ring scotoma from glaucoma. This patient developed inferior and superior arcuate defects in addition to a dense inferonasal step. Although the mean deviation is not severely depressed (ie, worse than −12 dB), more than 25% of the points are depressed at the *P* < 1% level and there is a point within 5° of fixation with < 0 dB sensitivity.

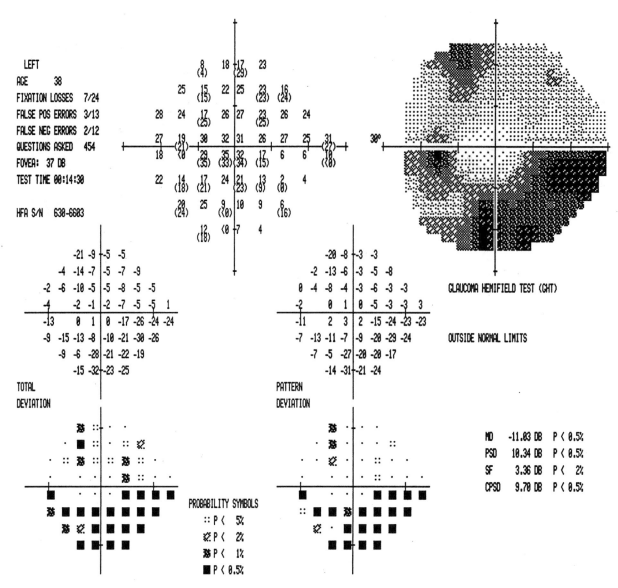

Figure 5-20. Severe inferior arcuate defect breaking into nasal step. Although this dense defect does not meet the mean deviation criteria (MD worse than − 12 dB) or have severely depressed points within 5° of fixation, more than 50% of the point in the field are depressed on the pattern deviation plot to the *P* < 5% level and more than 25% are depressed at the *P* < 1% level. The defect is, therefore, classified as severe.

CENTRAL 30 - 2 THRESHOLD TEST

DATE 03-22-93

STIMULUS III, WHITE, BCKGND 31.5 ASB BLIND SPOT CHECK SIZE III   FIXATION TARGET   CENTRAL   TIME 03:09:05 PM
STRATEGY FULL THRESHOLD   RX USED +4.75 DS +0.75 DCX 080 DEG   PUPIL DIAMETER 4.0 MM   VA 20/20

```
                                    11
                                   (9)   17  6   11

   LEFT                      20    16   20  7   11   15
                                  (20)     (11)
   AGE      58
                         23   23   25   24  15   17   6    0
   FIXATION LOSSES  0/26                  (21)      (21) (6) ((0))
   FALSE POS ERRORS  0/9   22   18  26   23   24 21  23   8   4   (0
                                (22)     (25)        (19) (12) ((0))
   FALSE NEG ERRORS  1/16   25  25  25   4   0  7   10   9   5   (0
   QUESTIONS ASKED  526              (0) (9) (4)  (0) (0)
                             24  24  (0   29  22 29   29   28  22   18
   FOVEA: 32 DB ::              (24) ((0))  (27)(28)
   TEST TIME 00:16:31        24  16   26  29   26 27   31   26  24   24
                                 (22)     (27)       (29)

   HFA S/N  630-6603          20  28   25  27 26  25   26   27
                             (24) (26)                (22)

                              24   26  22 25   24   27
```

```
       -12 -5 |-17 -12                               -9 -3 |-15 -9
    -5 -7 -6 |-17 -15 -10           25  25 23  20  -2 -5 -3 |-15 -12 -8
 -3 -4 -5 -4 |-13 -9 -21 -28                      -1 -1 -2 -1 |-11 -6 -19 -25
-5 -8 -2 -5 -6 |-9 -9 -19 -26 -27             -2 -5 0 -3 -3 |-7 -7 -16 -24 -24
-3 -4      -29 -33|-24 -24 -27 -26 -28        0 -1      -27 -31|-21 -22 -25 -23 -25
-5 -5    -2 -5 |-4 -3 -3 -7 -8               -2 -3    1 -2 |-1 0 0 -4 -6
-4 -10 -4 -3 -5 |-4 -1 -4 -4 -2              -2 -7 -1 0 -2 |-2 1 -1 -1 1
   -6 -2 -5 -3 |-4 -5 -4 0                     -4 0 -2 0 |-1 -2 -2 3
     -4 -3 -7 |-3 -4 0                          -2 0 -4 |-1 -1 3
TOTAL      -2 -2 |-3 -6                   PATTERN      1 0 |-1 -3
DEVIATION                                DEVIATION
```

GLAUCOMA HEMIFIELD TEST (GHT)

OUTSIDE NORMAL LIMITS

PROBABILITY SYMBOLS

:: P < 5%
⊠ P < 2%
▨ P < 1%
■ P < 0.5%

MD   - 8.88 DB   P < 0.5%
PSD   10.39 DB   P < 0.5%
SF   1.96 DB
CPSD   10.14 DB   P < 0.5%

Figure 5-21. Severe superior visual field defect encroaching on fixation. This field is classified as severe because of the single point within 5° of fixation with a sensitivity of < 0 dB. None of the other criteria for severe visual field loss are met.

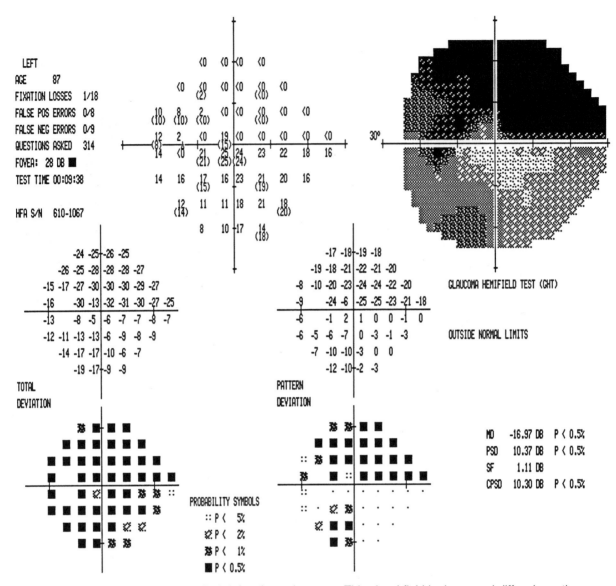

Figure 5-22. Superior altitudinal defect from glaucoma. This visual field is depressed diffusely on the graytone printout and total deviation plots. The pattern deviation plot shows a superior altitudinal defect, similar to that seen in ischemic optic neuropathy. Clinical correlation (amount of optic disc cupping versus pallor) is necessary to determine the cause of such a defect. The defect is classified as severe because the mean deviation is worse than −12 dB, there are more than 50% of points depressed at the $P < 5\%$ level and more than 25% depressed at the $P < 1\%$ level, and there is a point within 5° of fixation with a sensitivity of < 0 dB.

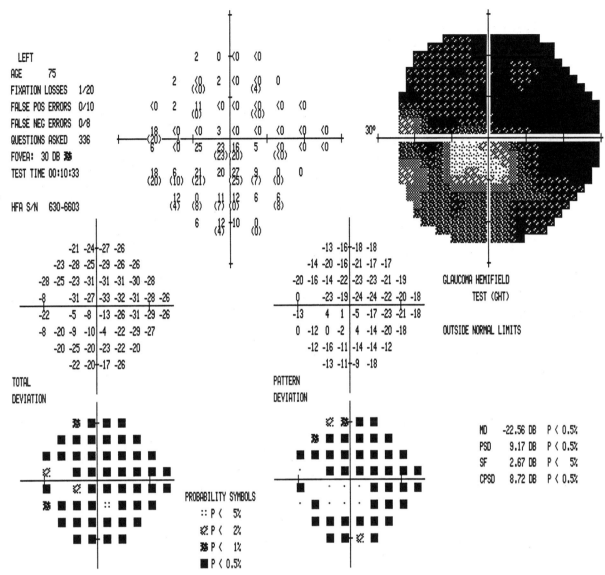

LEFT

AGE   75
FIXATION LOSSES   1/20
FALSE POS ERRORS 0/10
FALSE NEG ERRORS 0/8
QUESTIONS ASKED   336
FOVEA: 30 DB 🖩
TEST TIME 00:10:33

HFA S/N   630-6603

GLAUCOMA HEMIFIELD
TEST (GHT)

OUTSIDE NORMAL LIMITS

TOTAL
DEVIATION

PATTERN
DEVIATION

PROBABILITY SYMBOLS

:: P < 5%
🖉 P < 2%
🖩 P < 1%
■ P < 0.5%

MD	-22.56 DB	P < 0.5%
PSD	9.17 DB	P < 0.5%
SF	2.67 DB	P < 5%
CPSD	8.72 DB	P < 0.5%

Figure 5-23. Severe glaucomatous field defect. The central and temporal regions of the visual field are usually affected very late in glaucoma due to the relative resistance of the papillomaculary bundle and nasal nerve fibers to glaucomatous damage. This patient has only a small central island and a few temporal points remaining. The temporal island, which is typically spared until the last in progressive glaucoma, is usually beyond the central 24° or 30° measured by automated perimetry. All criteria for a severely depressed visual field are met except that only one hemifield (the superior one) contains a point with a sensitivity of less than 15 dB within 5° of fixation. Because there are so few remaining normal points to follow on this central 24° field, future field would best be performed using a central 10° field, which would provide more points to follow. (Courtesy of Kevin Coolbaugh, O.D.)

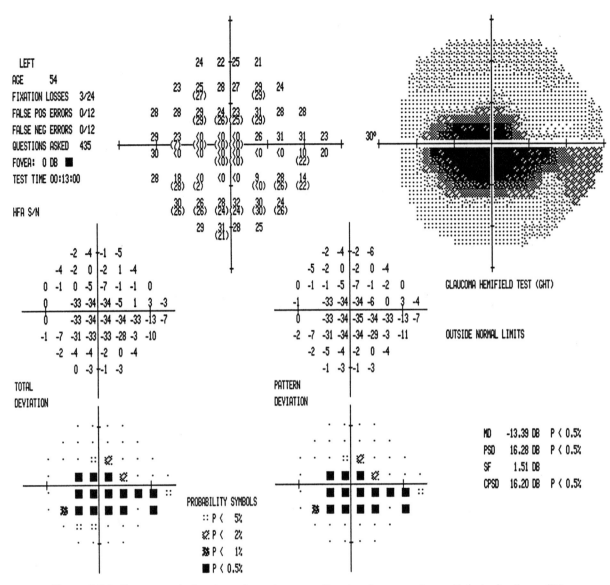

Figure 5-24. Severe central scotoma from glaucoma. Rarely, when superior and inferior fixation splitting defects are present in the same patient, a central scotoma results in glaucoma. Despite a foveal threshold of 0 dB, the normal tension glaucoma patient who had the above visual field had a visual acuity of 20/50. A central 10° or macular test with a 2° distance between test points may have revealed a small island of vision accounting for the 20/50 visual acuity. This defect is classified as severe because the mean deviation is worse than − 12 dB, and there are points adjacent to fixation that are 0 dB or worse.

JUDGING GLAUCOMATOUS PROGRESSION

The glaucomatous visual field may progress in three ways. First, a new defect may appear in a previously normal region, and it should fit Anderson's criteria for a minimal defect (see Table 5-1). Second, an existing defect may get deeper. And third, an existing defect may get larger. There is not general agreement on judging progressive deepening of a visual field defect, probably because there is no gold standard for comparison. There are two statistical programs that can be used to judge progression that come with the Humphrey Field Analyzer, glaucoma change probability and linear regression analysis.

A third statistical program, called Progressor Programme, performs pointwise linear regression analysis of each point in the field over time.[10,11] The interested reader is encouraged to review several articles on the relative values of these programs[11–13] or Anderson's criteria[15] in more detail than this text allows. Regardless of the criteria chosen for judging progression, one important rule should be followed: always confirm progression with a second visual field and even a third if important clinical decisions are being based on subtle changes in the visual field.[15] A summary of the criteria that I use for judging progression, based on criteria used by Anderson[14] and the Normal Tension Glaucoma Study,[15] is provided in Table 5-5.

Following an already poor visual field for signs of progression is a difficult but common problem in glaucoma management. Correct assessment of progression in these patients has enormous therapeutic impact because they are usually under consideration for surgical intervention. However, it is difficult to judge progression in the already poor visual field because there are fewer points with vision on which change may be judged and because variability in threshold determination is greater in areas with depressed sensitivity.

(References begin on page 193)

Table 5-5. *Judging Glaucoma Progression**

Pointwise comparison[16]	Defect has deepened or enlarged if two or more points† within or adjacent to an existing scotoma have worsened by at least 10 dB or 3 times the average of the short-term fluctuations, whichever is larger
Glaucoma change probability	Deterioration of two or more adjacent points† within or adjacent to an existing scotoma at the $P < 5\%$ level as indicated by a black triangle
Regression analysis of global indices	Deterioration of slope of mean deviation at the $P < 5\%$ level per year

* All criteria assume confirmation on at least one subsequent field and clinical correlation with no other explanation for deterioration.

† Edge points of a central 30° field are excluded from analysis.

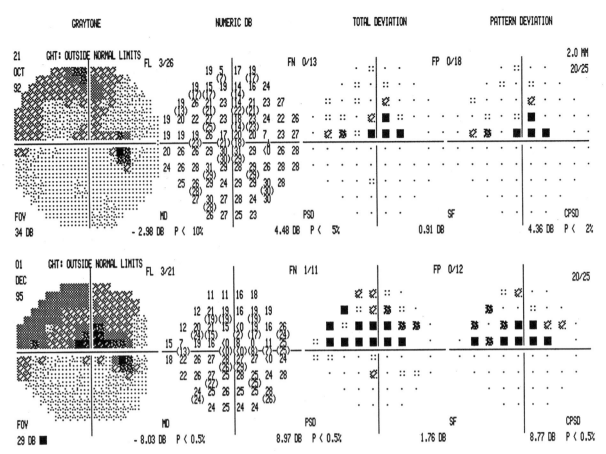

Figure 5-25. Worsening of glaucoma: pointwise comparison. This overview printout, shows the visual fields of a patient with worsening glaucoma over a 3-year period. The printout demonstrates deepening and enlargement of the existing superior arcuate scotoma that covered most of the upper hemifield and came close to fixation. There are at least two points that worsen by at least 10 dB within and adjacent to the scotoma. Note worsening of the MD and CPSD. The central visual acuity was unchanged, despite a 5-decibel reduction in foveal threshold. If the field had deteriorated because of media opacity, all points in the field would have deteriorated more-or-less equally, and although the MD would worsen with media opacity, the CPSD would not.

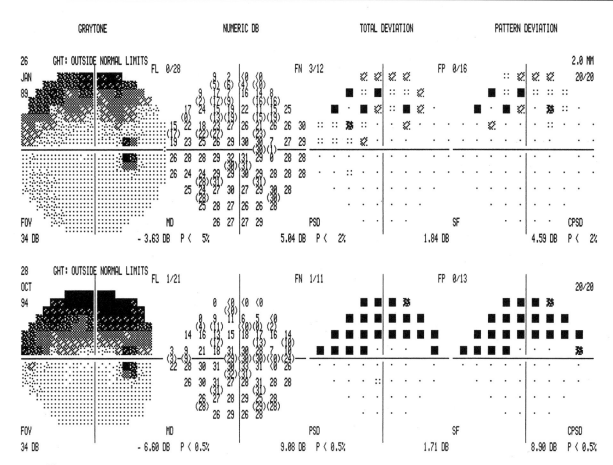

Figure 5-26. Worsening of glaucoma: pointwise comparison. Another example of a superior arcuate defect from glaucoma that deepened and enlarged with time. Using pointwise comparison, two or more points within the scotoma deepened by at least 10 dB and two or more points adjacent to the scotoma worsened by at least 10 dB. The MD and CPSD also worsened with a stable foveal threshold and visual acuity, which is consistent with worsening localized rather than diffuse depression.

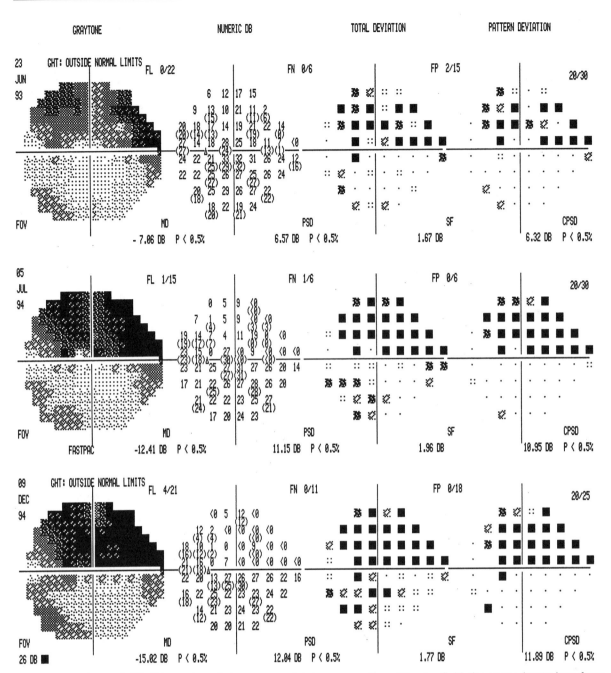

Figure 5-27. Worsening of glaucoma: pointwise comparison. The *top* field shows moderate loss from glaucoma superiorly. The field 1 year later (*center*) shows definite deepening of the superior defect and this defect would be classified as severe at this stage. The *bottom* field shows worsening at a single point superotemporal to fixation. This point was normal in the center field just 5 months previously. A confirmatory field was performed and demonstrated a sensitivity of <0 dB at this location, prompting escalation of glaucoma therapy. Although progression at a single point does not strictly fit criteria for calling progression, subtle change of this nature (ie, close to fixation) should be considered evidence of worsening if confirmed on repeat testing.

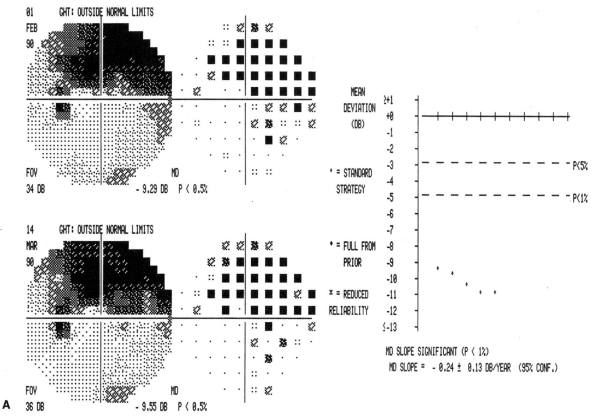

Figure 5-28. Worsening of glaucoma: glaucoma change probability. Serial visual fields of a patient with normal tension glaucoma. These two fields **(A)** are selected as baseline fields (either by the perimetrist or a default program) and the sensitivities are averaged by the computer and compared with all subsequent fields. The graph shows the change in mean deviation over time and gives the slope of the line connecting the mean deviations (MD slope) as well as the significance of the slope of the line. The subsequent fields **(B)** contain the glaucoma change probability plots. This plot is a pointwise comparison and indicates whether a particular point is worse (solid triangle) or better (open triangle) at the $P < 5\%$ level. There are four black triangles on the Glaucoma change Probability plots (*far right*), which were worse than baseline on all subsequent fields. The superior defect enlarged at two points and the inferior defect enlarged at two points. From 1994 to 1996, only one new black triangle appeared, which would not fit the criteria for worsening (at least two points must be worse), supporting the impression that the field has stabilized. The occasional open triangle in the change Glaucoma Probability plots indicates improvement in that particular point compared with the baseline fields, but these are not reproducible and are most likely an artifact of long-term fluctuation. The MD is not significantly worse over time. However, the pointwise comparison provided in the glaucoma change probability program demonstrates an important change over time and may be the most sensitive of the available methods for judging progression.

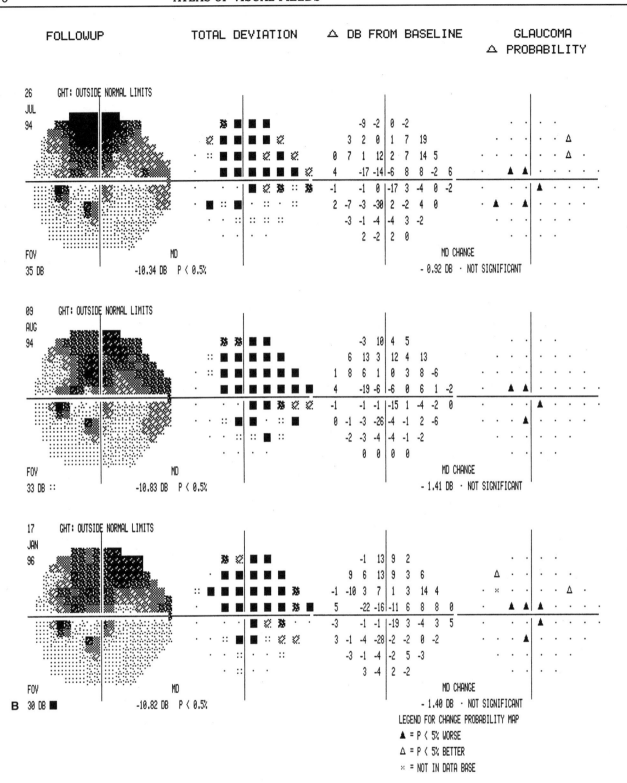

Figure 5-28. *Continued.*

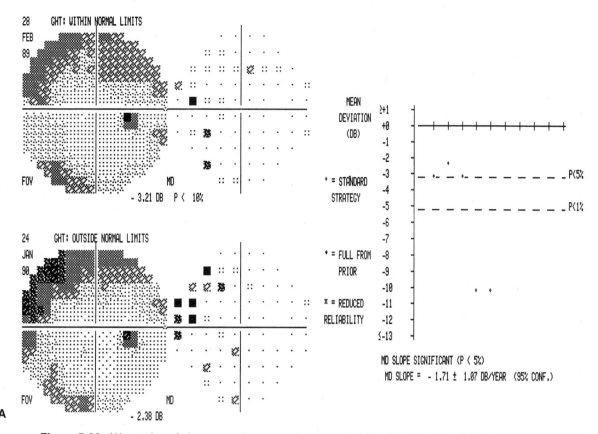

Figure 5-29. Worsening of glaucoma: glaucoma change probability. This series of fields shows worsening and expansion of the superonasal defect and development of an inferior defect **(A)** baseline, **(B)** follow-up. There are three new black triangles on the Glaucoma change Probability plot of October, 1990, and many new black triangles on the Glaucoma change Probability plot of May, 1993, which persist in the field done in April, 1994. Between 1993 and 1994, there are only two new adjacent black triangles and these are continuous with the blind spot temporally, a variable region of the field. The mean deviation graph worsens over time at a rate of -1.71 dB per year, and the slope of the worsening line is significant at the $P < 5\%$ level.

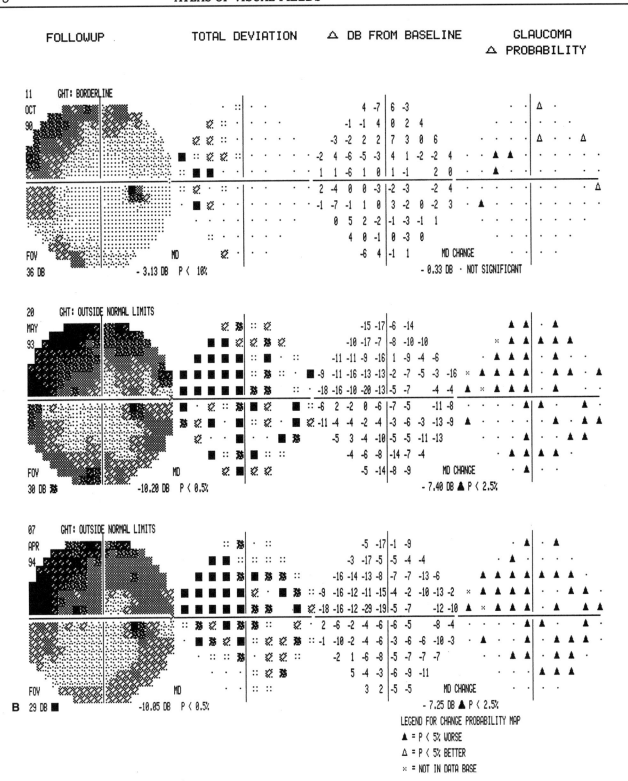

Figure 5-29. *Continued.*

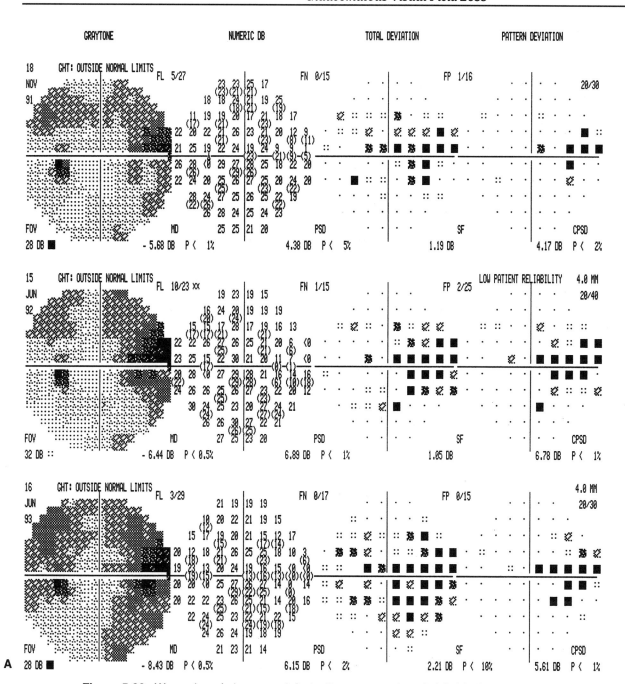

Figure 5-30. Worsening of glaucoma defects: linear regression of global indices. This series of fields shows deepening of an existing superonasal field defect and enlargement of an inferonasal step over a 3-year period. Using the global indices, the MD declines from −5.69 dB in November of 1991 **(A)** to −9.79 dB in October of 1994 **(B)**, whereas the visual acuity and foveal threshold are unchanged, indicating that the worsening MD is probably not from a process such as media opacity.

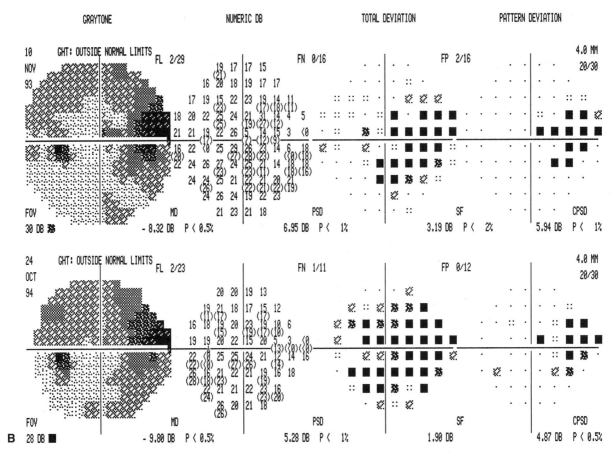

Figure 5-30. *Continued.*

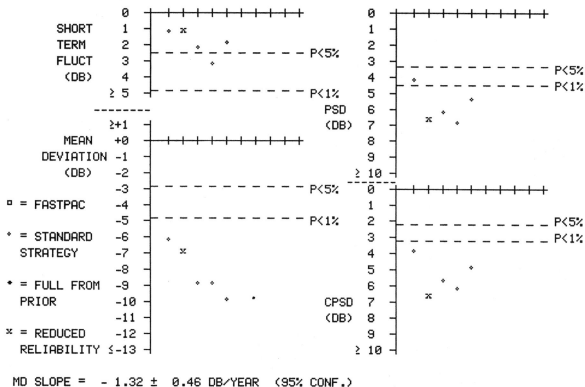

```
MD SLOPE =  - 1.32 ±  0.46 DB/YEAR  (95% CONF.)
```

C MD SLOPE SIGNIFICANT (P < 1%)

Figure 5-30. *Continued.* The change analysis printout for this patient **(C)** shows the change in global indices over time and the significance of the change in MD over time.* The MD worsens over time, and the slope of the line that shows this worsening is statistically significant at the *P* < 1% level. The short-term fluctuation also worsens, as is often the case when more of the double-determined points become adjacent to, or part of, a relative scotoma. The pattern deviation and CPSDs can increase over time as the localized defects become larger and deeper. As more of the field becomes involved, the pattern standard deviation and CPSD decrease.

    * Those experienced at looking at the Humphrey change analysis data will notice that the boxplot portion of the printout has been omitted. The interested reader is referred to Anderson DR. Automated static perimetry, St. Louis: Mosby–Year Book, 1992:214 for a full explanation of the boxplot analysis.

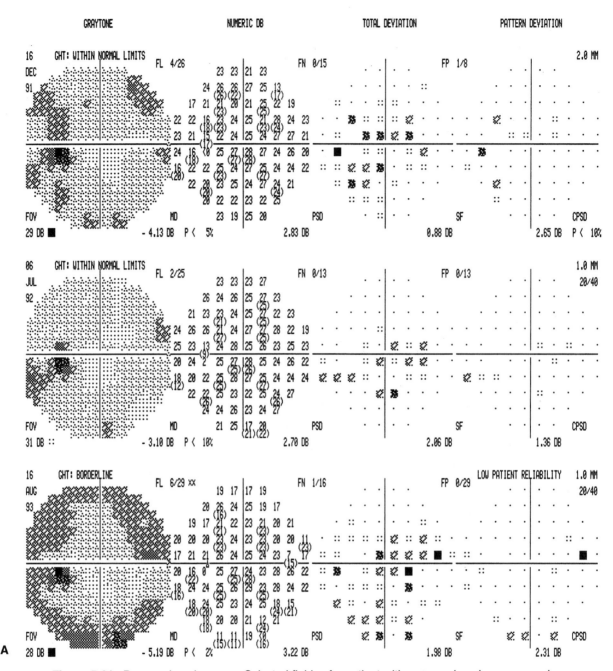

Figure 5-31. Progressive glaucoma. Selected fields of a patient with progressive glaucoma as shown by overview printout. **(A)** Baseline visual fields in December, 1991 and July, 1992 show mild generalized depression but normal GHT. The field of August, 1993 shows a borderline GHT with normal CPSD but probably an early glaucomatous superonasal defect which does not yet fit the criteria for minimal abnormality outlined in Table 5-1.

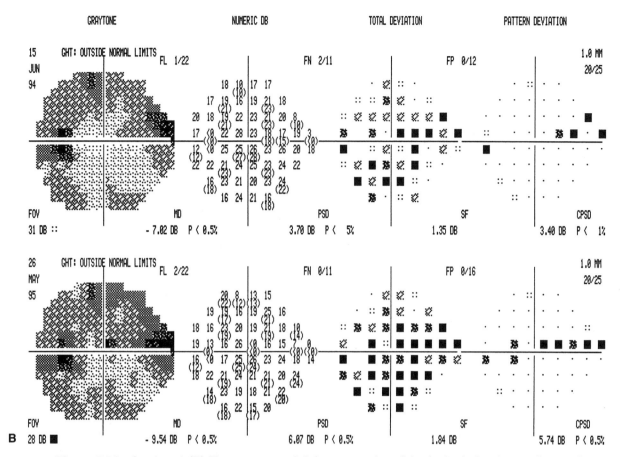

Figure 5-31. *Continued.* **(B)** The superonasal defect meets the minimal criteria for abnormality as of June, 1994 and worsens in May, 1995, encroaching on fixation. The MD declines from about −3.5 dB to −9.52 dB throughout this period, although the visual acuity and foveal threshold remain stable, an indication that the change in MD is not affecting fixation, as would a media opacity or central retinal process.

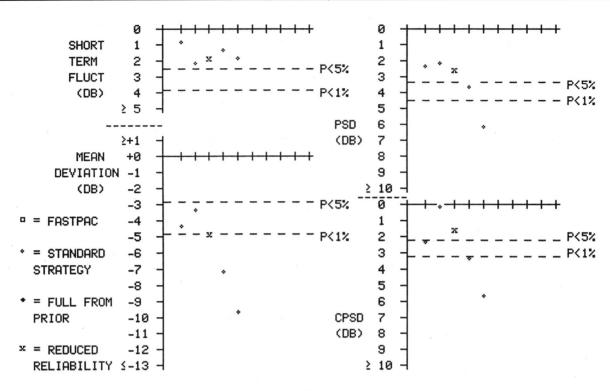

MD SLOPE = - 2.15 ± 1.04 DB/YEAR (95% CONF.)

C   MODIFIED MD SLOPE SIGNIFICANT (P < 5%)

Figure 5-31. *Continued.* (C) Plot of MD in the change analysis printout demonstrates worsening of the MD over time and the slope of the line is statistically significant at the $P < 5\%$ level. The PSD and CPSD also worsen with time, particularly from 1993 to 1995.

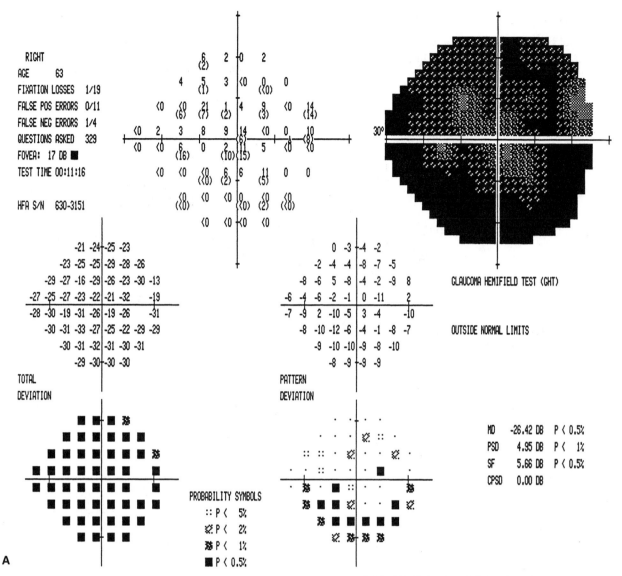

RIGHT

AGE 63
FIXATION LOSSES 1/19
FALSE POS ERRORS 0/11
FALSE NEG ERRORS 1/4
QUESTIONS ASKED 329
FOVEA: 17 DB ■
TEST TIME 00:11:16

HFA S/N 630-3151

GLAUCOMA HEMIFIELD TEST (GHT)

OUTSIDE NORMAL LIMITS

TOTAL
DEVIATION

PATTERN
DEVIATION

PROBABILITY SYMBOLS

:: P < 5%
▨ P < 2%
▩ P < 1%
■ P < 0.5%

MD   -26.42 DB   P < 0.5%
PSD   4.95 DB   P < 1%
SF   5.66 DB   P < 0.5%
CPSD 0.00 DB

A

Figure 5-32. Following the severely depressed glaucoma field. **(A)** This visual field of a glaucoma patient with poor central acuity and severe glaucomatous visual field damage does not provide any data to judge progression. Using a size III stimulus, all of the points in the absolute value plot have values of el5dB, which are too low to judge progression over time.

CENTRAL 24 - 2 THRESHOLD TEST

STIMULUS   V, WHITE, BCKGND 31.5 ASB
BLIND SPOT CHECK SIZE   III
FIXATION TARGET   CENTRAL   DATE 07-25-95 TIME 09:15:06 AM
STRATEGY   FULL THRESHOLD   PUPIL DIAMETER   VA 20/200
                                    RX USED -2.25 DS   DCX   DEG

RIGHT   FIXATION LOSSES 0/23
                                    FALSE POS ERRORS 0/16
                                    FALSE NEG ERRORS 1/10
                                       FLUCTUATION   5.06 DB
                                    QUESTIONS ASKED   438
                                          FOVEA: 30 DB
        30°   30°   TEST TIME 00:16:15
                                    HFA S/N 630-7462

o = WITHIN 4 DB OF EXPECTED   NO. = THRESHOLD IN DB
NO. = DEFECT DEPTH IN DB   (NO.) = 2ND TIME
33 DB   = CENTRAL REF LEVEL

Figure 5-32. *Continued.* **(B)** To counteract this problem, the visual field was repeated using a larger stimulus size (size V). This increases the range of the points to follow as the new values will have better sensitivities. A larger stimulus size is recommended when the majority of points are depressed to < 15 dB. Future comparisons may be based on pointwise comparison or by comparing quad totals. Statistical analysis is not available for fields performed with a size V test object.

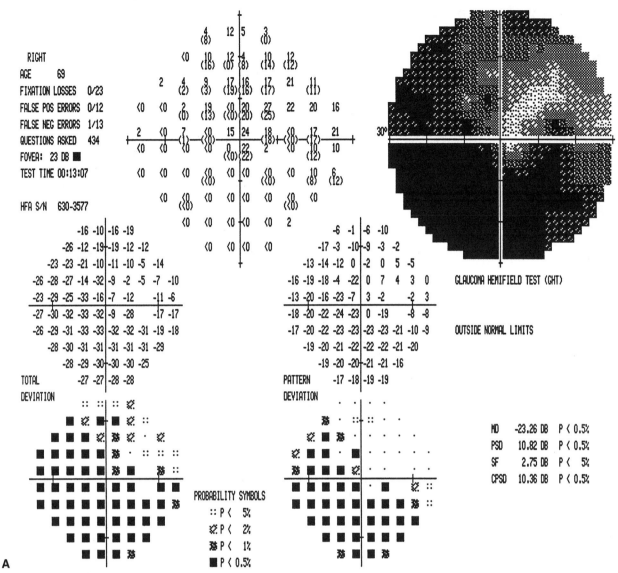

Figure 5-33. Following the severely constricted glaucoma field. **(A)** Visual field from a patient with severe long-standing glaucoma whose field has been reduced to the central 5°. Following this field for progression means relying on the interpretation of very few points. An alternative strategy may be employed, the macula program, **(B)**, which measures threshold at 16 points within 5° of fixation. Future comparisons must be made on a pointwise basis, and there is no statistical analysis available for the macula threshold or central 10° tests.

A

```
    MACULA THRESHOLD TEST

STIMULUS    III, WHITE, BCKGND 31.5 ASB
BLIND SPOT CHECK SIZE   III
FIXATION TARGET   CENTRAL          DATE  06-02-93  TIME  02:19:56 PM
STRATEGY    FULL THRESHOLD         PUPIL DIAMETER   2.0 MM  VA  20/40
                                   RX USED -2.25 DS +1.75 DCX 170 DEG
```

RIGHT

```
                                        FIXATION LOSSES  0/16
                                        FALSE POS ERRORS 0/5
                                        FALSE NEG ERRORS 0/5
                                          FLUCTUATION   1.41 DB
                                        QUESTIONS ASKED  247
                                                 FOVEA:    26 DB
                                             TEST TIME 00:07:18
                                             HFA S/N 630-3577
```

```
        17     25    25    23
      (19)   (23)  (23)  (23)

        17     24    26    27
10°   (19)   (24)  (24)  (27)              10°

        19     24    28    25
      (17)   (22)  (28)  (27)

         5     21    21    23
       (0)   (19)  (21)  (23)
```

```
                              NO.  = THRESHOLD IN DB
                              (NO.) = 2ND TIME
```

B

Figure 5-33. *Continued.*

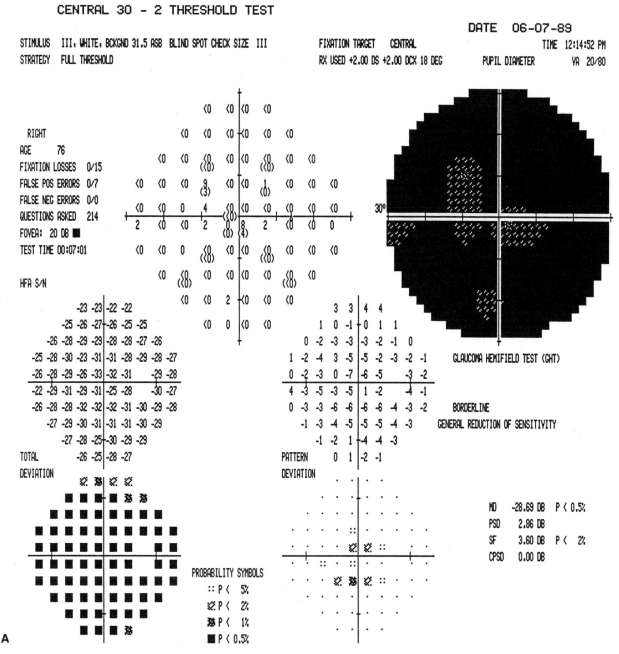

Figure 5-34. Following the severely depressed and constricted glaucoma field. The visual fields in this figure are from a patient with severe glaucoma and 20/80 visual acuity. Field **A**, covering the central 30° using a size III stimulus does not contain any points to follow for progression.

CENTRAL 10 - 2 THRESHOLD TEST

STIMULUS   III, WHITE, BCKGND 31.5 ASB   BLIND SPOT CHECK SIZE III   FIXATION TARGET   CENTRAL   DATE   06-07-89
STRATEGY   FULL THRESHOLD   RX USED +2.00 DS +2.00 DCX 18 DEG   TIME 12:32:58 PM
                                                                                                               PUPIL DIAMETER   VA 20/80

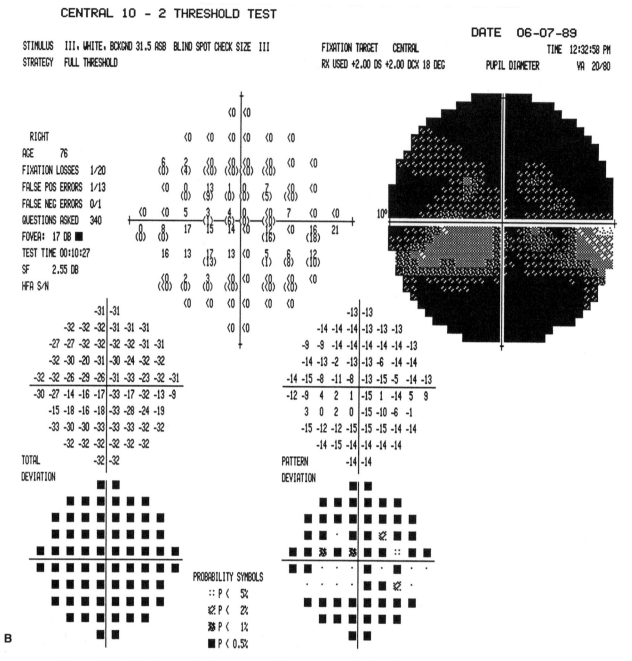

RIGHT

AGE   76
FIXATION LOSSES   1/20
FALSE POS ERRORS   1/13
FALSE NEG ERRORS   0/1
QUESTIONS ASKED   340
FOVEA: 17 DB ■
TEST TIME 00:10:27
SF   2.55 DB
HFA S/N

PROBABILITY SYMBOLS
:: P < 5%
▨ P < 2%
▩ P < 1%
■ P < 0.5%

Figure 5-34. *Continued.* Testing points within the central 10° in field **B** provide more points to follow but the sensitivities are all < 15 dB.

CENTRAL 10 - 2 THRESHOLD TEST

STIMULUS   V, WHITE, BCKGND 31.5 ASB
BLIND SPOT CHECK SIZE   III
FIXATION TARGET   CENTRAL   DATE   02-13-91   TIME   11:26:40 AM
STRATEGY   FULL THRESHOLD   PUPIL DIAMETER   2.0 MM   VA   20/80
                                     RX USED +2.00 DS 2.00 DCX 18 DEG

RIGHT

                                           FIXATION LOSSES   1/30
                                           FALSE POS ERRORS 0/12
                                           FALSE NEG ERRORS 3/17
                                           FLUCTUATION   2.71 DB
                                       QUESTIONS ASKED   586
10°   10°   FOVEA: 25 DB
                                           TEST TIME 00:19:22
                                           HFA S/N 630-4595

° = WITHIN 4 DB OF EXPECTED   NO.   = THRESHOLD IN DB
NO. = DEFECT DEPTH IN DB   (NO.) = 2ND TIME
30 DB ×× = CENTRAL REF LEVEL

```
                    25│ 24
           18  22  22│ 27  29  22
       18  10  24  23│ 22  21  25  24
       12  16  16  22│ 22  22  22  18
10° 11 11   °   °   5│ 10  22   °   5   9  10°
     5  °   °   °   °│  8  10   °   °  10
        9   °   °   °│ 10   6   8  12
       19  20  25  19│ 13  23  28  24
           26  28  27│ 27  29  26
                    28│ 28
```

```
QUAD TOTAL                    3 │ 6
  232                           │(2)
                  10   7   7 │ 2   0   6        QUAD TOTAL
                                │                  163
              10  24   3   5 │ 7   5   4   4
                 (14) (7) (8)│  (11)
              17  13  15   7 │ 7   7   7  10
                     (11)    │  (7)        (12)
10°  17  19  31  25  24 │14   7  22  23  20  10°
     23  27  31  27  28 │22  19  25  25
        (17)(27)(22)(26)│(26)      (25)(25)(18)
                                                (23)
         21  27  29  25 │19  25  21  11
        (19)    (27)    │   (21)      (23)
          8  12   5  19 │15   7   8   2
        (10) (6) (3)(1) │(17) (5) (2) (6)
              2   0   2 │ 2   0   2
QUAD TOTAL       (2)    │(2) ((0)      QUAD TOTAL
  273             0     │ 0 ((0)          220
```

C

Figure 5-34. *Continued.* Repeating the field with a larger spot size (size V), in field **C**, provides information on which progression can be judged.

```
CENTRAL 10 - 2 THRESHOLD TEST

STIMULUS    V. WHITE. BCKGND 31.5 ASB
BLIND SPOT CHECK SIZE   III
FIXATION TARGET   CENTRAL          DATE   02-07-96   TIME   09:11:12 AM
STRATEGY    FULL THRESHOLD         PUPIL DIAMETER   2.0 MM   VA   20/80
                                   RX USED +2.00 DS 2.00 DCX 015 DEG
```

RIGHT

FIXATION LOSSES 0/23
FALSE POS ERRORS 0/18
FALSE NEG ERRORS 1/10
 FLUCTUATION   2.00 DB
QUESTIONS ASKED 426
  FOVEA: 20 DB
 TEST TIME 00:14:27
  HFA S/N 630-7462

10°   10°

° = WITHIN 4 DB OF EXPECTED   NO. = THRESHOLD IN DB
NO. = DEFECT DEPTH IN DB   (NO.) = 2ND TIME
30 DB ×× = CENTRAL REF LEVEL

Left grid (defect depth in DB):

```
                28 | 28
            28  28  29 | 29  29  28
        28  23  24  26 | 26  29  27  28
        25  22  17  24 | 22  22  22  29
10°  28 29 18 16 16 | 18 18 22 26 28  10°
     28 29  6  °  6 | 14 22 18 26 28
        29 10  °  23 | 18 21 24 27
        28 27 29 27 | 24 29 29 28
            28 29 29 | 29 29 28
                28 | 28
```

Right grid (threshold in DB, (NO.) = 2nd time):

```
QUAD TOTAL                       <0 | <0                  QUAD TOTAL
81                                                        59
                  8     <0          <0   0    0    <0
                 (0)    (2)
            8     6     7    5    |3     8    2    8
           (0)        (3)  (2)       (0)      (0)
            4     7   13    5    |7     7    7    1
                     (11)  (5)      (7)        (0)
10°  <0  0  11  13  14 |12  11   7   3   <0  10°
     <0  0   23  27  24 |16   7  11   5   <0
        (0)            (16)         (1)
         1   19  27   3 |11   9   5   5
        (0)     (23) (3)     (7)     (0)
         8    4   8    4 |5    1    8    <0
        (0) (0) (0) (0)  (0)  (0)
            <0  <0  <0 |0    8   <0
QUAD TOTAL             (0) (0)        QUAD TOTAL
128         <0 | <0                    68
```

Figure 5-34. *Continued.* Field **D** is a follow-up field, 5 years later, which demonstrates progression. Either pointwise comparison can be performed to compare fields or the quad totals in the threshold printout can be compared to judge progression. No criteria have been established for judging progression in severely depressed fields so that clinical impression is used. Sensitivities in this range tend to be highly variable and progression is likely to be overcalled.

D

References

1. Stewart WC, Shields MB, Ollie AR. Peripheral visual field testing by automated kinetic perimetry in glaucoma. Arch Ophthalmol 1988;106:202.
2. Werner EB, Drance SM. Early visual field disturbances in glaucoma. Arch Ophthalmol 1977;95:1173.
3. Hart WM Jr, Becker B. The onset and evolution of glaucomatous visual field defects. Ophthalmology 1982;89:268.
4. Phelps CD, Hayreh SS, Montague PR. Visual fields in low-tension glaucoma, primary open angle glaucoma, and anterior ischemic optic neuropathy. Doc Ophthalmol Proc Ser 1983;35:113.
5. Drance SM. Diffuse visual field loss in open-angle glaucoma. Ophthalmology 1991;98:1533.
6. Åsman P, Heijl A. Diffuse visual field loss and glaucoma. Acta Ophthal 1994;72:303.
7. Flammer J, Drance SM, Zulauf M. Short and long term fluctuation in patients with glaucoma, normal controls and patients with suspected glaucoma. Arch Ophthalmol 1984;102:704.
8. Anctil J-L, Anderson DR. Early foveal involvement and generalized depression of the visual field in glaucoma. Arch Ophthalmol 1984;102:363.
9. Araia, M. Pattern of visual field defects in normal-tension and high-tension glaucoma. Cur Op Ophthalmol 1995 volume 6, number 2:36.
10. Noureddin BN, Poinoosawmy D, Fitzke FW, Hitchings RA. Regression analysis of visual field progression in low tension glaucoma. Br J Ophthalmol 1991;75:493
11. Fitzke FW, McNaught AI. The diagnosis of visual field progression in glaucoma. Curr Op Ophthalmol 1994 volume 5, number 2:110.
12. Morgan RK, Feuer WJ, Anderson DR. Statpac 2 glaucoma change probability. Arch Ophthalmol 1991;109:1690
13. Birch MK, Wishart PK, O'Donnell NP. Determining progressive visual field loss in serial Humphrey visual fields. Ophthalmology 1995;102:1227.
14. Anderson DR. Automated Static Perimetry. St. Louis: Mosby–Year Book, 1992:204.
15. Schulzer M. Errors in the diagnosis of visual field progression in normal-tension glaucoma. Ophthalmology 1994;101:1589.
16. Anderson DR. Automated Static Perimetry. St. Louis: Mosby–Year Book, 1992:182.

6

Nonglaucomatous Optic Nerve Disorders

Donald L. Budenz and
R. Michael Siatowski

Nonglaucomatous optic neuropathies may produce a wide spectrum of visual field defects. In addition to typical paracentral, arcuate, and altitudinal defects from disruption of the nerve fiber layer as described in Chapter 5, nonglaucomatous optic nerve disorders may also cause central and cecocentral scotomas.[1] With rare exception, primary optic neuropathies do not respect the vertical meridian unless they are caused by a pathologic process which also involves the optic chiasm.

Figures 6.1–6.38 follow on pages 196–255.

References appear on page 256.

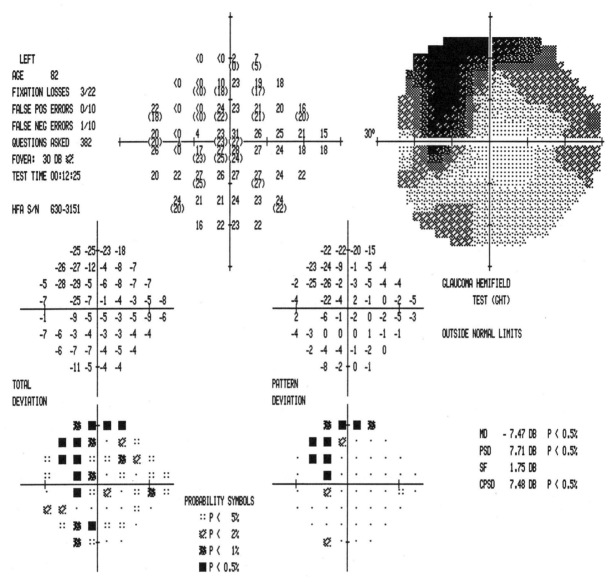

Figure 6-1. Optic nerve coloboma. Visual field from a patient with a small coloboma of the left optic nerve. There is a superior defect emanating from the blind spot that corresponds to an inferior defect in the optic nerve head. Because most optic nerve colobomas occur inferiorly, visual field defects are typically seen superiorly. Large colobomas may cause superior altitudinal defects.

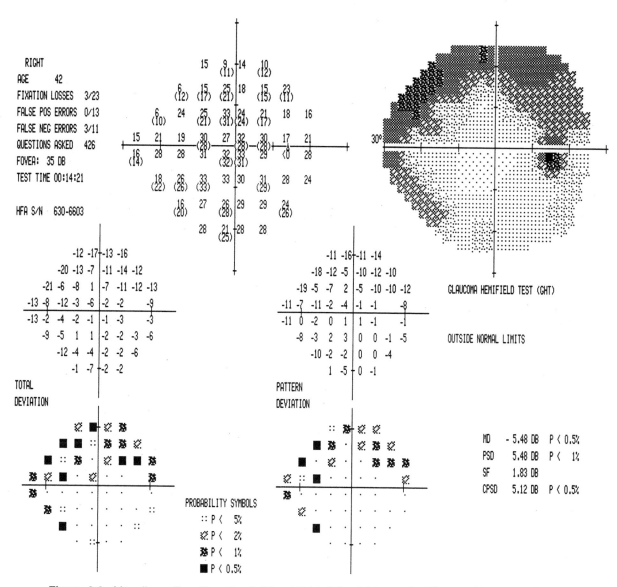

Figure 6-2. Megallopapilla with optic pit. Visual field of the right eye of a 42-year-old woman who was diagnosed with glaucoma. The field shows a superior arcuate defect which emanates from the blind spot and crosses the vertical and horizontal meridians. Ophthalmoscopy showed an optic disc that was 50% larger than that of the left eye and an optic pit inferotemporally, which corresponded to the nerve fiber layer defect superiorly. The defect was stable over time, lending support to the diagnosis of a congenital rather than an acquired optic nerve and visual field abnormality.

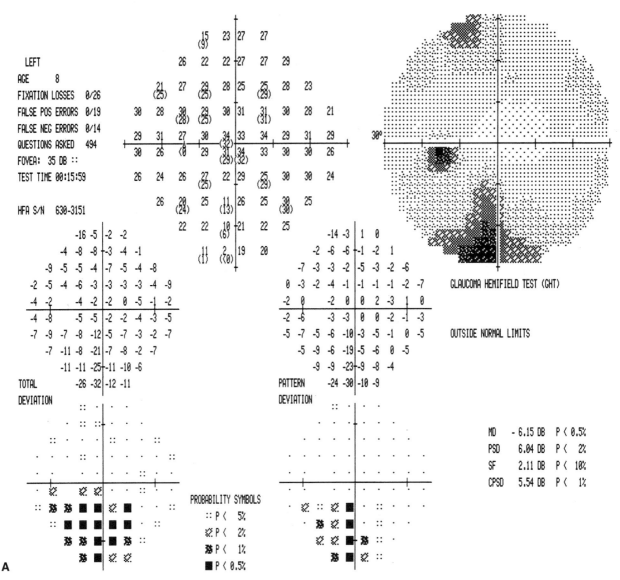

Figure 6-3. Congenitally anomalous nerves. Bilateral visual fields of a 9-year-old boy with anomalous optic nerves **(A)** left eye, **(B)** right eye. There are fairly similar inferior defects noted bilaterally. These defects cross the vertical meridian, allaying any concern of a chiasmal or posterior visual pathway lesion as the cause of the defects. A bilateral occipital lesion could conceivably cause this same visual field pattern, but this would be a most unusual presentation, and the fundus exam would be normal. (Courtesy of Norman J. Schatz, MD)

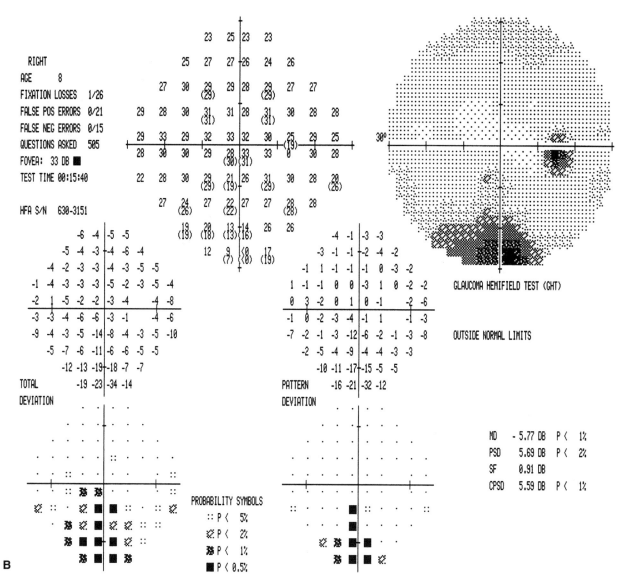

Figure 6-3. *Continued.*

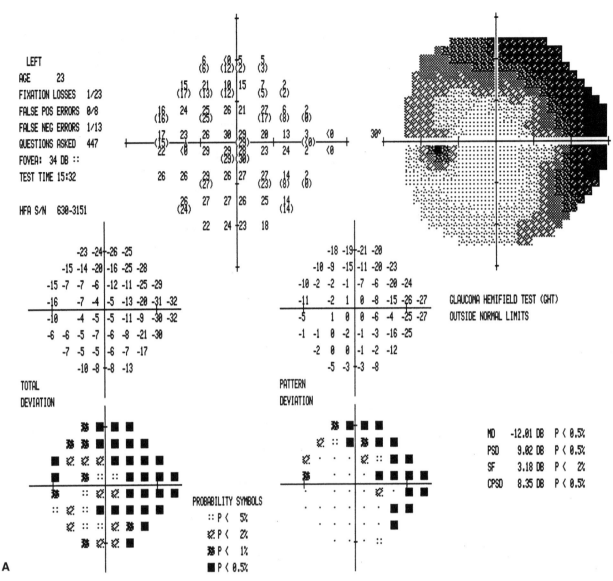

Figure 6-4. Tilted optic disc syndrome. Visual fields of a 22-year-old woman with high myopia and mildly elevated intraocular pressures **(A)** left eye, **(B)** right eye. The optic nerves appeared tilted and sloped temporally, and there was a temporal peripapillary crescent without focal cupping or pallor. The binasal visual field defects were contiguous across the horizontal meridian, which is highly atypical for glaucoma. However, if such a field defect changes over time, glaucoma must be considered as a contributing factor to the field loss, especially if accompanied by changes in the disc appearance.

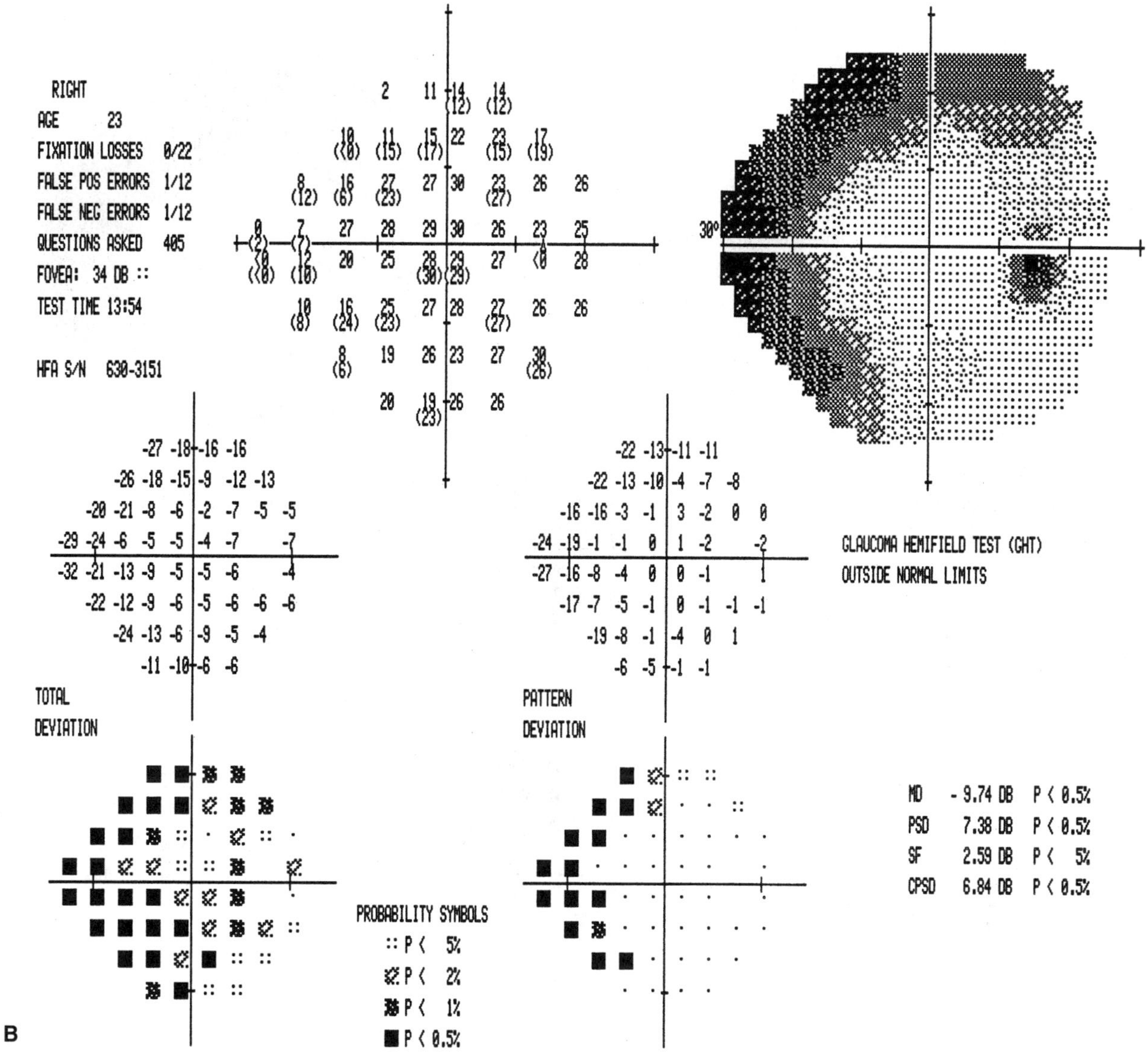
RIGHT
AGE 23
FIXATION LOSSES 0/22
FALSE POS ERRORS 1/12
FALSE NEG ERRORS 1/12
QUESTIONS ASKED 405
FOVEA: 34 DB ::
TEST TIME 13:54
HFA S/N 630-3151
30°
TOTAL DEVIATION
PATTERN DEVIATION
GLAUCOMA HEMIFIELD TEST (GHT)
OUTSIDE NORMAL LIMITS
MD - 9.74 DB P < 0.5%
PSD 7.38 DB P < 0.5%
SF 2.59 DB P < 5%
CPSD 6.84 DB P < 0.5%
PROBABILITY SYMBOLS
:: P < 5%
P < 2%
P < 1%
P < 0.5%
B

Figure 6-4. *Continued.*

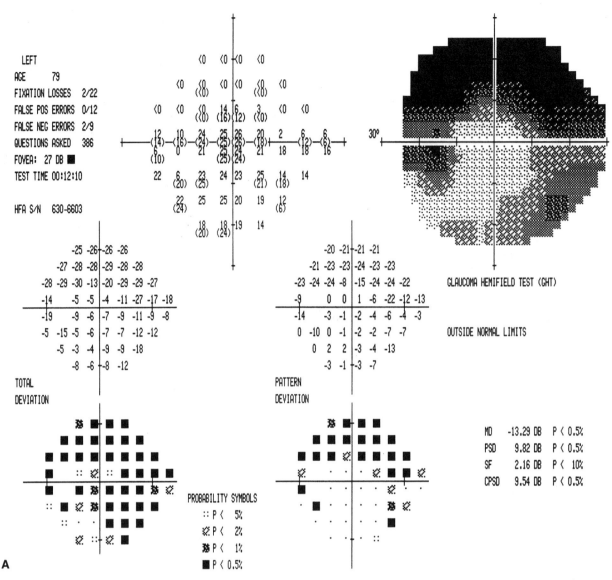

A

Figure 6-5. Tilted optic disc syndrome. Visual fields of a 79- year-old man with cataracts and elevated intraocular pressures **(A)** left eye, **(B)** right eye. Visual fields show diffuse depression OU (total deviation plot) with superimposed superior arcuate defects (pattern deviation plot). Optic nerves were tilted with peripapillary hypopigmentation, but no cupping.

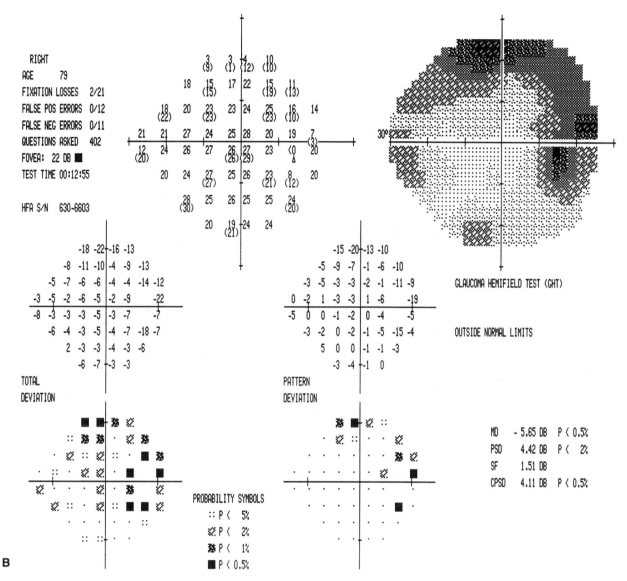

RIGHT
AGE   79
FIXATION LOSSES   2/21
FALSE POS ERRORS   0/12
FALSE NEG ERRORS   0/11
QUESTIONS ASKED   402
FOVEA: 22 DB ■
TEST TIME 00:12:55

HFA S/N   630-6603

```
              3   3  4  10
             (8) (1)(12)(10)
         18  15  17 22 15  11
            (15)       (19)(13)
         18  20  23 23 24 25 16  14
        (22)    (23)       (23)(10)
    21  21  27  24  25  28  20  19  7
                                  (3)
    12  24  26 '27  26  27  23 (0  20
   (20)           (26)(29)       A
        20  24  27 25 26 23 8  20
               (27)       (21)(12)
            28  25  26 25  25  24
           (30)                (20)
                20  19 24  24
                   (21)
```

```
        -18 -22 -16 -13
       -8 -11 -10 -4 -9 -13
     -5 -7 -6 -6 -4 -4 -14 -12
  -3 -5 -2 -6 -5 -2 -9    -22
   -8 -3 -3 -3 -5 -3 -7   -7
     -6 -4 -3 -5 -4 -7 -18 -7
        2 -3 -3 -4 -3 -6
          -6 -7 -3 -3
```

TOTAL
DEVIATION

```
        -15 -20 -13 -10
       -5 -9 -7 -1 -6 -10
     -3 -5 -3 -3 -2 -1 -11 -9
   0 -2  1 -3 -3  1 -6    -19
   -5  0  0 -1 -2  0 -4   -5
     -3 -2  0 -2 -1 -5 -15 -4
        5  0  0 -1 -1 -3
          -3 -4 -1  0
```

PATTERN
DEVIATION

GLAUCOMA HEMIFIELD TEST (GHT)

OUTSIDE NORMAL LIMITS

PROBABILITY SYMBOLS
:: P < 5%
▨ P < 2%
▩ P < 1%
■ P < 0.5%

MD   - 5.65 DB   P < 0.5%
PSD   4.42 DB   P < 2%
SF   1.51 DB
CPSD   4.11 DB   P < 0.5%

B

Figure 6-5. *Continued.*

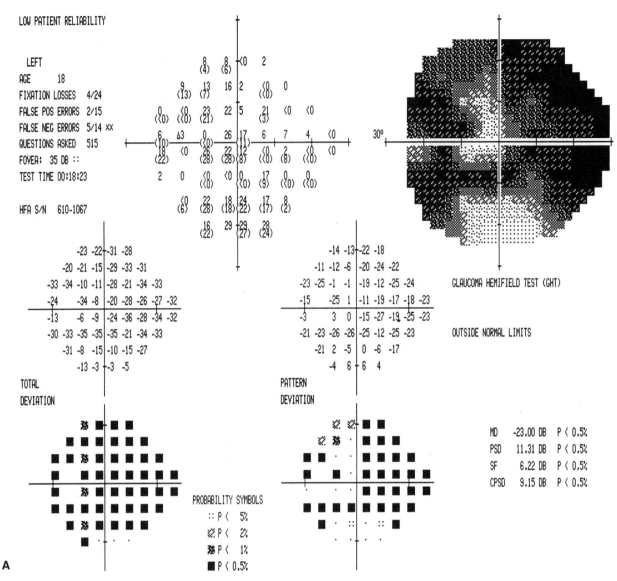

Figure 6-6. Optic disc drusen OU. Bilateral visual fields of an 18-year-old patient with optic disc drusen in both eyes. The right field **(B)** shows an inferior arcuate defect connected to a dense nasal defect that crosses the horizontal meridian as well as defect temporal to the blind spot. The left eye **(A)** shows similar, but more extensive, defects. Enlargement of the blind spot and arcuate scotomas (particularly inferonasal scotomas) are the most common defects seen with optic disc drusen,[2] although the majority of patients with optic disc drusen have no detectable field deficits. Only in rare cases do disc drusen result in progressive field loss.

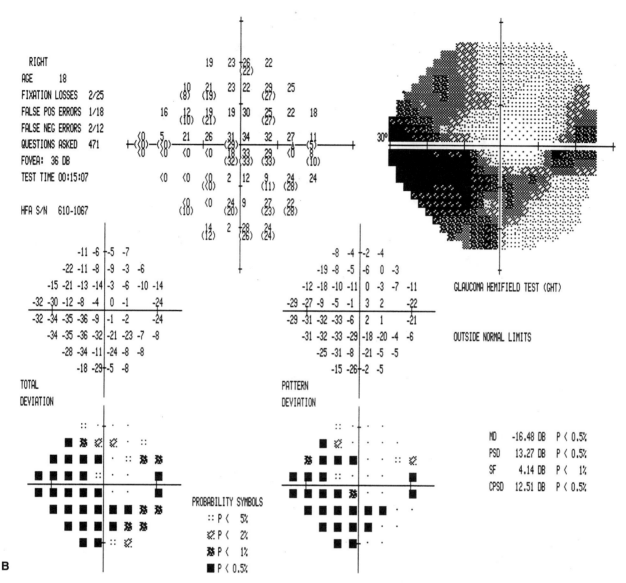

RIGHT

AGE   18

FIXATION LOSSES 2/25

FALSE POS ERRORS 1/18

FALSE NEG ERRORS 2/12

QUESTIONS ASKED 471

FOVEA: 36 DB

TEST TIME 00:15:07

HFA S/N 610-1067

GLAUCOMA HEMIFIELD TEST (GHT)

OUTSIDE NORMAL LIMITS

TOTAL
DEVIATION

PATTERN
DEVIATION

PROBABILITY SYMBOLS

:: P < 5%

▨ P < 2%

▧ P < 1%

■ P < 0.5%

MD	-16.48 DB	P < 0.5%
PSD	13.27 DB	P < 0.5%
SF	4.14 DB	P < 1%
CPSD	12.51 DB	P < 0.5%

B

Figure 6-6. *Continued.*

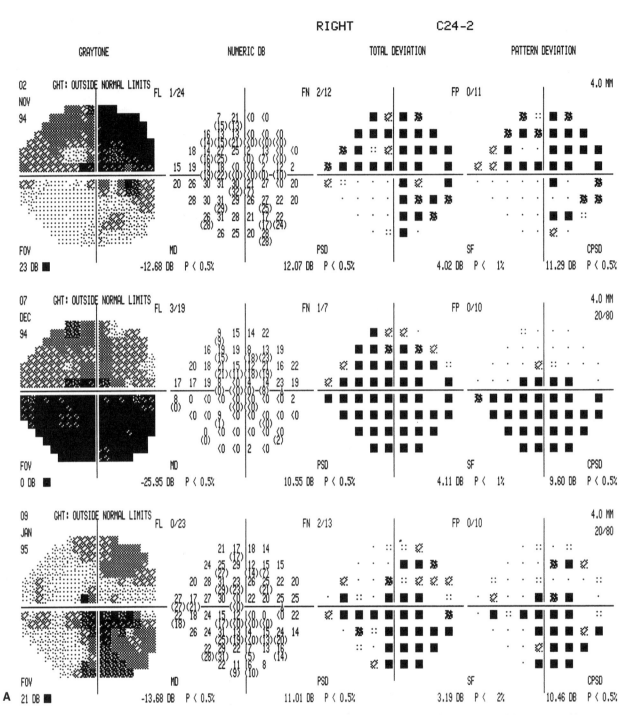

Figure 6-7. Optic neuritis Visual fields of the left **(A)** and right **(B)** eyes of a 35-year-old woman with multiple sclerosis and bilateral optic neuritis, which waxed and waned over a 3-month period. Serial visual fields show central, paracentral, and altitudinal field defects, demonstrating the wide variety of field defects that may occur in these patients.[3]

NAME

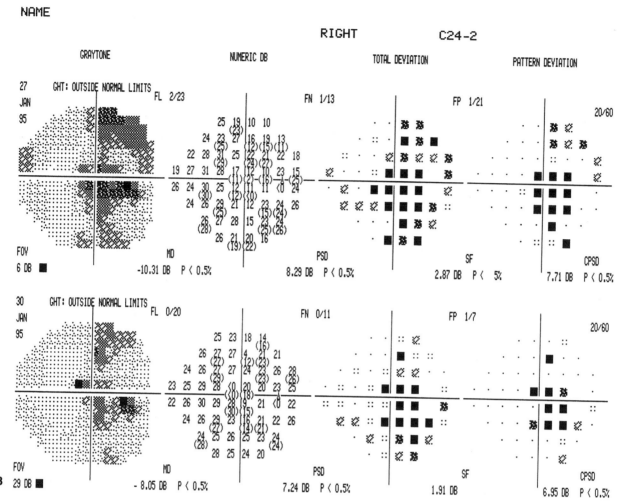

Figure 6-7. *Continued.*

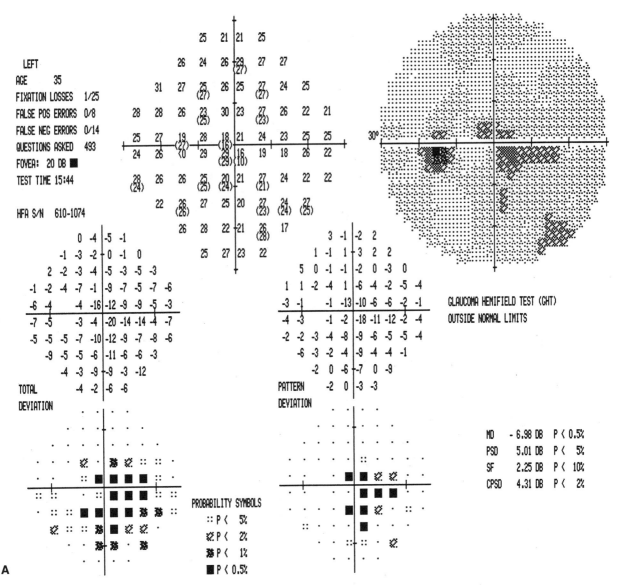

Figure 6-8. Bilateral optic neuritis. Visual fields of a 35-year- old man who presented with decreased visual acuity in both eyes and optic disc swelling secondary to demyelinating disease. Visual fields **(A)** left eye, **(B)** right eye, show bilateral central scotomas.

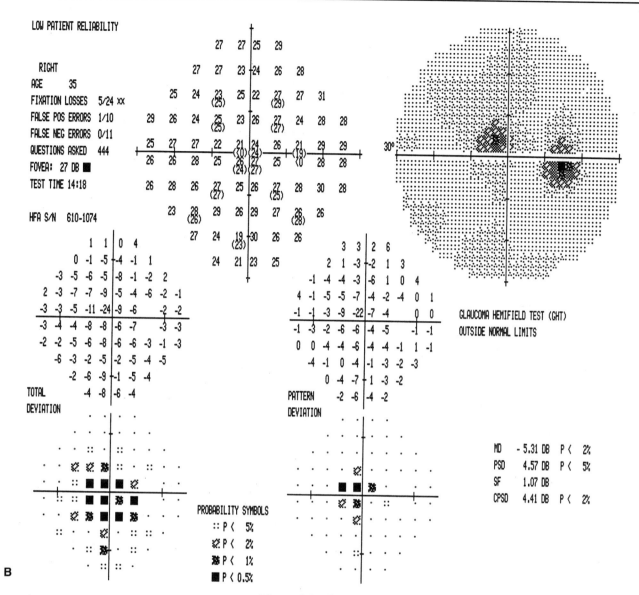

LOW PATIENT RELIABILITY

RIGHT

AGE 35
FIXATION LOSSES 5/24 xx
FALSE POS ERRORS 1/10
FALSE NEG ERRORS 0/11
QUESTIONS ASKED 444
FOVEA: 27 DB ■
TEST TIME 14:18

HFA S/N 610-1074

GLAUCOMA HEMIFIELD TEST (GHT)
OUTSIDE NORMAL LIMITS

PROBABILITY SYMBOLS
:: P < 5%
▨ P < 2%
▩ P < 1%
■ P < 0.5%

MD   - 5.31 DB   P < 2%
PSD   4.57 DB   P < 5%
SF   1.07 DB
CPSD 4.41 DB   P < 2%

B

Figure 6-8. *Continued.*

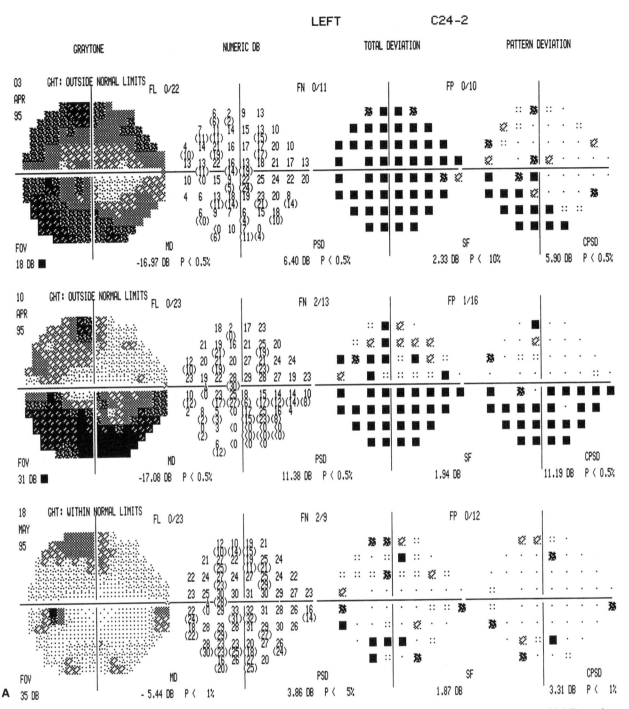

Figure 6-9. Bilateral optic neuritis. Serial visual fields of a 22-year-old man who presented with bilateral decreased visual acuity and optic nerve swelling **(A)** left eye, **(B)** right eye. Visual fields and vision gradually improved without treatment. MRI revealed enhancement of the intracanalicular portions of both optic nerves. Although atypical, this case was attributed to demyelinating disease. Visual fields were initially diffusely depressed, although the pattern deviation plot showed a predominance of inferior altitudinal changes.

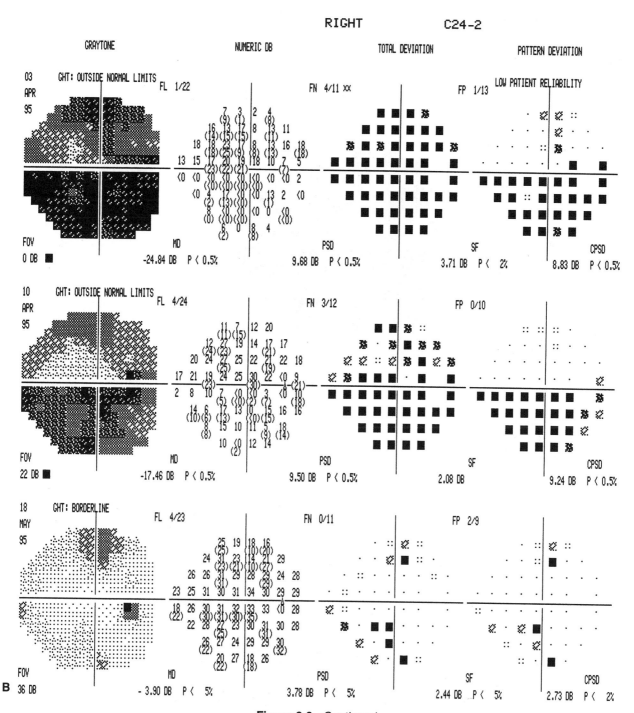

Figure 6-9. *Continued.*

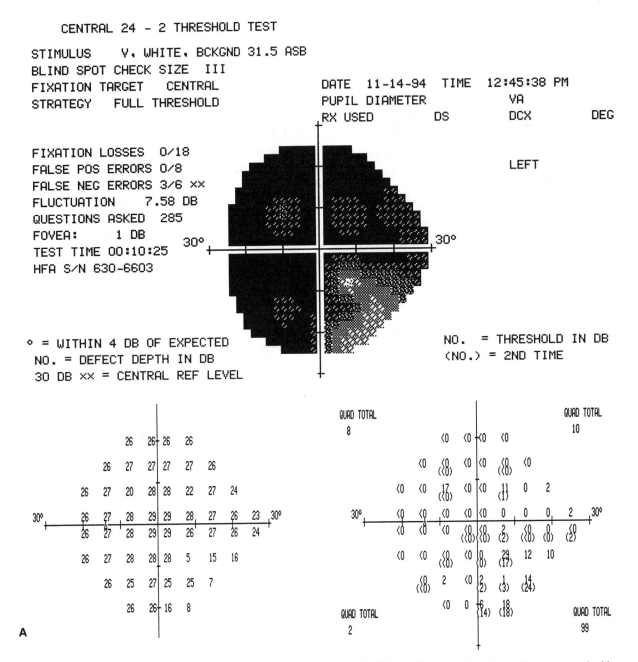

Figure 6-10. Severe retrobulbar optic neuritis. Visual fields of a 35-year-old patient who presented with a large central scotoma of the left eye with sudden profound visual acuity loss (2/200 "E") and an afferent pupillary defect. The optic nerve appeared normal, and the diagnosis of retrobulbar optic neuritis was made. The presenting field **(A)** was performed with a size V stimulus because the visual acuity was so poor. **(B)** The field and vision (20/300) improved somewhat, but the optic nerve turned pale over time and the patient was left with generalized depression of the central field, particularly in the cecocentral region.

CENTRAL 24 - 2 THRESHOLD TEST

STIMULUS III, WHITE, BCKGND 31.5 ASB BLIND SPOT CHECK SIZE III   FIXATION TARGET   CENTRAL   12-28-94
STRATEGY   FULL THRESHOLD   RX USED 000 DS   DCX   DEG   PUPIL DIAMETER   TIME 01:09:15 PM
                                                                                                                               VA

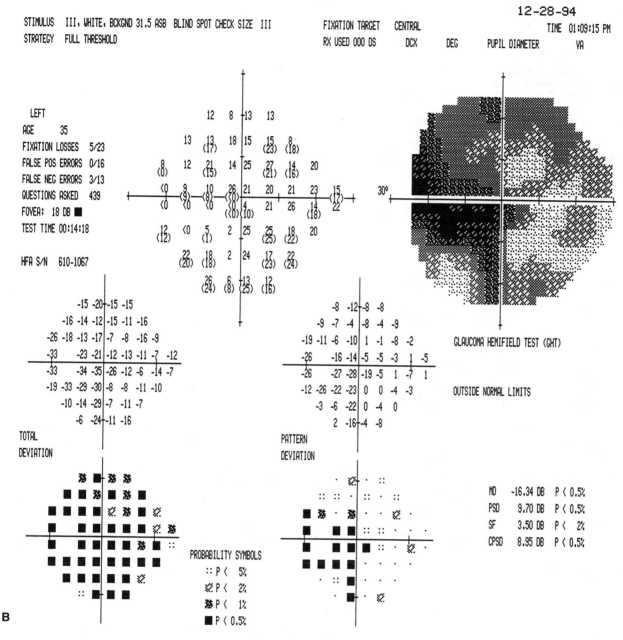

LEFT

AGE   35

FIXATION LOSSES   5/23

FALSE POS ERRORS   0/16

FALSE NEG ERRORS   3/13

QUESTIONS ASKED   439

FOVEA: 18 DB ■

TEST TIME 00:14:18

HFA S/N   610-1067

GLAUCOMA HEMIFIELD TEST (GHT)

OUTSIDE NORMAL LIMITS

TOTAL
DEVIATION

PATTERN
DEVIATION

MD   -16.34 DB   P < 0.5%

PSD   9.70 DB   P < 0.5%

SF   3.50 DB   P < 2%

CPSD   8.95 DB   P < 0.5%

PROBABILITY SYMBOLS

:: P < 5%

▨ P < 2%

▩ P < 1%

■ P < 0.5%

B

Figure 6-11. *Continued.*

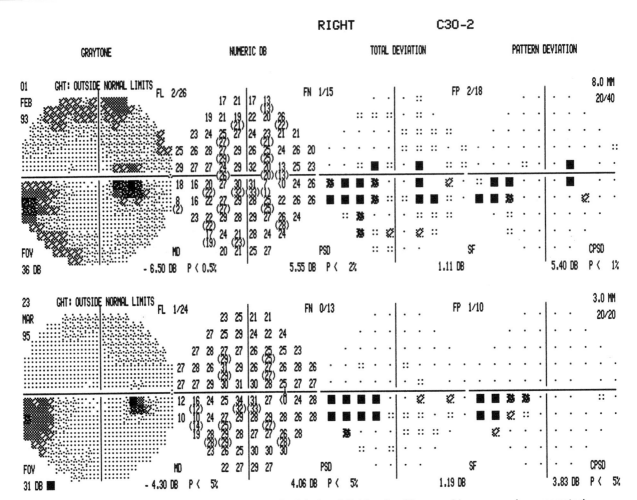

Figure 6-11. Vasculitic optic neuropathy. Serial visual fields of a 31-year-old woman who presented with distorted vision and optic disc swelling in the right eye. Work-up was consistent with systemic lupus erythomatosus. Initial field (*top*) shows an enlarged blind spot and an inferonasal step. The vision at presentation was 20/40. The disc edema resolved, as did the enlargement of the blind spot, but the inferonasal step persisted despite return of visual acuity to 20/20 (*bottom*). The foveal threshold actually worsened, which was contrary to the improvement in visual acuity.

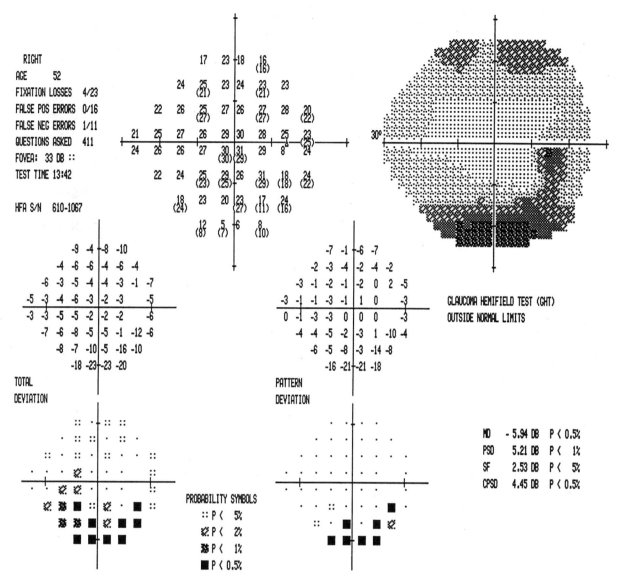

Figure 6-12. Optic atrophy secondary to nonarteritic ischemic optic neuropathy. Visual field of the right eye of a 52-year-old man with focal temporal optic nerve pallor presumed secondary to mild ischemic optic neuropathy. The field shows inferior arcuate defect emanating from the blind spot, seen best in the graytone printout and pattern deviation plot.

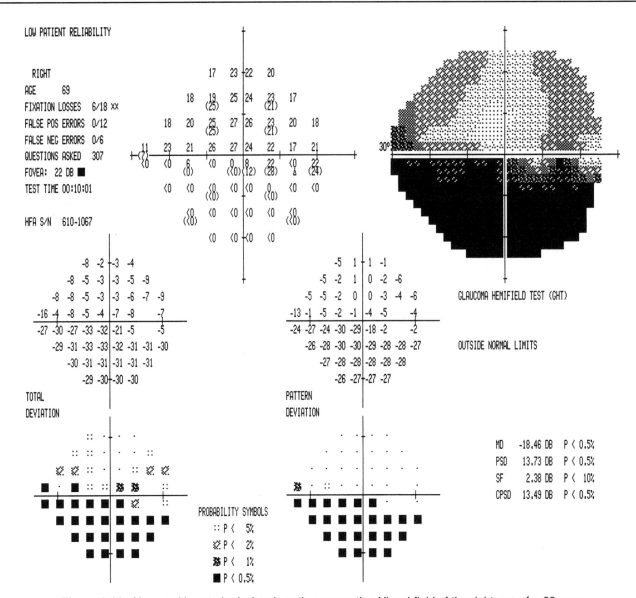

LOW PATIENT RELIABILITY

RIGHT

AGE   69

FIXATION LOSSES   6/18 xx

FALSE POS ERRORS   0/12

FALSE NEG ERRORS   0/6

QUESTIONS ASKED   307

FOVEA: 22 DB ■

TEST TIME 00:10:01

HFA S/N   610-1067

TOTAL
DEVIATION

PATTERN
DEVIATION

GLAUCOMA HEMIFIELD TEST (GHT)

OUTSIDE NORMAL LIMITS

PROBABILITY SYMBOLS

:: P < 5%

▨ P < 2%

▩ P < 1%

■ P < 0.5%

MD	-18.46 DB	P < 0.5%
PSD	13.73 DB	P < 0.5%
SF	2.38 DB	P < 10%
CPSD	13.49 DB	P < 0.5%

Figure 6-13. Nonarteritic anterior ischemic optic neuropathy. Visual field of the right eye of a 68-year-old patient who awakened with decreased vision in the right eye. An inferior altitudinal visual field defect was apparent on the visual field and ophthalmoscopy revealed optic nerve swelling consistent with anterior ischemic optic neuropathy. Although altitudinal defects are classically described in anterior ischemic optic neuropathy, central scotomas and nerve fiber layer defects can be seen as well.

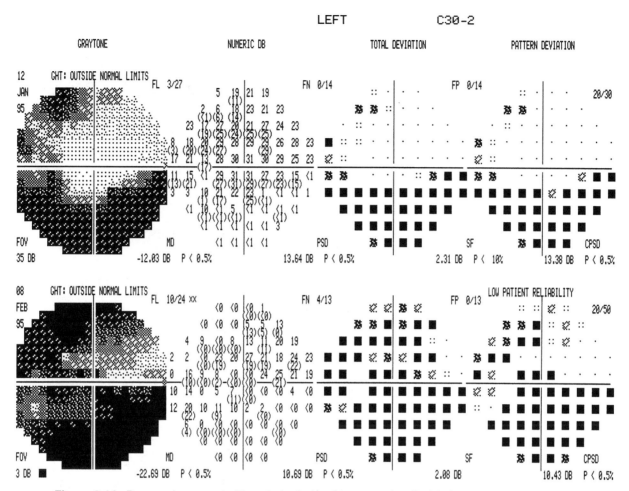

Figure 6-14. Progressive nonarteritic anterior ischemic neuropathy. Serial visual fields of the left eye of a 68-year-old man with anterior ischemic optic neuropathy that progressed over a 1-month period. The *top* visual field shows an incomplete inferior altitudinal defect and the *bottom* field (obtained several weeks later) shows worsening of the inferior altitudinal defect and a new superior arcuate and central defect. (Courtesy of Michael A. Schaffer, M.D.)

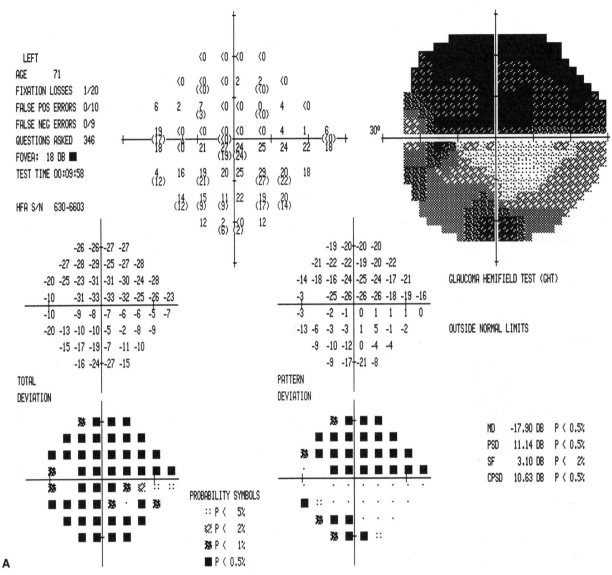

```
LEFT                              <0    <0  <0    <0
AGE      71
FIXATION LOSSES  1/20         <0   <8   <0  2     2   <0
                                   (<0)             (<0)
FALSE POS ERRORS  0/10     6    2    7   <0  <0   8   4   <0
                                   (3)              (<0)
FALSE NEG ERRORS  0/9     19  <0  <0  <8 <0   <0   4    1    6
QUESTIONS ASKED   346    (17) <0      (<0)                   (<0)
                          18  <0   21        22   24  25  24  22  18
FOVEA: 18 DB ■                            (19)(24)
                                                  29  20
TEST TIME 00:09:58         4  16  19  20  25  (27)(22)  18
                          (12)    (21)
                                                  19  20
HFA S/N   630-6603         14  15  11  22  (17)(14)
                          (12) (9) (9)
                              12   2  <0  12
                                  (6) (2)
```

```
TOTAL DEVIATION                        PATTERN DEVIATION

    -26 -26 -27 -27                      -19 -20 -20 -20
  -27 -28 -29 -25 -27 -28             -21 -22 -22 -19 -20 -22
-20 -25 -23 -31 -31 -30 -24 -28     -14 -18 -16 -24 -25 -24 -17 -21
-10    -31 -33 -33 -32 -25 -26 -23   -3    -25 -26 -26 -26 -18 -19 -16
-10     -9  -8 -7  -6  -6  -5  -7    -3    -2  -1  0   1   1   1   0
-20 -13 -10 -10 -5  -2  -8  -9      -13 -6  -3  -3  1   5  -1  -2
  -15 -17 -19 -7 -11 -10              -9 -10 -12 0  -4  -4
    -16 -24 -27 -15                      -9 -17 -21 -8
```

TOTAL
DEVIATION

PATTERN
DEVIATION

GLAUCOMA HEMIFIELD TEST (GHT)

OUTSIDE NORMAL LIMITS

```
PROBABILITY SYMBOLS
 ::  P < 5%
 ▨  P < 2%
 ▩  P < 1%
 ■  P < 0.5%
```

```
MD    -17.90 DB   P < 0.5%
PSD    11.14 DB   P < 0.5%
SF      3.10 DB   P <  2%
CPSD   10.63 DB   P < 0.5%
```

A

Figure 6-15. Bilateral nonarteritic anterior ischemic optic neuropathy. Visual fields of a 71-year-old man with hypertension and bilateral, sequential anterior ischemic optic neuropathy. Visual fields show an inferior altitudinal defect on the right **(B)** and superior altitudinal defect on the left **(A)**.

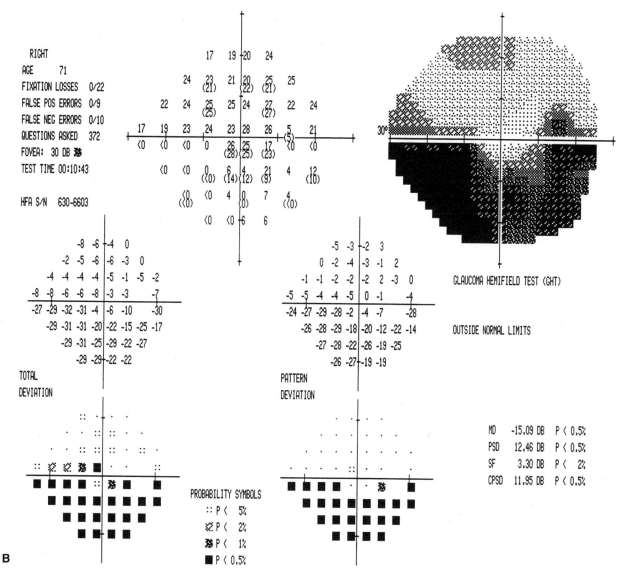

RIGHT

AGE   71

FIXATION LOSSES   0/22

FALSE POS ERRORS   0/9

FALSE NEG ERRORS   0/10

QUESTIONS ASKED   372

FOVEA: 30 DB

TEST TIME 00:10:43

HFA S/N   630-6603

TOTAL DEVIATION

PATTERN DEVIATION

GLAUCOMA HEMIFIELD TEST (GHT)

OUTSIDE NORMAL LIMITS

MD   -15.09 DB   P < 0.5%

PSD   12.46 DB   P < 0.5%

SF   3.30 DB   P < 2%

CPSD 11.95 DB   P < 0.5%

PROBABILITY SYMBOLS

:: P < 5%

P < 2%

P < 1%

■ P < 0.5%

B

Figure 6-15. *Continued.*

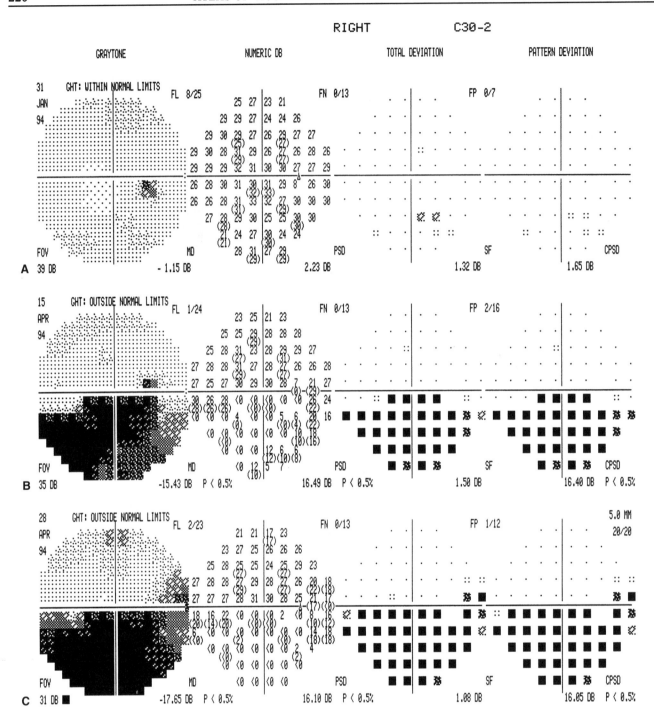

Figure 6-16. Progressive nonarteritic anterior ischemic optic neuropathy. Serial visual fields of the right eye of a 50-year-old man with hypertension and renal failure of 15 years duration. Field **A**, which is normal, was obtained at the time of presentation for visual complaints in the opposite eye from a superior altitudinal defect involving fixation causing finger counting vision. The visual field in the right eye developed an inferior altitudinal defect (Field **B**) which progressed (Field **C**). A superior altitudinal defect also developed (Field **D**), although the patient maintained excellent central visual acuity.

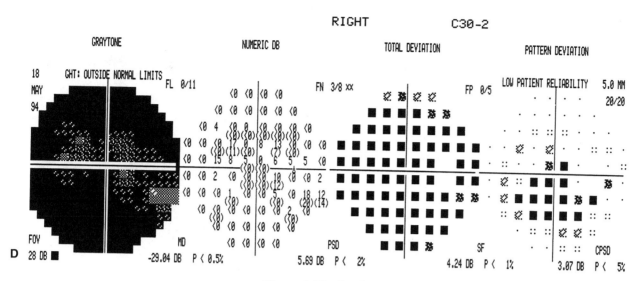

Figure 6-16. *Continued.*

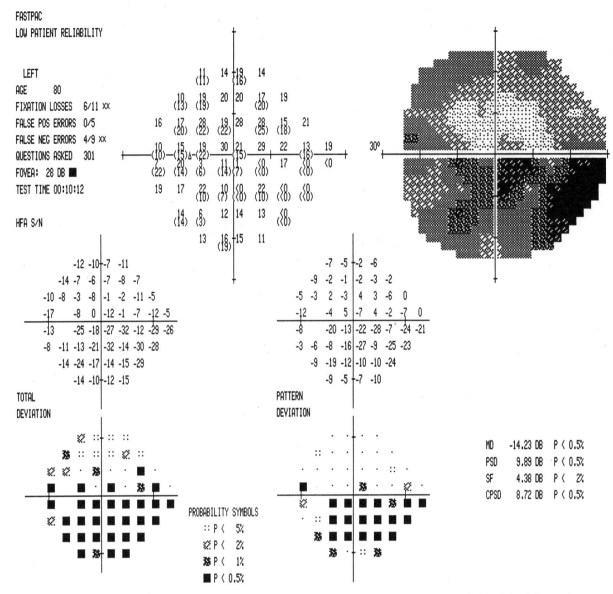

```
FASTPAC
LOW PATIENT RELIABILITY


   LEFT                              11   14  19   14
                                    (11)      (16)
AGE      80                       10   19   20  20   17   19
FIXATION LOSSES   6/11 xx        (13) (19)         (20)
FALSE POS ERRORS  0/5      16   17   28   19 28  28   15   21
FALSE NEG ERRORS  4/9 xx       (20) (22) (22)    (25) (18)
QUESTIONS ASKED   301      10  15  19   30  21   29   22  13   19
                          (10)(15)Δ(22)    (15)      (18)   (0)
FOVEA: 28 DB ■                 20   8    11       8   17   8
                          (22)(14)(6)  (14)(7)  (0)      (0)
TEST TIME 00:10:12      19   17  22   10  8   22   8   8
                               (10) (7)(8)  (10) (8)  (8)
HFA S/N                      14   6   12  14   13   8
                            (14) (3)              (0)
                                 13  16  15   11
                                    (19)
```

```
          -12 -10 -7 -11                         -7 -5 -2 -6
       -14 -7 -6 -7 -8 -7                      -9 -2 -1 -2 -3 -2
    -10 -8 -3 -8 -1 -2 -11 -5                 -5 -3  2 -3  4  3 -6  0
    -17    -8  0 -12 -1 -7 -12 -5             -12   -4  5 -7  4 -2 -7  0
    -13    -25 -18 -27 -32 -12 -29 -26        -8    -20 -13 -22 -28 -7 -24 -21
     -8 -11 -13 -21 -32 -14 -30 -28           -3 -6 -8 -16 -27 -9 -25 -23
       -14 -24 -17 -14 -15 -29                  -9 -19 -12 -10 -10 -24
          -14 -10 -12 -15                        -9 -5 -7 -10

TOTAL                                        PATTERN
DEVIATION                                    DEVIATION
```

```
                                                     MD    -14.23 DB   P < 0.5%
                                                     PSD     9.89 DB   P < 0.5%
                                                     SF      4.38 DB   P < 2%
                                                     CPSD    8.72 DB   P < 0.5%
```

PROBABILITY SYMBOLS

:: P < 5%

▨ P < 2%

▩ P < 1%

■ P < 0.5%

Figure 6-17. Ischemic optic neuropathy secondary to giant-cell arteritis. Visual field of the left eye in a patient with sudden onset of acute visual loss in the left eye associated with headaches, temporal scalp pain, 20/400 vision, afferent pupillary defect, swollen optic nerve, and elevated Westergren erythrocyte sedimentation rate. Visual field testing showed a central scotoma breaking out into an inferonasal step. A temporal artery biopsy was positive for giant cell arteritis. Although the visual acuity and visual field loss are often worse in arteritic than nonarteritic ischemic optic neuropathy, there are no field characteristics that distinguish between the two types.

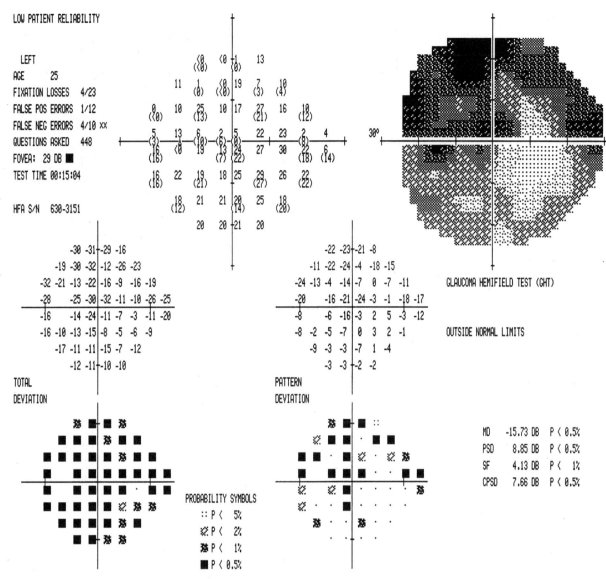

LOW PATIENT RELIABILITY

LEFT
AGE   25
FIXATION LOSSES   4/23
FALSE POS ERRORS 1/12
FALSE NEG ERRORS 4/10 xx
QUESTIONS ASKED   448
FOVEA: 29 DB ■
TEST TIME 00:15:04

HFA S/N   630-3151

GLAUCOMA HEMIFIELD TEST (GHT)

OUTSIDE NORMAL LIMITS

TOTAL DEVIATION

PATTERN DEVIATION

PROBABILITY SYMBOLS
:: P < 5%
▨ P < 2%
▩ P < 1%
■ P < 0.5%

MD	-15.73 DB	P < 0.5%
PSD	8.85 DB	P < 0.5%
SF	4.13 DB	P < 1%
CPSD	7.66 DB	P < 0.5%

Figure 6-18. Traumatic optic neuropathy. Visual field of the left eye of a 25-year-old man who sustained blunt head trauma. The field shows diffuse depression on the total deviation plot. A central scotoma and a superior altitudinal defect are noted on the graytone printout and pattern deviation plot. Nine weeks after the accident, when the field was obtained, the optic nerve was mildly pale nasally and moderately pale temporally, particularly in the region subserving the papillomacular bundle. Blunt head trauma and direct injury to the optic nerve may cause traumatic optic neuropathy, resulting in a variety of visual field defects.

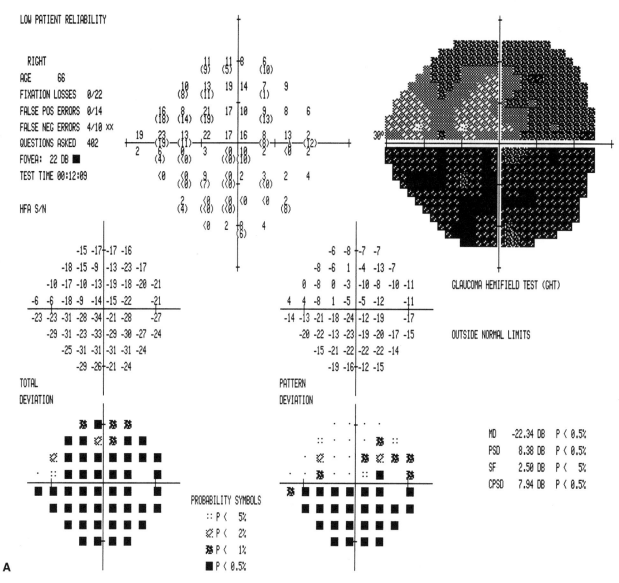

LOW PATIENT RELIABILITY

RIGHT

AGE   66

FIXATION LOSSES   0/22

FALSE POS ERRORS   0/14

FALSE NEG ERRORS   4/10 xx

QUESTIONS ASKED   402

FOVEA: 22 DB ■

TEST TIME 00:12:09

HFA S/N

GLAUCOMA HEMIFIELD TEST (GHT)

OUTSIDE NORMAL LIMITS

TOTAL
DEVIATION

PATTERN
DEVIATION

PROBABILITY SYMBOLS

:: P < 5%

⩔ P < 2%

▨ P < 1%

■ P < 0.5%

MD	-22.34 DB	P < 0.5%
PSD	8.38 DB	P < 0.5%
SF	2.50 DB	P < 5%
CPSD	7.94 DB	P < 0.5%

A

Figure 6-19. Infiltrative optic neuropathy. Visual fields of a 66-year-old-man with bilateral infiltrative optic neuropathy from lymphoproliferative disorder, diagnosed by MRI and ceresospinal spinal fluid cytology **(A)** left eye, **(B)** right eye. Visual acuity was 20/60 in the right eye and 20/40 in the left. Although diffuse depression is noted on the total deviation plot of both eyes, the pattern deviation plots show denser field loss inferiorly than superiorly. Field defects vary widely in patients with infiltrative optic neuropathy secondary to lymphoproliferative disease. This case is unusual in that there is simulating of the bilateral involvement. (Courtesy of Norman J. Schatz, M.D.)

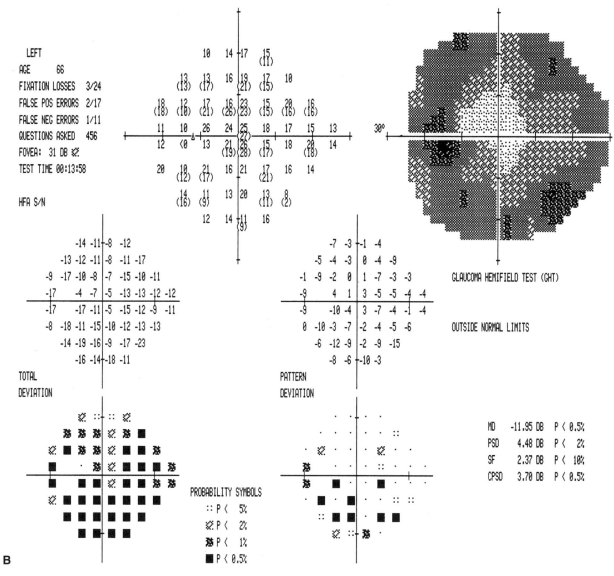

Figure 6-19. *Continued.*

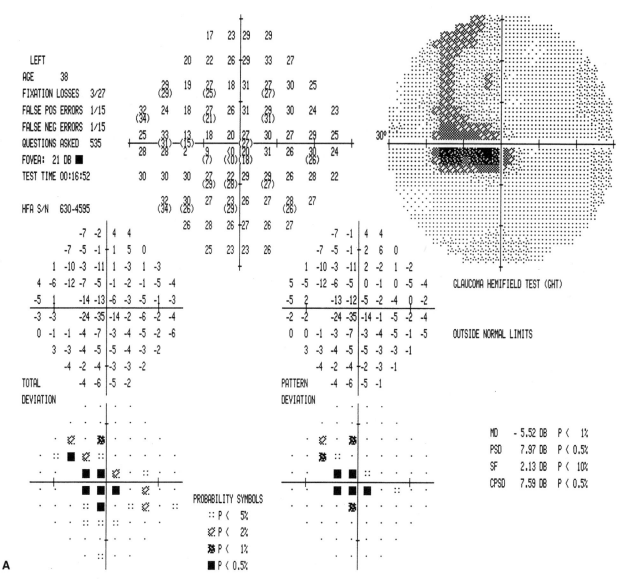

Figure 6-20. Leber's hereditary optic neuropathy. Visual fields of a 38-year-old woman who presented with gradual "hazy" vision over a 1- month period **(A)** left eye, **(B)** right eye. Visual fields showed bilateral cecocentral scotomas with visual acuities of 20/100 in the right eye and 20/40 in the left. After an extensive work-up, testing of mitochondrial DNA revealed a point mutation at position 11778, consistent with Leber's hereditary optic neuropathy. Patients with Leber's optic neuropathy typically present with central or cecocentral scotomas.[4] (Courtesy of Norman J. Schatz, M.D.)

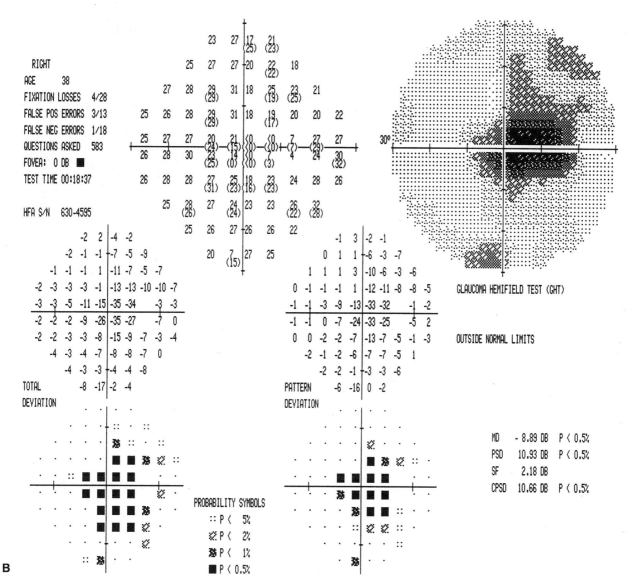

Figure 6-20. *Continued.*

B

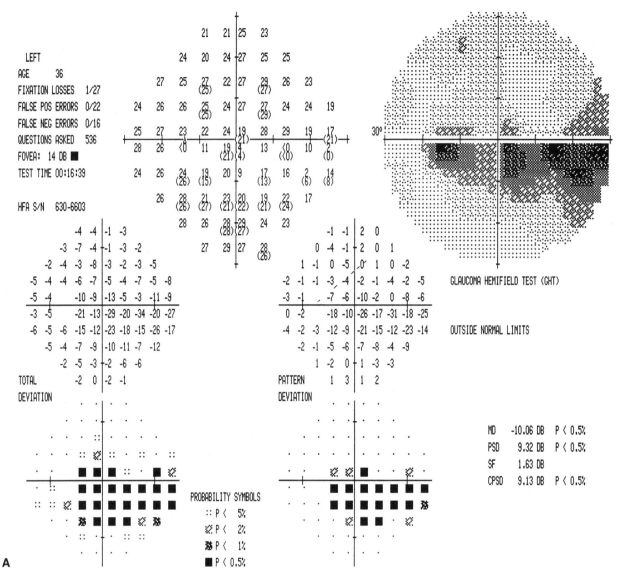

Figure 6-21. Advanced Leber's hereditary optic neuropathy. Visual fields of a 36-year-old woman with vision loss OU. The visual acuities were 8/200 "E" in the right eye and 20/80 in the left eye. Color vision was poor, and an afferent pupillary defect was present in the right eye. The visual field shows cecocentral scotomas and inferonasal defects in both eyes. Scotomas from Leber's can break out into the peripheral field later in the disease,[4] as in this case, which was confirmed via mitochondrial DNA analysis.

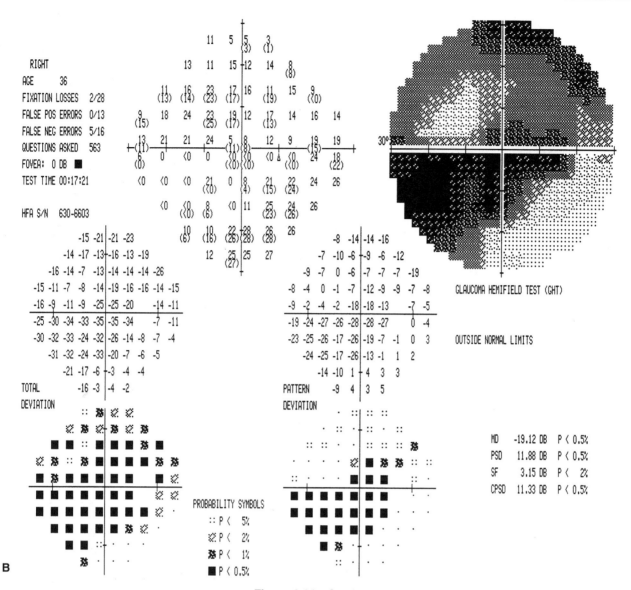

Figure 6-21. *Continued.*

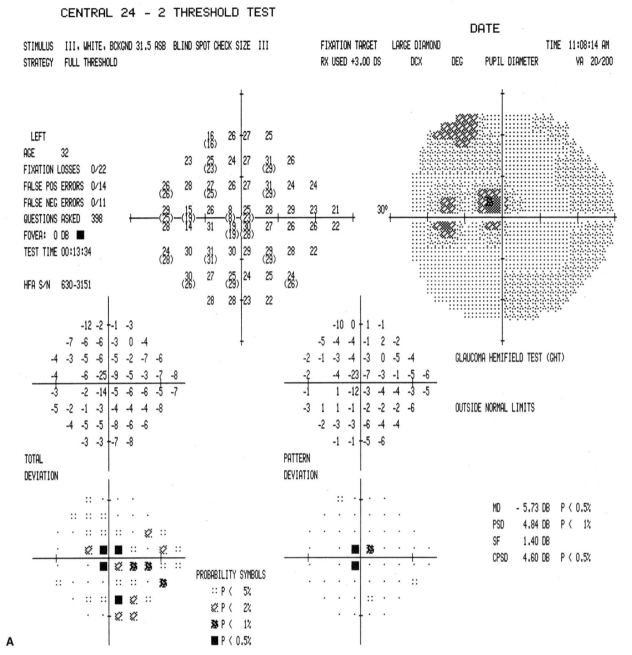

Figure 6-22. Dominant optic atrophy. Visual fields of a 32-year-old man with bilateral decreased vision (20/200 OU) since childhood and symmetric temporal optic nerve pallor of both eyes **(A)** left eye, **(B)** right eye. Diagnosis of dominant (Kjer's) optic atrophy was made. Atrophy of the temporal portion of the optic nerves, which subserves is seen with the papillomacular bundles, central scotomas due to deviant optic atrophy. Cecocentral and paracentral scotomas have also been described in this condition, as well as tritanopic (blue-yellow axis) color defects.[5] Note that the fixation target was changed to the large diamond because of poor fixation centrally from the scotoma. (Courtesy of David Greenfield, M.D.)

CENTRAL 24 - 2 THRESHOLD TEST

STIMULUS III, WHITE, BCKGND 31.5 ASB BLIND SPOT CHECK SIZE III   FIXATION TARGET   LARGE DIAMOND   ID   TIME 10:51:13 AM
STRATEGY   FULL THRESHOLD   RX USED +3.00 DS   DCX   DEG   PUPIL DIAMETER   VA 20/200

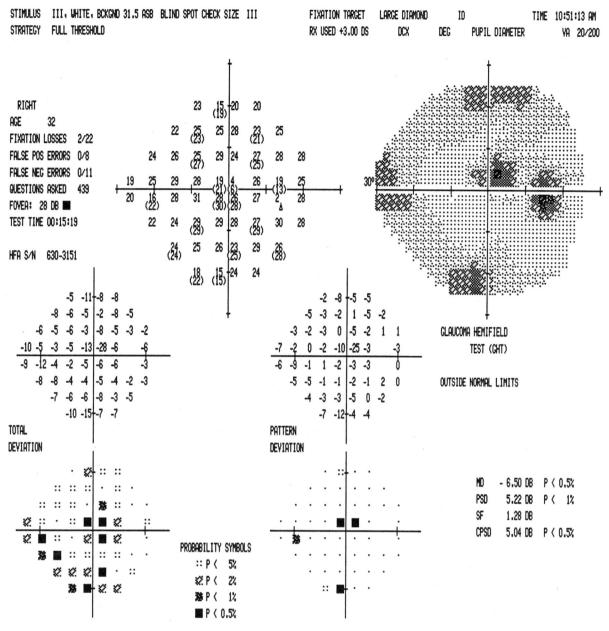

RIGHT

AGE   32
FIXATION LOSSES   2/22
FALSE POS ERRORS 0/8
FALSE NEG ERRORS 0/11
QUESTIONS ASKED   439
FOVEA: 28 DB ■
TEST TIME 00:15:19

HFA S/N   630-3151

TOTAL
DEVIATION

PATTERN
DEVIATION

GLAUCOMA HEMIFIELD

TEST (GHT)

OUTSIDE NORMAL LIMITS

PROBABILITY SYMBOLS
:: P < 5%
▨ P < 2%
▦ P < 1%
■ P < 0.5%

MD   - 6.50 DB   P < 0.5%
PSD   5.22 DB   P < 1%
SF   1.28 DB
CPSD 5.04 DB   P < 0.5%

B

Figure 6-22. *Continued.*

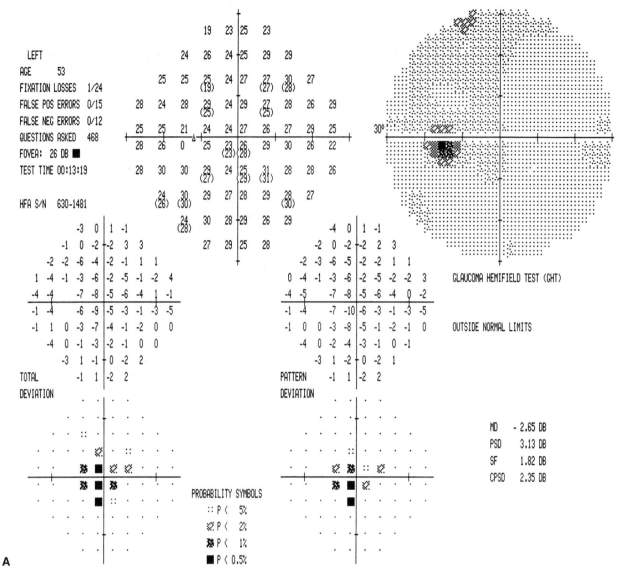

Figure 6-23. Nutritional/toxic optic neuropathy. Visual fields of a 53-year-old man who presented with slowly progressive visual loss to 20/100 OU, **(A)** left eye, **(B)** right eye. Bilateral cecocentral scotomas were found, as well as dyschromatopsia and temporal optic nerve pallor. The patient had a history of poor dietary intake, heavy alcohol use, and moderate smoking. Visual acuities slowly improved to the 20/50 level OU 2 years after vitamin supplementation was introduced. Nutritional optic neuropathy may present as either slowly progressive or acute bilateral visual loss associated with central or cecocentral scotomas.[6] (Courtesy of John McSoley, O.D.)

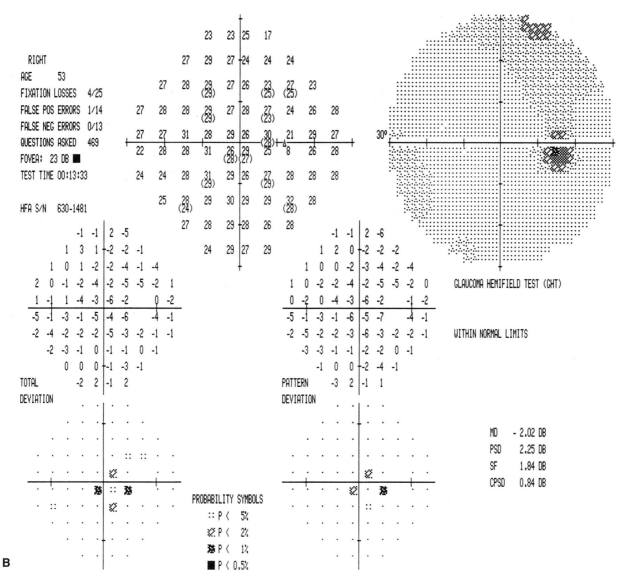

RIGHT

AGE   53
FIXATION LOSSES   4/25
FALSE POS ERRORS 1/14
FALSE NEG ERRORS 0/13
QUESTIONS ASKED   469
FOVEA: 23 DB ■
TEST TIME 00:13:33

HFA S/N   630-1481

GLAUCOMA HEMIFIELD TEST (GHT)

WITHIN NORMAL LIMITS

TOTAL DEVIATION

PATTERN DEVIATION

MD   - 2.02 DB
PSD   2.25 DB
SF   1.84 DB
CPSD   0.84 DB

PROBABILITY SYMBOLS
:: P < 5%
▨ P < 2%
▩ P < 1%
■ P < 0.5%

B

Figure 6-23. *Continued.*

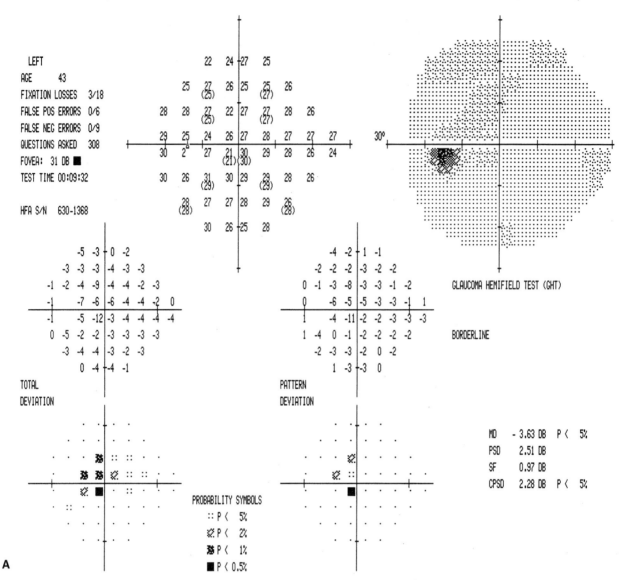

HFA S/N   630-1368

Figure 6-24. Nutritional/toxic optic neuropathy. Bilateral visual fields of a 43-year-old man who presented with a 3- to 6-month history of progressive visual loss OU **(A)** left eye, **(B)** right eye. Dyschromatopsia, mild temporal pallor, and mild cecocentral visual field defects were noted on examination. A history of heavy tobacco and alcohol use was elicited, as well as poor dietary intake. Vitamin B_{12} and folate levels were normal. Visual acuity and fields improved over a 3-month period following cessation of alcohol consumption and nutritional therapy.

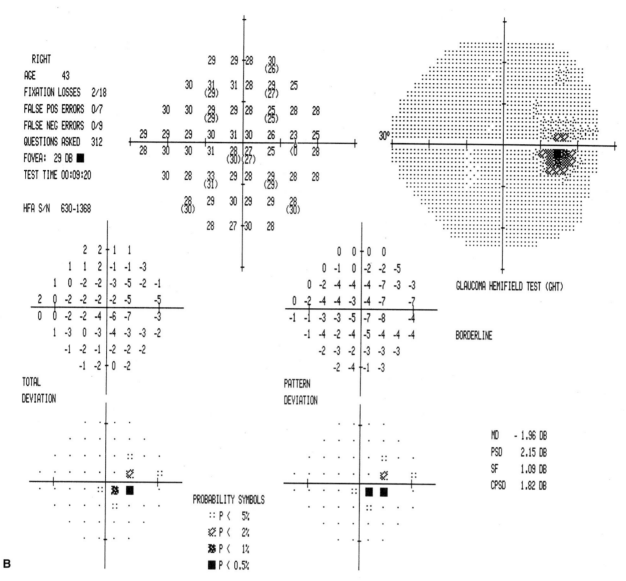

```
RIGHT                          29   29  28   30
                                              (26)
AGE      43
FIXATION LOSSES  2/18     30    31   31  28   29   25
                               (29)           (27)
FALSE POS ERRORS  0/7      30   30   29   29  28  25   28   28
                                    (28)          (25)
FALSE NEG ERRORS  0/9
QUESTIONS ASKED   312   29  29  29   30   31  30   26   23   25
                        28  30  30   31   28  27   25   (0   28
FOVEA:  29 DB ■                          (30)(27)
TEST TIME 00:09:20        30   28   33   29  28   29   28   28
                                    (31)          (29)
HFA S/N   630-1368             28   29   30  29   29   28
                               (30)                  (30)

                                28   27  30   28
```

```
          2   2   1   1                          0   0   0   0
      1   1   2  -1  -1  -3                   0  -1   0  -2  -2  -5
    1  0  -2  -2  -3  -5  -2  -1            0  -2  -4  -4  -4  -7  -3  -3
  2  0  -2  -2  -2  -2  -5       -5       0  -2  -4  -4  -3  -4  -7       -7
  0  0  -2  -2  -4  -6  -7       -3      -1 -1  -3  -3  -5  -7  -8       -4
    1 -3   0  -3  -4  -3  -3  -2           -1 -4  -2  -4  -5  -4  -4  -4
     -1  -2  -1  -2  -2  -2                   -2  -3  -2  -3  -3  -3
         -1  -2   0  -2                           -2  -4  -1  -3

TOTAL                                    PATTERN
DEVIATION                                DEVIATION
```

GLAUCOMA HEMIFIELD TEST (GHT)

BORDERLINE

PROBABILITY SYMBOLS
:: P < 5%
▨ P < 2%
▩ P < 1%
■ P < 0.5%

MD   - 1.96 DB
PSD   2.15 DB
SF   1.09 DB
CPSD   1.82 DB

B

Figure 6-24. *Continued.*

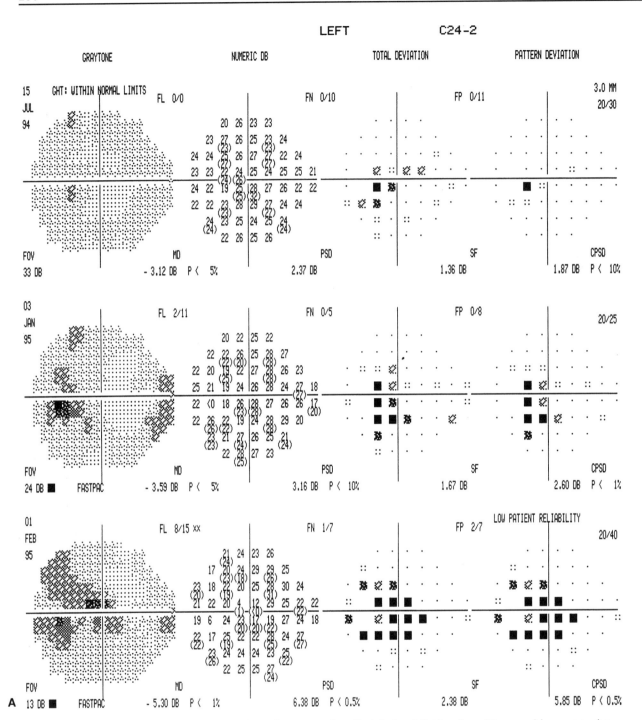

Figure 6-25. Drug-induced toxic optic neuropathy. Serial visual fields of an 81-year-old woman who developed central scotomas (middle fields) 3 months after starting therapy with isoniazid and ethambutol for *Mycobacterium intracellulare infection of the lungs,* **(A)** left eye, **(B)** right eye. Drug-induced retrobulbar optic neuropathy was diagnosed, and both possible offending agents were discontinued. However, the vision and fields continued to worsen. Both of these antituberculous drugs typically produce bilateral central scotomas and ethambutol may also produce peripheral constriction[7] or even bitemporal hemianopia, thought due to chiasmal involvement.[8] Drug withdrawal may or may not result in visual field improvement.

RIGHT   C24-2

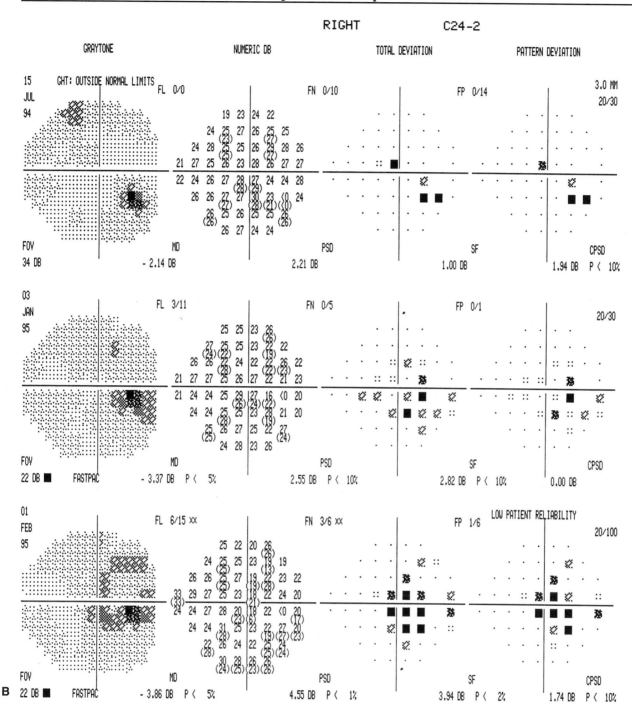

Figure 6-25. *Continued.*

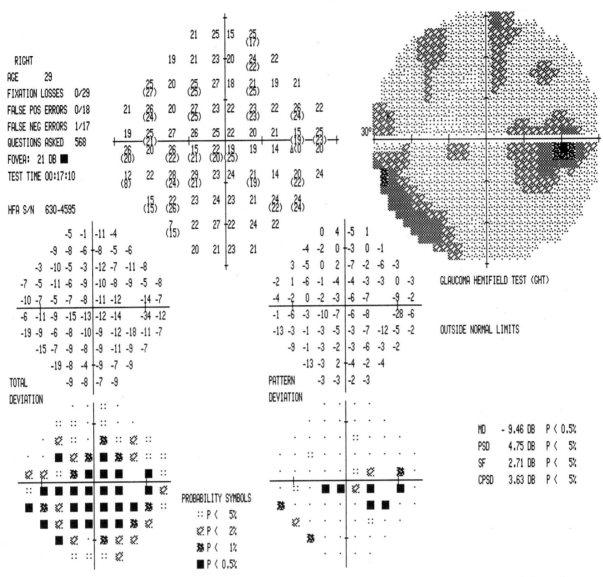

```
                              21  25 |15   25
                                          (17)
   RIGHT                    19  21  23 +20  24   22
                                            (22)
AGE      29                       25      25         21
                               20     27 |18        19  21
FIXATION LOSSES   0/29        (27)    (25)         (25)
                          21   26   20  27 |23  22  23   22   26   22
FALSE POS ERRORS  0/18        (24)      (25)       (23)      (24)
FALSE NEG ERRORS  1/17    19  25   27  26 |25  22  20  21   15   25
                              (21)                          (19) (23)
QUESTIONS ASKED   568     +   26   20  26 |15  22  19  19   14  10  20+
                              (20)    (22)(21)(20)(25)          (20)
FOVEA:  21 DB ■
                              12   22  28 |29  23 |24  21   14   20   24
TEST TIME 00:17:10            (8)      (24)(21)     (19)    (22)

HFA S/N  630-4595             15   22   23  24 |23  21  24   24
                             (15) (26)                  (22) (24)
                                                7
                      -5  -1 |-11 -4          (15)   22  27 +22  24   22            0  4 |-5  1
                -9  -8  -6 +-8  -5  -6                20  21 |23  21            -4  -2  0 +-3  0  -1
            -3  -10  -5  -3 |-12  -7  -11  -8                +                3  -5  0  2 |-7  -2  -6  -3
       -7  -5  -11  -6  -9 |-10  -8  -9  -5  -8                          -2   1  -6  -1  -4 |-4  -3  -3  0  -3
      -10  -7  -5  -7  -8 |-11 -12      -14  -7                          -4  -2  0  -2  -3 |-6  -7      -9  -2     GLAUCOMA HEMIFIELD TEST (GHT)
       -6  -11  -9  -15 -13 |-12 -14      -34 -12                        -1  -6  -3  -10 -7 |-6  -8      -28 -6
      -19  -9  -6  -8  -10 |-9  -12 -18 -11  -7                         -13  -3  -1  -3  -5 |-3  -7  -12 -5  -2    OUTSIDE NORMAL LIMITS
          -15  -7  -9  -8 |-9  -11  -9  -7                                 -9  -1  -3  -2 |-3  -6  -3  -2
             -19  -8  -4 +-9  -7  -9                                         -13 -3   2 +-4  -2  -4
TOTAL          -9  -8 |-7  -9                                      PATTERN       -3  -3 |-2  -3
DEVIATION                                                         DEVIATION

                 .   . |::   .                                                       .   . |
              ::  ::  . +::   .   .                                                 .   . |                      MD   - 9.46 DB  P < 0.5%
           .  ▨  ::  . |▩  ::  ▨  ::                                       .   . |::                             PSD    4.75 DB  P <  5%
          .  ▨  ::  ■  ▨ ▩ |■  ▨  ▨  ::  ::                              ::  .                                   SF     2.71 DB  P <  5%
       ▨  ▨  ::  ▩  ■ |■  ■  ■      ■                              .   .     |      ::  ▨       ▩               CPSD    3.63 DB  P <  5%
       ::  ■  ■  ■  ■ |■  ■  ■  ■  ▨                         .   .  ::  . |■  ■  ▨   ■  ■
          ■  ▩  ▨  ■  ■ |■  ■  ■  ▩  ::           PROBABILITY SYMBOLS    ▩  .   . | .      ■  ■
             ■  ▨  ▨  ■ |■  ■  ▩  ▨              :: P <  5%                  ▨  .   . | .  ::
                ■  ▨  . +■  ▨  ▨                 ▨ P <  2%                      ▩  .   . | .  .
                   ::  ::  :: ▨                  ▩ P <  1%                         .   . | .
                                                ■ P < 0.5%
```

Figure 6-26. Compressive optic neuropathy. Visual field of the right eye of a patient with a right optic nerve sheath meningioma. The foveal threshold is markedly reduced although the visual acuity was 20/30. A large central defect is seen on the total deviation plot. On the pattern deviation plot, the defect is noted to be worse in the area of the blind spot and in the paracentral region.

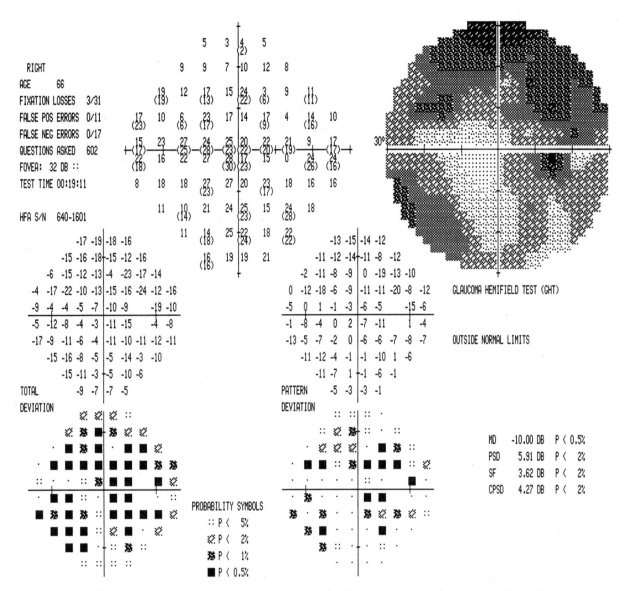

RIGHT

AGE 66
FIXATION LOSSES 3/31
FALSE POS ERRORS 0/11
FALSE NEG ERRORS 0/17
QUESTIONS ASKED 602
FOVEA: 32 DB ::
TEST TIME 00:19:11

HFA S/N 640-1601

```
                    5   3  4   5
                              (2)
                 9   9   7  10  12   8
            19  12  17  15  24  3   9   11
           (19)    (13)    (22)(8)     (11)
       17  10  6   23  17  14  17  4   14  10
      (23)    (6) (17)        (9)    (16)
    15  23  27  24  25  20  22  21  9   17
   (17)    (22)(28)(23)(22)(20)(19)    (17)
    22  16  22  27  30 17  15  0   24  24
   (18)                (30)(23)    (26)(16)
    8   18  18  27  27  20  23  18  16  16
           (23)        (17)
    11  10  21  24  25  15  24  18
       (14)        (23)    (28)
    11  14  25  22  18  22
       (18)    (24)    (22)
           16  19  19  21
          (16)
```

TOTAL DEVIATION

```
 -17 -19 -18 -16
 -15 -16 -18 -15 -12 -16
  -6 -15 -12 -13 -4 -23 -17 -14
  -4 -17 -22 -10 -13 -15 -16 -24 -12 -16
  -9 -4  -4  -5  -7 -10 -9     -19 -10
  -5 -12 -8  -4  -3 -11 -15    -4  -8
 -17 -9 -11  -6  -4 -11 -10 -11 -12 -11
 -15 -16 -8  -5 -5 -14 -3 -10
 -15 -11 -3 -5 -10 -6
 -9 -7 -7 -5
```

PATTERN DEVIATION

```
                   -13 -15 -14 -12
               -11 -12 -14 -11 -8 -12
            -2 -11 -8  -9  0 -19 -13 -10
     0 -12 -18 -6  -9 -11 -11 -20 -8 -12
    -5  0   1  -1  -3 -6 -5     -15 -6
    -1 -8  -4   0   2 -7 -11    1   -4
   -13 -5  -7  -2   0 -6 -6 -7 -8 -7
       -11 -12 -4  -1 -1 -10 1 -6
       -11 -7   1 -1 -6 -1
       -5 -3 -3 -1
```

PROBABILITY SYMBOLS

:: P < 5%
⌘ P < 2%
⅗ P < 1%
■ P < 0.5%

GLAUCOMA HEMIFIELD TEST (GHT)

OUTSIDE NORMAL LIMITS

MD   -10.00 DB   P < 0.5%
PSD   5.91 DB   P < 2%
SF   3.62 DB   P < 2%
CPSD   4.27 DB   P < 2%

Figure 6-27. Compressive optic neuropathy. Visual field of the right eye of a patient with a right optic nerve sheath meningioma. The central field and acuity are relatively spared, but there are extensive areas of peripheral field involvement. Compressive lesions of the optic nerve may cause almost any pattern of visual field defect although prolonged preservation of central acuity is rare.[9]

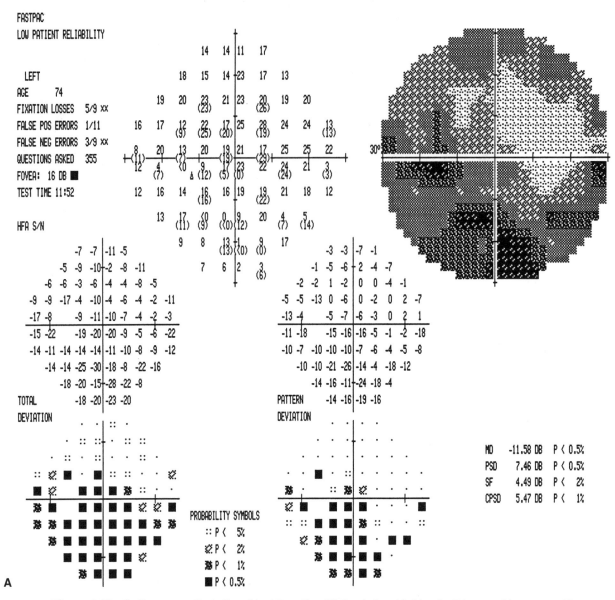

Figure 6-28. Optic neuropathy in thyroid orbitopathy. Bilateral visual fields of a 74-year-old woman with compressive optic neuropathy from thyroid eye disease. Visual fields show diffuse depression but worse loss inferiorly in the left eye **(A)** and diffuse depression with worse loss nasally in the right eye **(B)**.

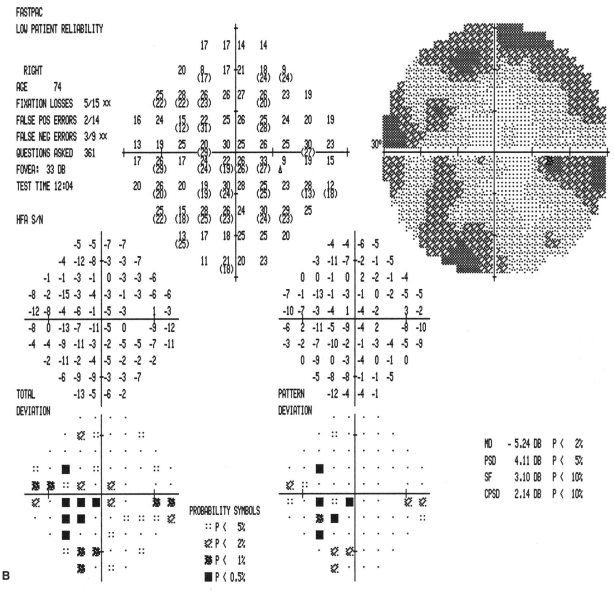

```
FASTPAC
LOW PATIENT RELIABILITY

                                      17   17 |14   14

   RIGHT                          20   8    17 |21   18    9
                                      (17)           (24) (24)
AGE        74
FIXATION LOSSES   5/15 xx            25   28   26   26 27   26   23   19
                                     (22) (22) (23)          (20)
FALSE POS ERRORS  2/14         16  24   15   22   25 |26   25   24   20   19
                                        (12) (31)          (28)
FALSE NEG ERRORS  3/9 xx
                               13  19   25   20   30 |25   26   25   30   23
QUESTIONS ASKED   361                        (23)               (27)
                               17  26   17   24   22 |26   33   9    19   15
FOVEA:  33 DB                      (23)      (24) (19)|(26) (27)  A
TEST TIME 12:04                20  26   20   19   30 |28   25   23   28   12
                                   (20)      (19) (24)     (25)      (13) (18)

HFA S/N                           25   15   28   26 |24   30   28   25
                                  (22) (18) (25) (23)     (24) (23)
          -5  -5 |-7  -7          13   17   18 |25   25   20              -4  -4 |-6  -5
                                  (25)
       -4 -12 -8 |-3  -3  -7           11   21 |20   23            -3 -11 -7 |-2  -1  -5
                                          (18)
    -1  -1  -3 |-1   0  -3  -3  -6                              0   0  -1  0 |2  -2  -1  -4
   -8  -2 -15 -3 |-4  -3  -1  -3  -6  -6                       -7  -1 -13 -1 |-3  -1   0  -2  -5  -5
  -12 -8  -4  -6 |-1  -5  -3       1  -3                      -10 -7  -3  -4 |1  -4  -2        3  -2
   -8   0 -13 -7 |-11 -5   0      -9 -12                       -6   2 -11 -5 |-9  -4   2      -8 -10
   -4  -4  -9 -11 |-3  -2  -5  -5  -7 -11                      -3  -2  -7 -10 -2 |-1  -3  -4  -5  -9
       -2 -11 -2 |-4  -5  -2  -2  -2                               0  -9   0 -3 |-4   0  -1   0
          -6  -9 |-9 -3  -3  -7                                   -5  -8  -8 |-1  -1  -5
TOTAL            -13 -5 |-6  -2                       PATTERN         -12 -4 |-4  -1
DEVIATION                                            DEVIATION
```

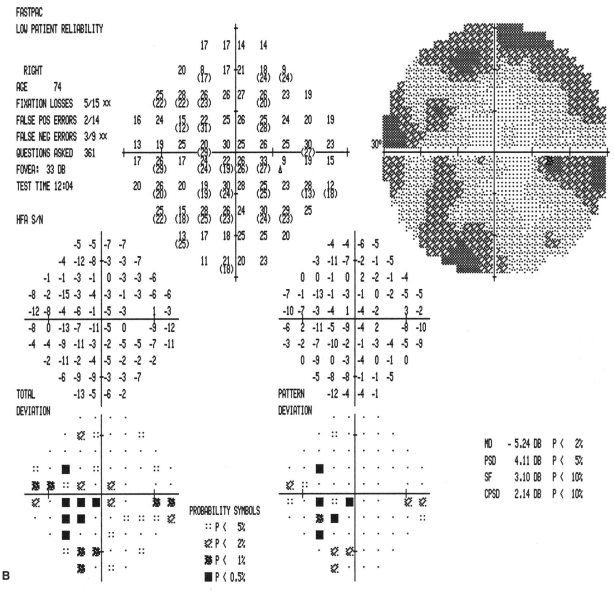

PROBABILITY SYMBOLS

:: P < 5%
✷ P < 2%
▨ P < 1%
■ P < 0.5%

MD   - 5.24 DB   P < 2%
PSD   4.11 DB   P < 5%
SF   3.10 DB   P < 10%
CPSD   2.14 DB   P < 10%

B

Figure 6-28. *Continued.*

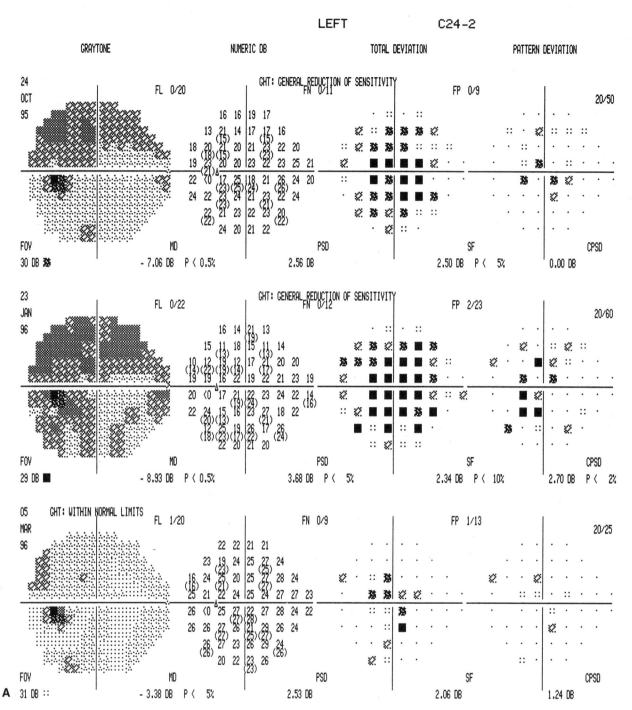

Figure 6-29. Thyroid-related compressive optic neuropathy. Serial visual fields of a 75-year-old woman with difficulty seeing after treatment for hyperthyroidism, **(A)** left eye, **(B)** right eye. Initial visual fields (*top*) show diffuse depression, which is worse centrally on the pattern deviation plot. The visual acuity and field worsened despite radiation and steroid therapies, particularly in the right eye (*center*), and orbital decompression was performed. The visual acuity and visual field 5 weeks later improved dramatically. Serial visual fields are critical in determining the course of the disease as well as the need for, and response to, various treatment modalities.

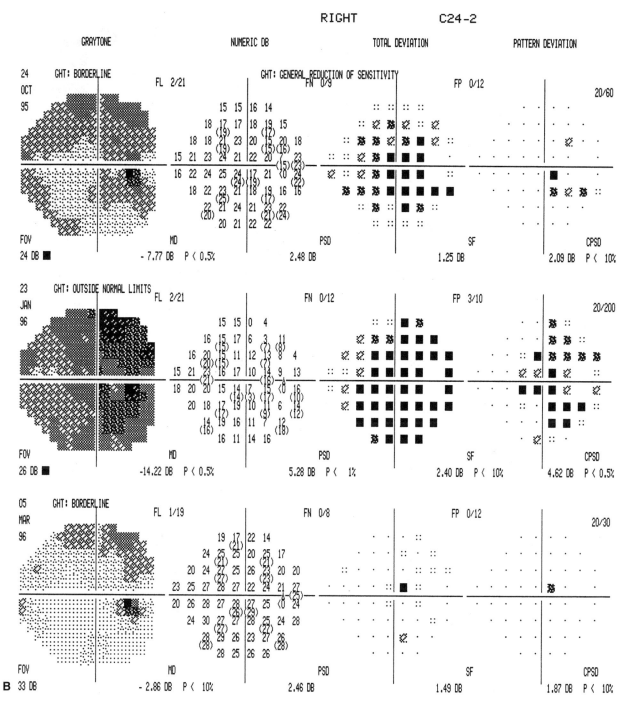

Figure 6-29. *Continued.*

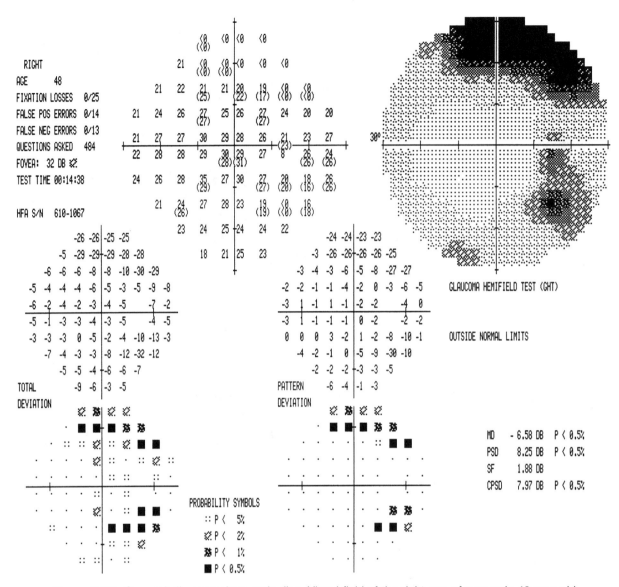

RIGHT

AGE   48

FIXATION LOSSES   0/25

FALSE POS ERRORS 0/14

FALSE NEG ERRORS 0/13

QUESTIONS ASKED   484

FOVEA: 32 DB ✂

TEST TIME 00:14:38

HFA S/N   610-1067

TOTAL DEVIATION

PATTERN DEVIATION

PROBABILITY SYMBOLS

:: P < 5%

✂ P < 2%

▩ P < 1%

■ P < 0.5%

GLAUCOMA HEMIFIELD TEST (GHT)

OUTSIDE NORMAL LIMITS

MD   - 6.58 DB   P < 0.5%

PSD   8.25 DB   P < 0.5%

SF   1.88 DB

CPSD   7.97 DB   P < 0.5%

Figure 6-30. Congenitally anomalous optic disc. Visual field of the right eye of a myopic 48-year-old woman referred for glaucoma evaluation. The optic nerve appeared tilted and the retinal vascular pattern was anomalous. The field shows a defect in the inferotemporal quadrant, just below the blind spot, and a superior defect that is mostly temporal but does not respect the vertical meridian. Neither defect worsened over time, an important feature of visual field defects secondary to congenital disc anaomalies.

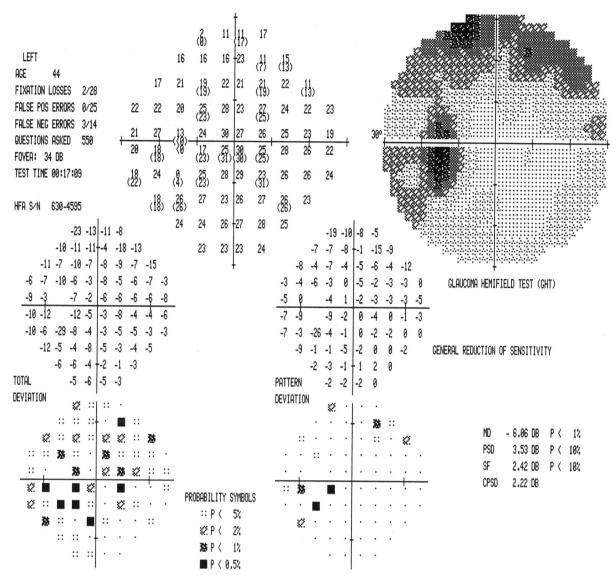

Figure 6-31. Papilledema. Visual field of the left eye of a 44-year-old woman with acute papilledema secondary to malignant hypertension. Field shows concentric enlargement of the blind spot, which is the earliest and most common visual field defect noted in papilledema.[10] The contralateral eye of this patient had a normal visual field, despite optic nerve head swelling.

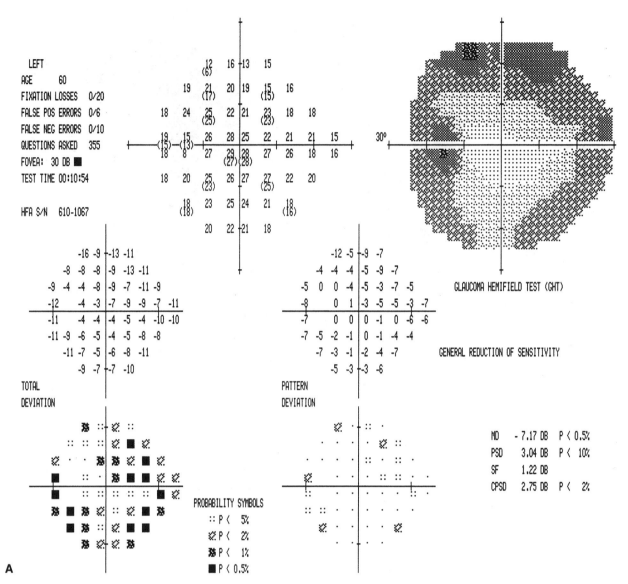

A

Figure 6-32. Chronic papilledema. Visual fields of a 68-year-old woman with an olfactory groove meningioma of the causing increased intracranial pressure and papilledema, **(A)** left eye, **(B)** right eye. Visual fields show diffuse depression OU and nasal defect OD.

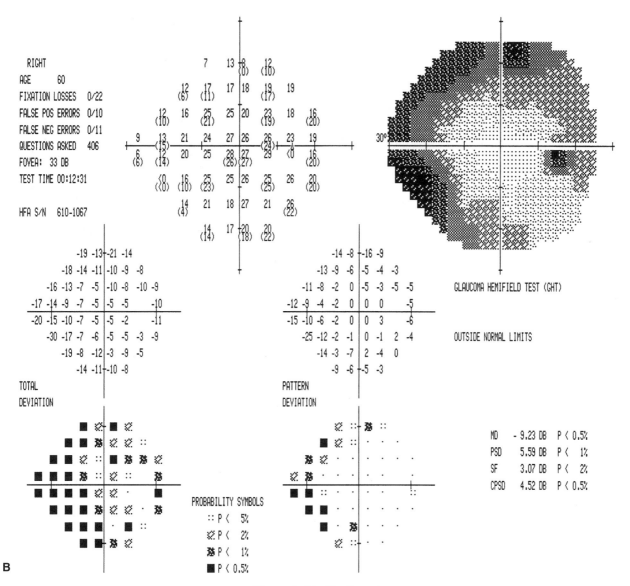

RIGHT

AGE   60

FIXATION LOSSES   0/22

FALSE POS ERRORS   0/10

FALSE NEG ERRORS   0/11

QUESTIONS ASKED   406

FOVEA: 33 DB

TEST TIME 00:12:31

HFA S/N   610-1067

```
                    7    13   8    12
                              (0)  (10)
                12   17   17  18   19   19
                (6)  (11)             (17)
           12   16   25   25  20   23   18   16
           (10)     (21)          (19)          (20)
      9    13   21   24   27  26   26   23   19
           (15)                      (24)    (0)
      8    12   20   25   28  27   26   16
      (6)  (14)          (26) (27) (29)     (20)
           8    16   25   25  26   25   26   20
           (0)  (10) (23)          (25)    (20)
                14   21   18  27   21   26
                (4)                 (22)
                     14   17  20   20
                     (14)     (18) (22)
```

```
        -19 -13 -21 -14                    -14  -8 -16  -9
     -18 -14 -11 -10  -9  -8            -13  -9  -6  -5  -4  -3
  -16 -13  -7  -5 -10  -8 -10  -9    -11  -8  -2   0  -5  -3  -5  -5
-17 -14  -9  -7  -5  -5  -5     -10  -12  -9  -4  -2   0   0   0      -5
-20 -15 -10  -7  -5  -5  -2     -11  -15 -10  -6  -2   0   0   3      -6
  -30 -17  -7  -6  -5  -5  -3  -9    -25 -12  -2  -1   0  -1   2  -4
     -19  -8 -12  -3  -9  -5            -14  -3  -7   2  -4   0
        -14 -11 -10  -8                     -9  -6  -5  -3
```

TOTAL
DEVIATION

PATTERN
DEVIATION

GLAUCOMA HEMIFIELD TEST (GHT)

OUTSIDE NORMAL LIMITS

PROBABILITY SYMBOLS

:: P < 5%

▨ P < 2%

▩ P < 1%

■ P < 0.5%

MD	- 9.23 DB	P < 0.5%
PSD	5.59 DB	P < 1%
SF	3.07 DB	P < 2%
CPSD	4.52 DB	P < 0.5%

B

Figure 6-32. *Continued.*

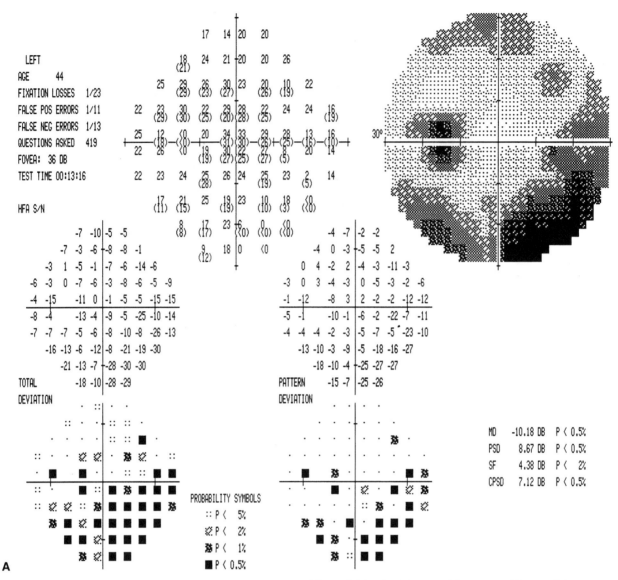

LEFT
AGE   44
FIXATION LOSSES   1/23
FALSE POS ERRORS   1/11
FALSE NEG ERRORS   1/13
QUESTIONS ASKED   419
FOVEA: 36 DB
TEST TIME 00:13:16

HFA S/N

PROBABILITY SYMBOLS
:: P < 5%
⊠ P < 2%
▩ P < 1%
■ P < 0.5%

MD   -10.18 DB   P < 0.5%
PSD   8.67 DB   P < 0.5%
SF   4.38 DB   P < 2%
CPSD   7.12 DB   P < 0.5%

A

Figure 6-33. Idiopathic intracranial hypertension. Visual fields of a 44-year-old woman with pseudotumor cerebri. The right eye **(B)** shows a typical early visual field defect of enlargement of the blind spot and the left eye **(A)** shows enlargement of the blind spot and a moderate inferior arcuate scotoma. Defects in automated perimetry are found in the majority of patients with pseudotumor cerebri.[12] The most frequent field defects found in one study were an enlarged blind spot (80%), generalized depression (43%), and inferonasal depression (23%).[12]

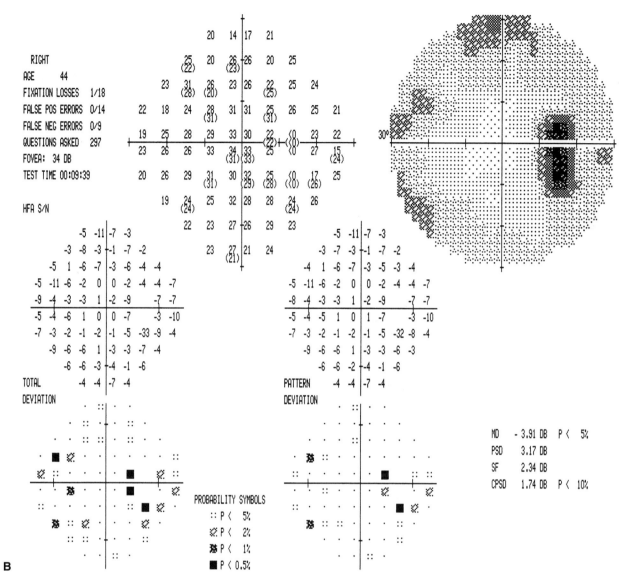

RIGHT
AGE   44
FIXATION LOSSES   1/18
FALSE POS ERRORS   0/14
FALSE NEG ERRORS   0/9
QUESTIONS ASKED   297
FOVEA: 34 DB
TEST TIME 00:09:39

HFA S/N

TOTAL
DEVIATION

PATTERN
DEVIATION

PROBABILITY SYMBOLS

:: P < 5%

▨ P < 2%

▨ P < 1%

■ P < 0.5%

MD   - 3.91 DB   P < 5%
PSD   3.17 DB
SF   2.34 DB
CPSD 1.74 DB   P < 10%

B

Figure 6-33. *Continued.*

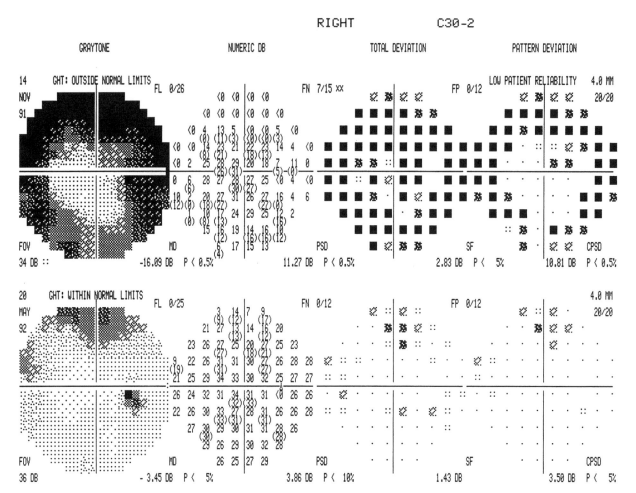

Figure 6-34. Improvement in idiopathic intracranial hypertension. Severe concentric constriction (*top*) of the right visual field in a 27-year-old woman with chronic papilledema secondary to pseudotumor cerebri that improved with medical treatment (*bottom*).

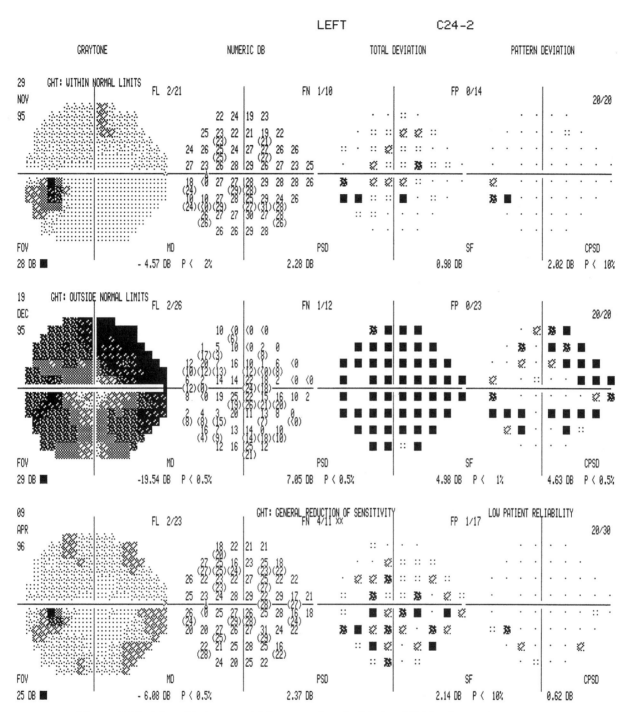

Figure 6-35. Idiopathic intracranial hypertension. Serial visual fields of the left eye in a 41-year-old woman with papilledema secondary to pseudotumor cerebri. The initial visual field (*top*) showed the earliest change seen in papilledema, diffuse depression (best seen in the total deviation plot), and enlargement of the blind spot (seen best in the pattern deviation plot). Follow-up field was worse (*middle*) and, after confirmation of the worsening with a second field, optic nerve sheath fenestration was performed. The visual field improved over the next few months (*bottom*).

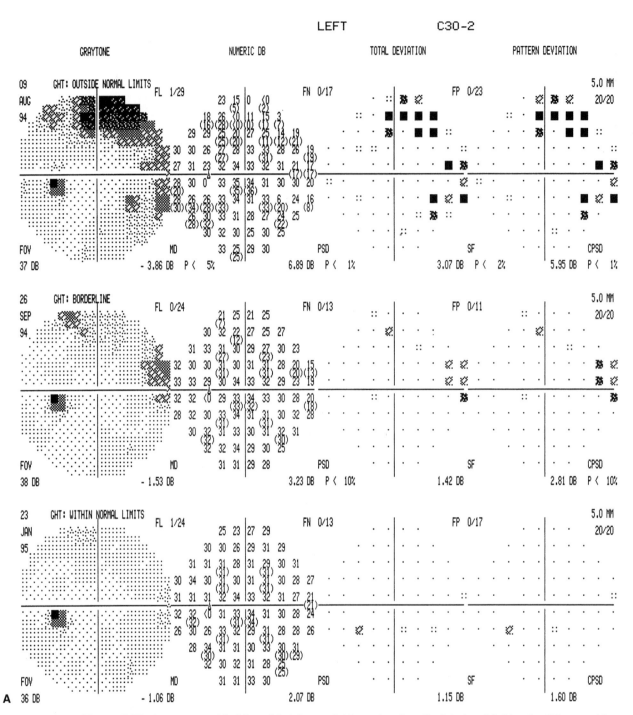

Figure 6-36. Improvement in idiopathic intracranial hypertension. Serial visual fields of a 26-year-old woman who presented with bilateral disk edema and transient visual obscuration. Visual fields show superior and nasal loss in the left eye **(A)** and an enlarged blind spot, superior, and nasal field loss in the right eye **(B)** (*top fields*). Visual fields improved with diet and pharmacologic reduction of intracranial pressure. (*center, bottom*).

RIGHT C30-2

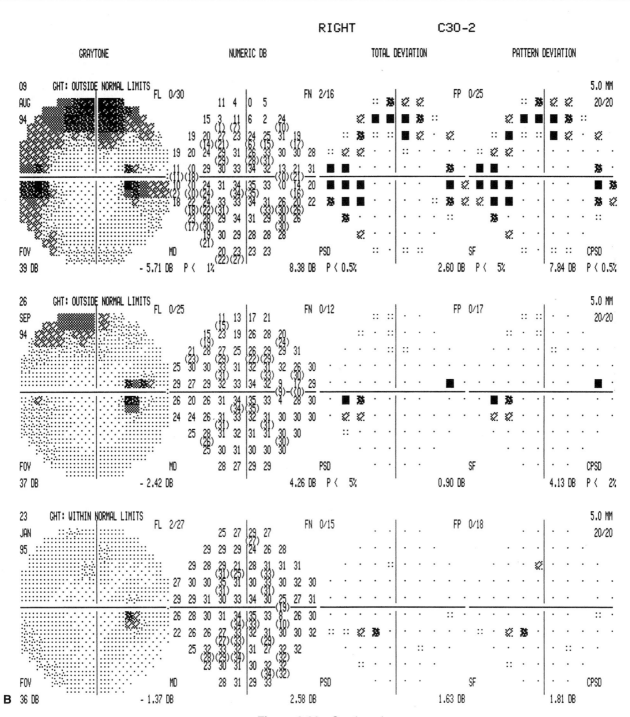

Figure 6-36. *Continued.*

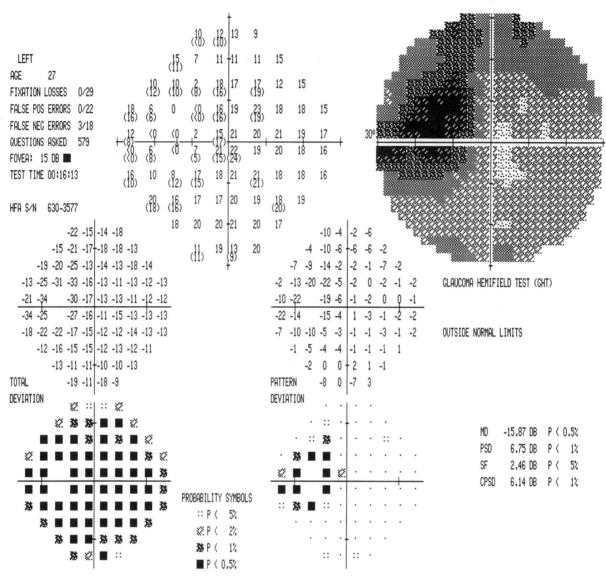

LEFT

AGE	27	
FIXATION LOSSES	0/29	
FALSE POS ERRORS	0/22	
FALSE NEG ERRORS	3/18	
QUESTIONS ASKED	579	
FOVEA: 15 DB ■		
TEST TIME	00:16:13	

HFA S/N   630-3577

```
              10  12  13   9
             (<0)(<10)
                  15    7  11 +11  11  15
                 (11)
              10  10   2  10  17  17  12  15
             (12)(10)  (8)(10)      (19)
         10   6   0  <0  16  19  23  18  18  15
        (10) (6)     (<0)(10)     (19)
         12  <0  <0   2  15  21  20  21  19  17
        (<0)     (<0)(<7)(17)
         -30 -25     -27        22  19  20  18  16
        (<0)  (8)     (5) (15)(24)
         16  10   8  17  18  21  21  18  18  16
        (10)     (12)(15)      (21)
              20  16  17  17  20  19  18  19
             (18)(16)              (20)
                 18  20  20 +21  20  17
```

TOTAL DEVIATION					PATTERN DEVIATION				
-22 -15	-14 -18				-10 -4	-2 -6			
-15 -21 -17	-18 -18 -13				-4 -10 -6	-6 -6 -2			
-19 -20 -25 -13	-14 -13 -18 -14				-7 -9 -14 -2	-2 -1 -7 -2			
-13 -25 -31 -33 -16	-13 -11 -13 -12 -13				-2 -13 -20 -22 -5	-2 0 -2 -1 -2			
-21 -34 -30 -17	-13 -13 -11 -12 -12				-10 -22 -19 -6	-1 -2 0 0 -1			
-34 -25 -27 -16	-11 -15 -13 -13 -13				-22 -14 -15 -4	1 -3 -1 -2 -2			
-18 -22 -22 -17 -15	-12 -12 -14 -13 -13				-7 -10 -10 -5 -3	-1 -1 -3 -1 -2			
-12 -16 -15 -15	-12 -13 -12 -11				-1 -5 -4 -4	-1 -1 -1 1			
-13 -11 -11	-10 -10 -13				-2 0 0	2 1 -1			

TOTAL DEVIATION   -19 -11 | -18 -9

PATTERN DEVIATION   -8 0 | -7 3

GLAUCOMA HEMIFIELD TEST (GHT)

OUTSIDE NORMAL LIMITS

MD	-15.87 DB	P < 0.5%
PSD	6.75 DB	P < 1%
SF	2.46 DB	P < 5%
CPSD	6.14 DB	P < 1%

PROBABILITY SYMBOLS

:: P < 5%

⊠ P < 2%

▨ P < 1%

■ P < 0.5%

Figure 6-37. Neuroretinitis. Visual field of the left eye of a 27- year-old man with unilateral optic nerve swelling and circinate lipid exudate in the macula. Field shows diffuse depression from macular edema and enlargement of the blind spot from optic nerve swelling.

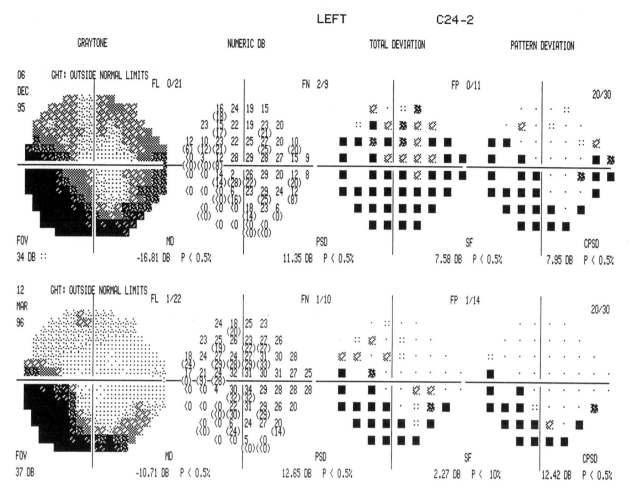

Figure 6-38. Neuroretinitis. Visual field of the left eye in a 21-year-old man with unilateral optic disc swelling, macular edema, and vitreous cells. The *top* visual field, performed on presentation, shows diffuse depression on the total deviation plot. The pattern deviation plot demonstrates enlargement of the blind spot with an inferior arcuate defect emanating from the blind spot. Oral steroids resulted in overall improvement although the inferior arcuate defect persisted (*bottom*). Visual field evaluation is critical in following patients with optic nerve disease to judge treatment benefits.

References

1. Mills RP. Automated perimetry in neuro-ophthalmology. Int Ophthalmol Clin 1991;vol 31, number 4:51.
2. Savino PJ, Glaser JS, Rosenberg MA. A clinical analysis of pseudopapilledema: II. Visual field defects. Arch Ophthalmol 1979;97:71.
3. Keltner JL. Johnson CA, Spurr JO, Beck RW. Baseline visual field profile of optic neuritis. The experience of the optic neuritis treatment trial. Optic Neuritis Study Group. Arch Ophthalmol 1993;111:231.
4. Miller NR. Clinical Neuro-ophthalmology. 4th ed. Baltimore: Williams and Wilkins, vol 1:1982:312.
5. Miller NR. Clinical Neuro-ophthalmology. 4th ed. Baltimore: Williams and Wilkins, vol 1:1982:318.
6. Miller NR. Clinical Neuro-ophthalmology. 4th ed. Baltimore: Williams and Wilkins, vol 1:1982:290.
7. Leibold JE. Drugs having toxic effect on the optic nerve. Int Ophthalmol Clin 1971:11;137.
8. Grant WM, Schuman JS. Toxicology of the eye. 4th ed. Springfield, Illinois: Charles C. Thomas, 1993: 649.
9. Miller NR. Clinical Neuro-ophthalmology. 4th ed. Baltimore: Williams and Wilkins, 1:1982:284.
10. Miller NR. Clinical Neuro-ophthalmology. 4th ed. Baltimore: Williams and Wilkins, 1:1982:194.
12. Smith TJ, Baker RS. Perimetric findings in pseudotumor cerebri using automated techniques. Ophthalmology 1986;93:887.

7

Chiasmal Visual Field Loss

Donald L. Budenz
R. Michael Siatowski

Visual field defects caused by lesions of the optic chiasm and retrochiasmal visual pathways have certain characteristic features which distinguish them from visual field loss due to prechiasmal pathology. First, visual field defects resulting from chiasmal and retrochiasmal lesions are, with rare exception, present in both eyes. These exceptions are the rare cases of chiasmal lesions causing monocular temporal defects and the temporal crescent syndrome from lesions that involve the most anterior portion of the occipital lobe (Chapter 8). Second, such defects tend to respect the vertical meridian. Third, these defects originate from fixation, as opposed to field defects from optic nerve disorders, which originate from the blind spot. It is often possible to localize an intracranial lesion involving the visual pathways based solely on the visual field appearance. Lesions of the anterior chiasm may involve the ipsilateral intracranial optic nerve, and cause extensive ipsilateral central visual field loss and contralateral temporal field loss. Lesions of the body of the chiasm usually cause bitemporal hemianopias. Lesions of the posterior chiasm may cause bitemporal hemianopia in addition to homonomous hemianopic defects due to involvement of the optic tract. Precise localization of parachiasmal tumors lesions requires neuroimaging, particularly because the position of the chiasm varies considerably from individual to individual.

Figures 7.1–7.9 follow on pages 258–273.

References appear on page 274.

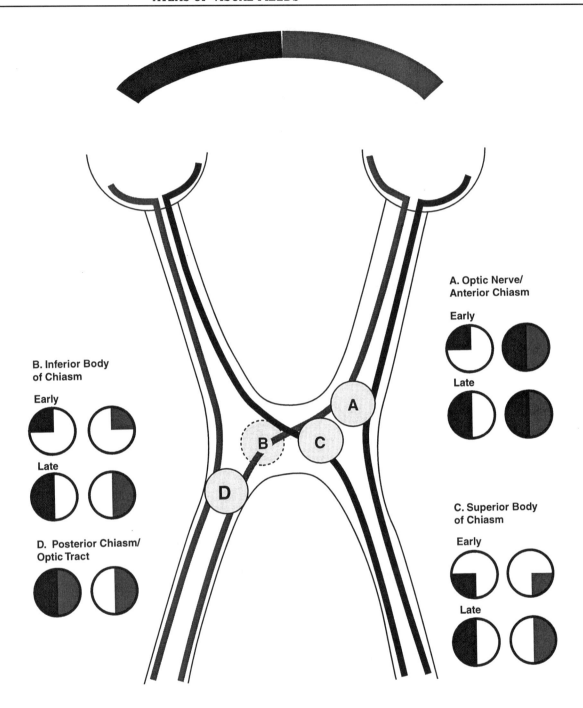

J. Graeber Fuentes

Figure 7-1. Anatomic basis of chiasmal visual field defects. Schematic representation of the anterior visual pathways (retina, optic nerves, optic chiasm). Lesions that affect the anterior chiasm (*A*) generally affect the ipsilateral optic nerve causing a "junctional" scotoma. Lesions compressing the body of the chiasm from below (*B*) cause a bitemporal hemianopia, which begins superiorly. Lesions compressing the body of the chiasm from above (*C*) cause a bitemporal hemianopia, which begins inferiorly. And lesions that affect the posterior chiasm (*E*) often affect the ipsilateral optic tract.

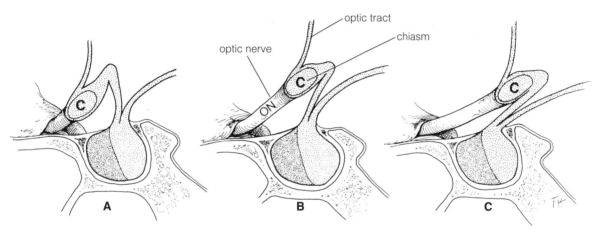

Figure 7-2. Relationship between sella turcica and optic chiasm. The optic chiasm usually lies directly superior to the sella turcica, which houses the pituitary gland (normal chiasm). Tumors of the pituitary most often affect the inferior optic chiasm, which causes a superior bitemporal hemianopic field defect early and complete bitemporal hemianopia as the tumor enlarges. If the optic chiasm is prefixed, pituitary tumors compress the optic tract and posterior chiasm. If the chiasm is postfixed, pituitary tumors affect the optic nerve and anterior chiasm. (From Miller NR. Clinical Neuro-ophthalmology. 4th ed. Baltimore: Williams and Wilkins, vol 1:1982:62; Redrawn from Rhoton AL, Harris FS, Renn WH. Microsurgical anatomy of the sellar region and cavernous sinus. In: Glaser JS, ed. Neuro-ophthalmology symposium of the University of Miami and the Bascom Palmer Eye Institute. St. Louis: CV Mosby, 1977:75).

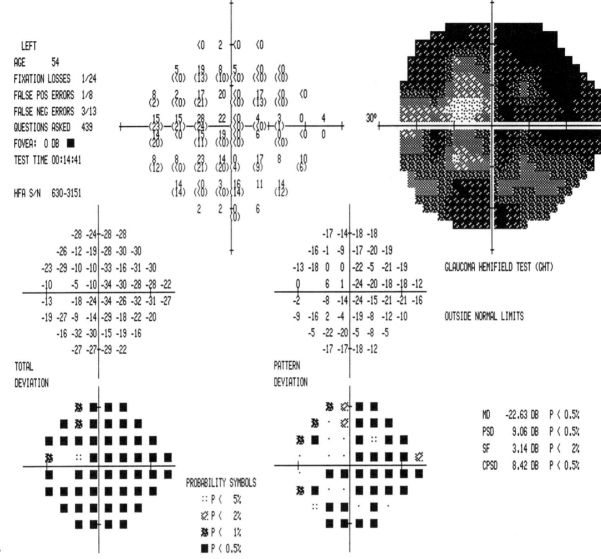

LEFT

AGE   54

FIXATION LOSSES 1/24

FALSE POS ERRORS 1/8

FALSE NEG ERRORS 3/13

QUESTIONS ASKED   439

FOVEA: 0 DB ■

TEST TIME 00:14:41

HFA S/N   630-3151

<0   2 <0   <0

5   19   8 5 <8 <8
(<0) (13) (10)(<0) (<8) (<8)

8   2   17   20 <8 <17 <8   <0
(<8) (<0) (21)   (<8) (13) (<8)

15   15   28   22 <8 -4 -3 0   4
(<23)(<21)(<15) (<0)(<1) (<0) 0

14   <0   11 <8 <8   6 <0   0
(<20)   (11)(<8)(<8)   (<0)

8   8   23   14 9   17   8   10
(12) (<0) (21) (20)(4) (9)   (6)

14   <8   3 16   11   14
(14) (<8) (<0)(14)   (12)

2   2 +0   6
        (0)

TOTAL DEVIATION

-28 -24 -28 -28
-26 -12 -19 -28 -30 -30
-23 -29 -10 -10 -33 -16 -31 -30
-10   -5 -10 -34 -30 -28 -28 -22
-13   -18 -24 -34 -26 -32 -31 -27
-19 -27 -9 -14 -29 -18 -22 -20
-16 -32 -30 -15 -19 -16
-27 -27 -29 -22

PATTERN DEVIATION

-17 -14 -18 -18
-16 -1 -9 -17 -20 -19
-13 -18 0 0 -22 -5 -21 -19
0   6 1 -24 -20 -18 -18 -12
-2   -8 -14 -24 -15 -21 -21 -16
-9 -16 2 -4 -19 -8 -12 -10
-5 -22 -20 -5 -8 -5
-17 -17 -18 -12

PROBABILITY SYMBOLS
:: P < 5%
▨ P < 2%
▩ P < 1%
■ P < 0.5%

GLAUCOMA HEMIFIELD TEST (GHT)

OUTSIDE NORMAL LIMITS

MD   -22.63 DB   P < 0.5%
PSD   9.06 DB   P < 0.5%
SF   3.14 DB   P < 2%
CPSD   8.42 DB   P < 0.5%

A

Figure 7-3. Anterior chiasmal lesion. Visual fields of a 54-year- old man with a 10-month history of poor vision in the left eye. The visual acuity was 20/100 in the left eye **(A)** and 20/20 in the right **(B)**. An afferent pupillary defect and mild temporal disc pallor led to testing by automated perimetry. The left eye shows severe diffuse depression. The right eye shows a superotemporal defect that respects the vertical meridian. These findings are characteristic of the junctional scotoma, that is, poor vision and extensive central field loss in the eye insulated to the lesion and a temporal defect (which typically starts superiorly) in the fellow eye. The temporal defect is due to the crossing inferonasal fibers, which have been thought to traverse slightly anteriorly into the contralateral optic nerve before entering the optic chiasm.* Neuroimaging showed a large left sphenoid wing meningioma intracranial compressing the left optic nerve. In evaluating a patient with unexplained poor vision in one eye, it is important to examine the visual field in the opposite eye, which may reveal a junctional scotoma, as in this case.

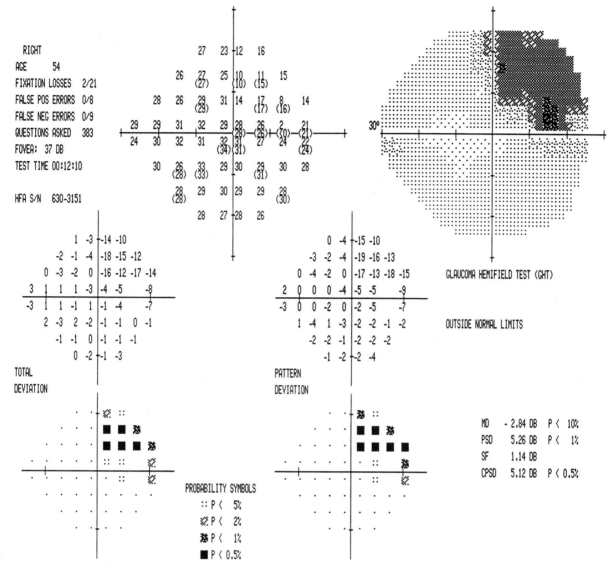

RIGHT

AGE   54

FIXATION LOSSES 2/21

FALSE POS ERRORS 0/8

FALSE NEG ERRORS 0/9

QUESTIONS ASKED   383

FOVEA: 37 DB

TEST TIME 00:12:10

HFA S/N   630-3151

```
                  27  23 +12  16
              26  27  25 |10   11  15
                 (27)    |10  (15)
          28  26  29  31 |14   17   8  14
                 (28)    |    (17) (16)
   29  29  31  32  29 |28   26   2   21
   24  30  32  31  32 |31   27  24   22
                 (34)(31)         (24)
          30  26  33  29 |30   29  30  28
                 (28)(33)        (31)
              28  29  30 |29  29   28
             (28)                 (30)
                  28  27 +28  26
```

```
        1  -3 +-14 -10                      0  -4 +-15 -10
    -2  -1  -4 |-18 -15 -12              -3 -2 -4 |-19 -16 -13
 0  -3 -2  0 |-16 -12 -17 -14        0  -4 -2  0 |-17 -13 -18 -15
 3  1  1  1  -3 |-4  -5      -8      2  0  0  0 |-5 -5      -9
-3  1  1 -1  1 |-1  -4      -7      -3  0  0 -2  0 |-2 -5      -7
 2 -3  2 -2 |-1  -1  0 -1          1 -4  1 -3 |-2 -2 -1 -2
   -1 -1  0 |-1  -1 -1             -2 -2 -1 |-2 -2 -2
        0 -2 +-1 -3                    -1 -2 +-2 -4
```

TOTAL
DEVIATION

PATTERN
DEVIATION

GLAUCOMA HEMIFIELD TEST (GHT)

OUTSIDE NORMAL LIMITS

MD   - 2.84 DB   P < 10%

PSD   5.26 DB   P < 1%

SF   1.14 DB

CPSD   5.12 DB   P < 0.5%

PROBABILITY SYMBOLS

:: P < 5%

▧ P < 2%

▨ P < 1%

■ P < 0.5%

B

Figure 7-3. *Continued.*   * The existence of these fibers in normal individuals has recently been called into question. It has been postulated that the so-called Wilbrand's knee occurs from herniation of the crossing chiasmal fibers into the posterior optic nerve only after the normal anatomy has been disrupted, for example, as an artifact after enucleation.

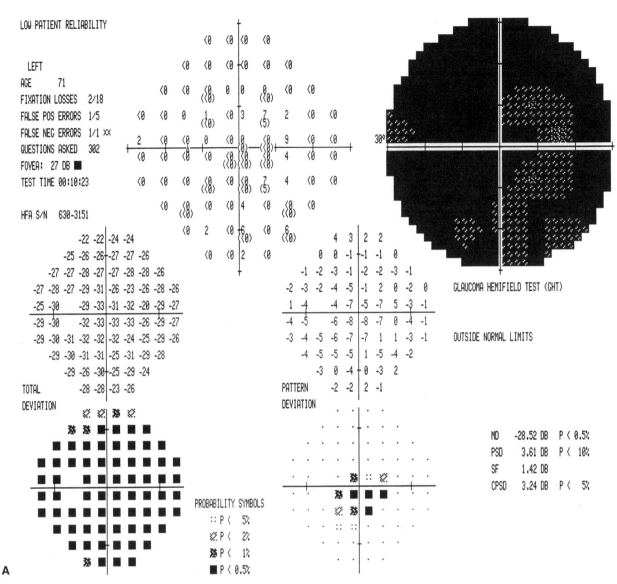

Figure 7-4. Anterior chiasmal lesion. Bilateral visual fields of a 71-year-old man with pituitary adenoma compressing the posterior optic nerve and anterior optic chiasm on the left side. The visual field of the left eye **(A)** shows severe diffuse depression, and the visual field of the right eye **(B)** shows a temporal defect that respects the vertical meridian. Pituitary tumors may cause compression of the optic nerve, optic chiasm, or optic tract depending on where the chiasm is in relation to the sella tursica (Figure 7-2). In this case, the chiasm was postfixed and the pituitary tumor compressed the optic nerve as it entered the anterior chiasm. (Courtesy of David Greenfield, M.D.)

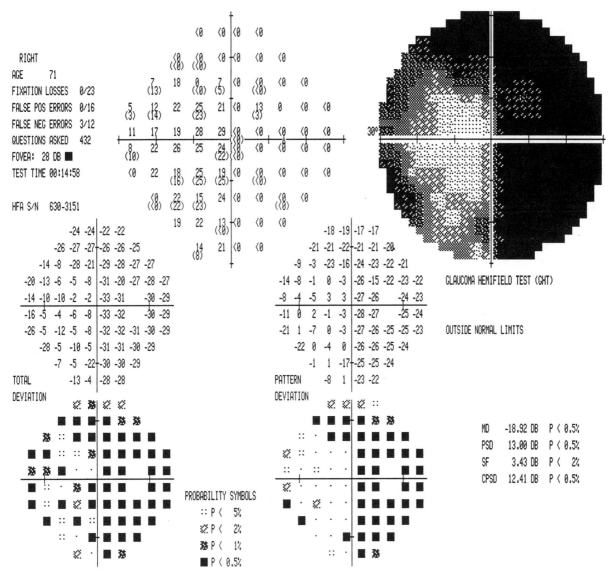

RIGHT

AGE 71

FIXATION LOSSES 0/23

FALSE POS ERRORS 0/16

FALSE NEG ERRORS 3/12

QUESTIONS ASKED 432

FOVEA: 28 DB ■

TEST TIME 00:14:58

HFA S/N 630-3151

GLAUCOMA HEMIFIELD TEST (GHT)

OUTSIDE NORMAL LIMITS

TOTAL DEVIATION

PATTERN DEVIATION

PROBABILITY SYMBOLS

:: P < 5%

⚡ P < 2%

▩ P < 1%

■ P < 0.5%

MD   -18.92 DB   P < 0.5%

PSD   13.00 DB   P < 0.5%

SF   3.43 DB   P < 2%

CPSD 12.41 DB   P < 0.5%

B

Figure 7-4. *Continued.*

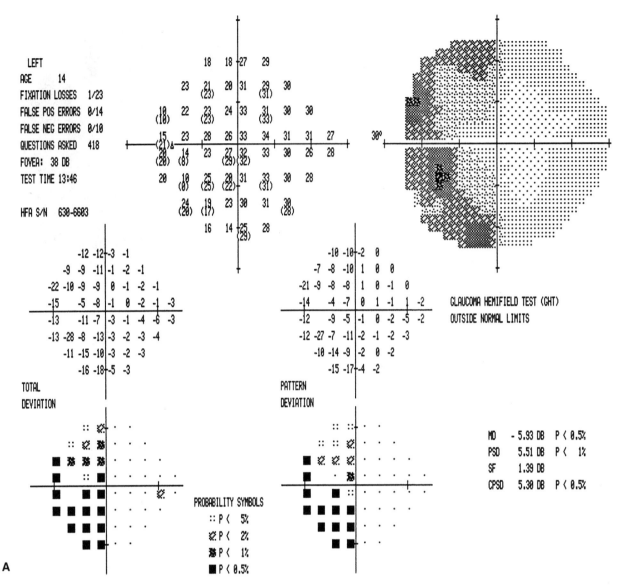

LEFT

AGE   14

FIXATION LOSSES   1/23

FALSE POS ERRORS   0/14

FALSE NEG ERRORS   0/10

QUESTIONS ASKED   418

FOVEA: 38 DB

TEST TIME 13:46

HFA S/N   630-6603

GLAUCOMA HEMIFIELD TEST (GHT)

OUTSIDE NORMAL LIMITS

TOTAL

DEVIATION

PATTERN

DEVIATION

MD   - 5.93 DB   P < 0.5%

PSD   5.51 DB   P < 1%

SF   1.39 DB

CPSD   5.30 DB   P < 0.5%

PROBABILITY SYMBOLS

:: P < 5%

▨ P < 2%

▩ P < 1%

■ P < 0.5%

A

Figure 7-5. Bitemporal defect from anterior suprachiasmal lesion. Visual fields of a 14-year-old boy 1 year following incomplete removal of a craniopharyngioma. There is a bitemporal hemianopia, which is worse inferiorly in the left eye **(A)**, and diffuse depression in the right eye **(B)**. The tumor compressed the anterior chiasm and right optic nerve from above. Tumors originating from above the chiasm (eg, craniopharyngiomas) typically cause bitemporal field defects that are denser inferiorly, in contrast to tumors that compress the chiasm from below (eg, pituitary tumors), which produce bitemporal defects that are denser superiorly.

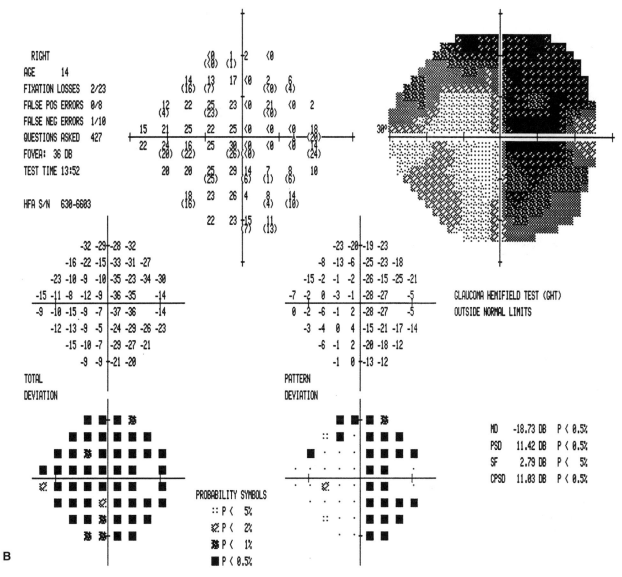

RIGHT

AGE   14

FIXATION LOSSES   2/23

FALSE POS ERRORS 0/8

FALSE NEG ERRORS 1/10

QUESTIONS ASKED   427

FOVEA: 36 DB

TEST TIME 13:52

HFA S/N 630-6603

GLAUCOMA HEMIFIELD TEST (GHT)
OUTSIDE NORMAL LIMITS

TOTAL
DEVIATION

PATTERN
DEVIATION

PROBABILITY SYMBOLS

:: P < 5%

▨ P < 2%

▩ P < 1%

■ P < 0.5%

MD	-18.73 DB	P < 0.5%
PSD	11.42 DB	P < 0.5%
SF	2.79 DB	P < 5%
CPSD	11.03 DB	P < 0.5%

B

Figure 7-5. *Continued.*

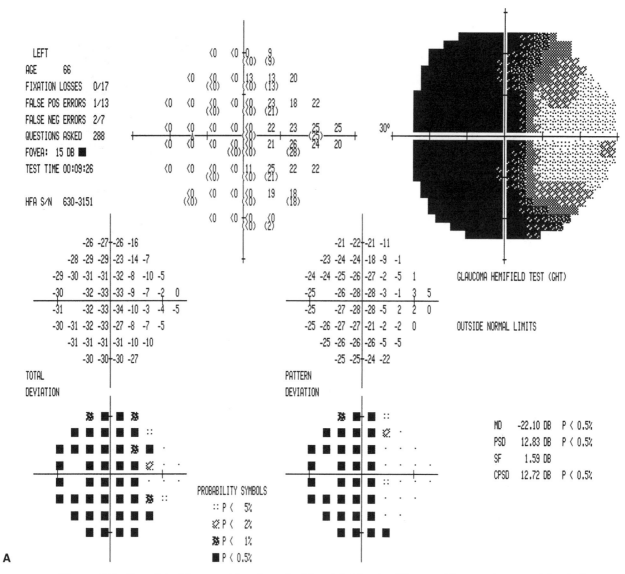

Figure 7-6. Complete bitemporal hemianopia. Visual fields of a 66-year-old man who complained of difficulty with night driving, **(A)** left eye, **(B)** right eye. Complete eye examination revealed a bitemporal hemianopia, afferent pupillary defect in the left eye, and optic disc pallor bilaterally. Neuroimaging showed a large pituitary tumor compressing the optic chiasm. The defect does not respect the vertical meridian in the left eye because the patient is not able to fixate well centrally due to poor central acuity (20/200). The fixation losses, however, are not measured as high because the hemifield that includes the blind spot is an absolute scotoma.

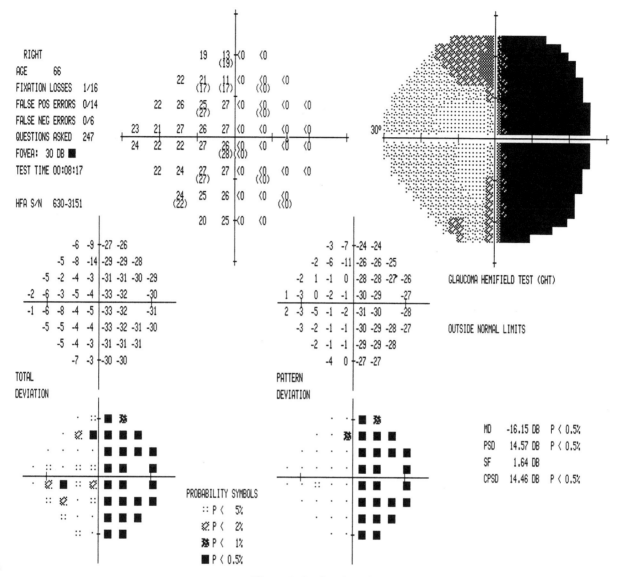

RIGHT

AGE   66
FIXATION LOSSES   1/16
FALSE POS ERRORS   0/14
FALSE NEG ERRORS   0/6
QUESTIONS ASKED   247
FOVEA: 30 DB ■
TEST TIME 00:08:17

HFA S/N   630-3151

```
                    19  13 <0  <0
                       (19)
                22  21  11 <0  <0  <0
                   (17) (17)   (8)
            22  26  25  27 <0  <8  <0  <0
               (27)         (8)
        23  21  27  26  27 <0  <0  <0  <0
        24  22  22  27  26 <8  <0  <0  <0
                       (28)(0) (8)
            22  24  27  27 <0  <8  <0  <0
               (27)          (8)
                24  25  26 <0  <0  <8
               (22)              (8)
                    20  25 <0  <0
```

```
           -6  -9 |-27 -26                        -3  -7 |-24 -24
       -5  -8 -14 |-29 -29 -28                 -2  -6 -11 |-26 -26 -25
   -5  -2  -4  -3 |-31 -31 -30 -29         -2   1  -1   0 |-28 -28 -27 -26
-2 -6  -3  -5  -4 |-33 -32     -30        1 -3   0  -2  -1 |-30 -29     -27
-1 -6  -8  -4  -5 |-33 -32     -31        2 -3  -5  -1  -2 |-31 -30     -28
   -5  -5  -4  -4 |-33 -32 -31 -30        -3  -2  -1  -1 |-30 -29 -28 -27
       -5  -4  -3 |-31 -31 -31                 -2  -1  -1 |-29 -29 -28
           -7  -3 |-30 -30                         -4   0 |-27 -27
```

TOTAL   PATTERN
DEVIATION   DEVIATION

GLAUCOMA HEMIFIELD TEST (GHT)

OUTSIDE NORMAL LIMITS

PROBABILITY SYMBOLS

∷ P < 5%
⊠ P < 2%
▩ P < 1%
■ P < 0.5%

MD   -16.15 DB   P < 0.5%
PSD   14.57 DB   P < 0.5%
SF   1.64 DB
CPSD   14.46 DB   P < 0.5%

B

Figure 7-6. *Continued.*

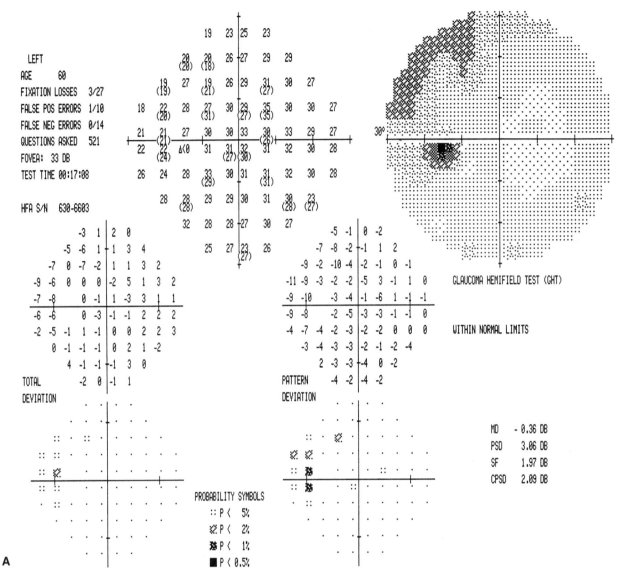

A

PROBABILITY SYMBOLS
:: P < 5%
⊠ P < 2%
▦ P < 1%
■ P < 0.5%

Figure 7-7. Inferior chiasmal compression. Visual fields of a 60-year-old woman who presented with headaches following a motor vehicle accident, **(A)** left eye, **(B)** right eye. Desaturation to red test object was noted bitemporally and formal visual fields showed an early bitemporal field defect. MRI revealed a pituitary adenoma. Subtle superotemporal defects of this nature may be the first sign of inferior chiasmal compression.

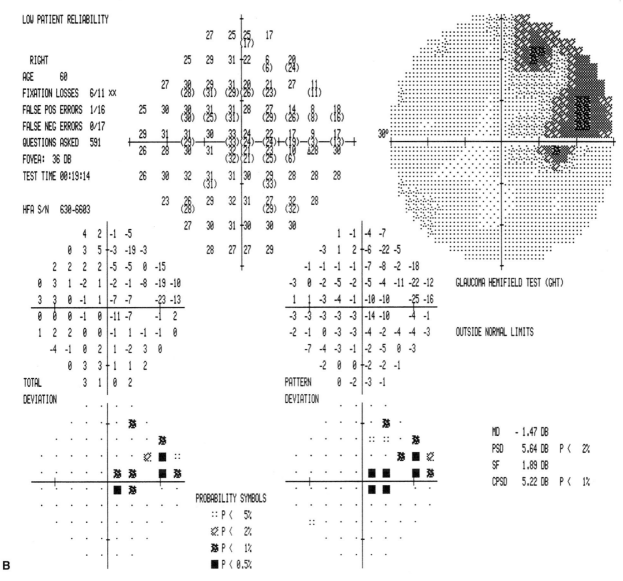

LOW PATIENT RELIABILITY

RIGHT

AGE 60
FIXATION LOSSES 6/11 XX
FALSE POS ERRORS 1/16
FALSE NEG ERRORS 0/17
QUESTIONS ASKED 591
FOVEA: 36 DB
TEST TIME 00:19:14

HFA S/N 630-6603

TOTAL DEVIATION

PATTERN DEVIATION

30°

GLAUCOMA HEMIFIELD TEST (GHT)

OUTSIDE NORMAL LIMITS

MD - 1.47 DB
PSD 5.64 DB P < 2%
SF   1.89 DB
CPSD 5.22 DB P < 1%

PROBABILITY SYMBOLS
:: P < 5%
▨ P < 2%
▩ P < 1%
■ P < 0.5%

B

Figure 7-7. *Continued.*

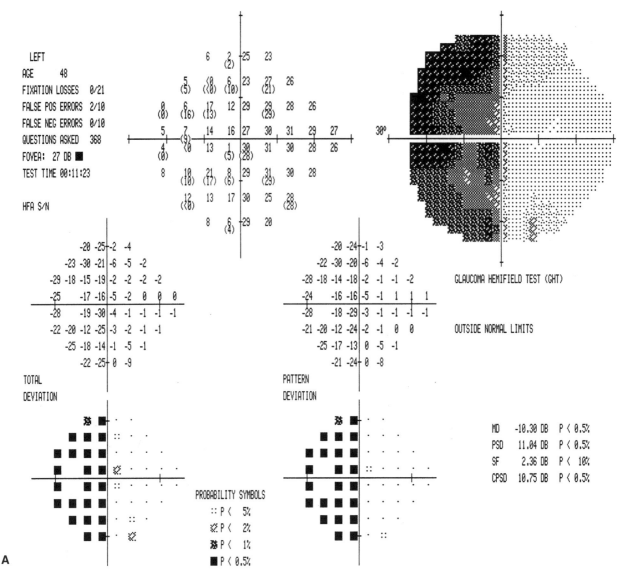

LEFT
AGE   48
FIXATION LOSSES   0/21
FALSE POS ERRORS 2/10
FALSE NEG ERRORS 0/10
QUESTIONS ASKED   368
FOVEA: 27 DB ■
TEST TIME 00:11:23

HFA S/N

GLAUCOMA HEMIFIELD TEST (GHT)

OUTSIDE NORMAL LIMITS

TOTAL DEVIATION

PATTERN DEVIATION

PROBABILITY SYMBOLS
:: P < 5%
※ P < 2%
※ P < 1%
■ P < 0.5%

MD   -10.30 DB   P < 0.5%
PSD   11.04 DB   P < 0.5%
SF   2.36 DB   P < 10%
CPSD 10.75 DB   P < 0.5%

A

Figure 7-8. Inferior chiasmal compression. Visual fields of a 48- year-old man who presented with tilted disc syndrome. A complete temporal hemianopic defect is noted on the visual field of the left eye **(A)**, and a superotemporal quadrantanopic defect is noted on the visual field of the right eye **(B)**.

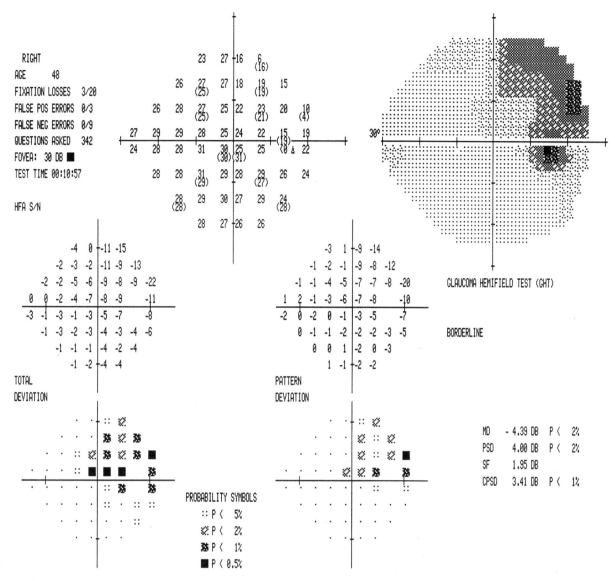

RIGHT

AGE   48

FIXATION LOSSES   3/20

FALSE POS ERRORS 0/3

FALSE NEG ERRORS 0/9

QUESTIONS ASKED   342

FOVEA: 30 DB ■

TEST TIME 00:10:57

HFA S/N

TOTAL
DEVIATION

PATTERN
DEVIATION

GLAUCOMA HEMIFIELD TEST (GHT)

BORDERLINE

PROBABILITY SYMBOLS

:: P < 5%

▨ P < 2%

▩ P < 1%

■ P < 0.5%

MD   - 4.39 DB   P < 2%

PSD   4.00 DB   P < 2%

SF   1.95 DB

CPSD 3.41 DB   P < 1%

B

Figure 7-8. *Continued.* Tilted disc syndrome characteristically causes bitemporal field defects that may resemble chiasmal defects but cross the vertical meridian.[2] However, the defect respects the vertical meridian in this case, which prompted neuroimaging. A pituitary tumor, compressing the optic chiasm from below, was diagnosed. (Courtesy of David Greenfield, M.D.)

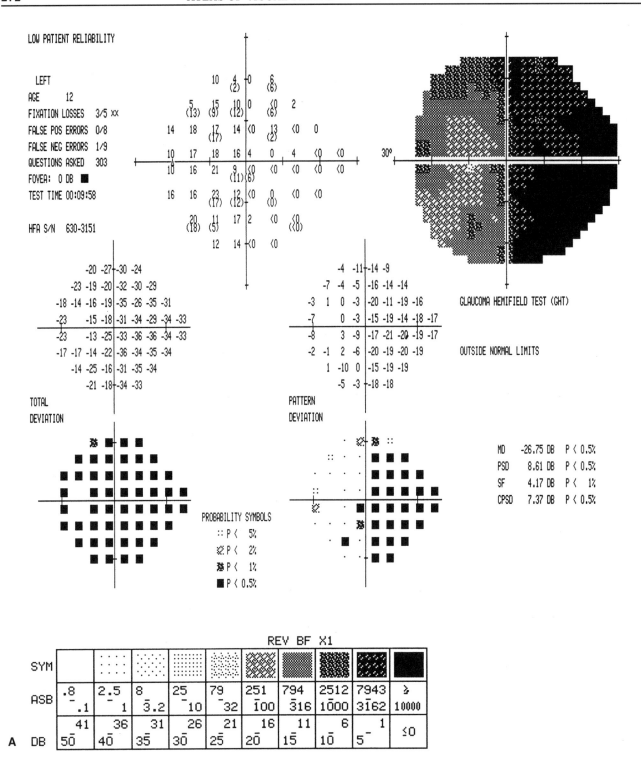

LOW PATIENT RELIABILITY

LEFT

AGE   12

FIXATION LOSSES   3/5 xx

FALSE POS ERRORS 0/8

FALSE NEG ERRORS 1/9

QUESTIONS ASKED   303

FOVEA: 0 DB ■

TEST TIME 00:09:58

HFA S/N   630-3151

30°

GLAUCOMA HEMIFIELD TEST (GHT)

OUTSIDE NORMAL LIMITS

TOTAL
DEVIATION

PATTERN
DEVIATION

PROBABILITY SYMBOLS

:: P < 5%

▨ P < 2%

▩ P < 1%

■ P < 0.5%

MD   -26.75 DB   P < 0.5%

PSD   8.61 DB   P < 0.5%

SF   4.17 DB   P < 1%

CPSD   7.37 DB   P < 0.5%

REV BF X1

SYM										
ASB	.8 .1	2.5 1	8 3.2	25 10	79 32	251 100	794 316	2512 1000	7943 3162	≥ 10000
DB	41 50	36 40	31 35	26 30	21 25	16 20	11 15	6 10	1 5	≤0

A

Figure 7-9. Posterior intrinsic chiasmal lesion. Visual fields of a 12-year-old boy with neurofibromatosis and a chiasmal glioma. The lesion primarily involves the posterior chiasm on the left side. The visual field in the left eye **(A)** is diffusely depressed, although the pattern deviation plot is worse in the right hemifield.

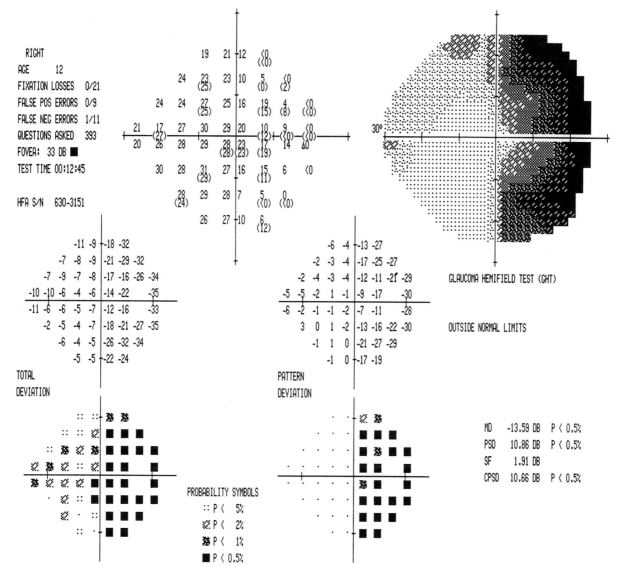

Figure 7-9. *Continued.* The visual field of the right eye **(B)** shows a right hemianopic defect. Thus the tumor is affecting the left optic tract as well as crossing nasal fibers of the left eye, which subserve the left hemifield of the left eye.

References

1. Horton JC. Wilbrand's knee of the optic chiasm is an artifact of long-term monocular enucleation [Abstract], Proceedings of the North American Neuro-Ophthalmology Society meeting, Feb. 1996.
2. Miller NR. Clinical Neuro-ophthalmology. 4th ed. Baltimore: Williams and Wilkins, vol 1:1982:349.

8

Retrochiasmal Visual Field Loss

Donald L. Budenz and
R. Michael Siatowski

Vascular, neoplastic, and inflammatory disorders that affect the visual pathways from the optic tracts to the occipital lobes are characterized by homonomous hemianopic visual field defects, ie, ones that respect the vertical meridian and occur in the same hemifield in each eye. Because of the hemidecussation of the visual fibers at the chiasm, the field defect is always in the hemifield contralateral to the intracranial pathology. Intracranial lesions that affect all of the visual fibers unilaterally are termed "complete" in that they affect the entire hemifield (Figures 8-11, 8-14). Complete (total) homonymous hemianopic defects are nonlocalizing, as they may be caused by lesions of the optic tract, lateral geniculate nucleus, optic radiations, or visual cortex. Complete homonymous hemianopic defects, however, are seen more commonly in posterior lesions of the retrochiasmal visual pathway. Incomplete hemianopic defects may help localize the pathology to the optic tract, lateral geniculate, optic radiations (which traverse the temporal and parietal lobes), or visualcortex (occipital lobe). Such localization is based on the congruity (that is, the similar of the field defects in the two eyes), location, and appearance of the field defects. Localization of intracranial pathology by visual field interpretation helps to direct neuroimaging studies to the area of interest.

Testing the central 24° to 30°, using static automated perimetry is adequate to characterize the majority of visual field defects from retrochiasmal disease. However, two exceptions must be considered. First, lesions that involve the most anterior portion of the occipital lobe, which receives projections from the most peripheral nasal fibers, produce field defects in the contralateral peripheral temporal visual field (60° to 90°). This clinical situation has been called the "temporal crescent syndrome," and is the only situation in which a retrochiasmal lesion produces a monocular field defect, because the peripheral extent of the temporal hemifield is larger than the nasal hemifield. Isolated defects such as these are rare, but may precede a more central homonymous hemianopia when caused by a mass lesion. Such defects would be missed by testing only the central 30° field. Any visual field program which tests the temporal periphery between 60° and 90° could be used. The Humphrey Visual Field Analyzer has a temporal crescent threshold program that can be employed for this purpose.

Second, occipital lobe lesions may cause a hemianopic defect to static stimulus presentation that is not present to kinetic stimulus presentation (statokinetic dissociation, otherwise known as the Riddoch phenomenon). These patients would have a deficit that appears more profound on automated static perimetry as opposed to manual kinetic perimetry. (Figures 8.1–8.21 follow on pages 277–316. References appear on page 317.)

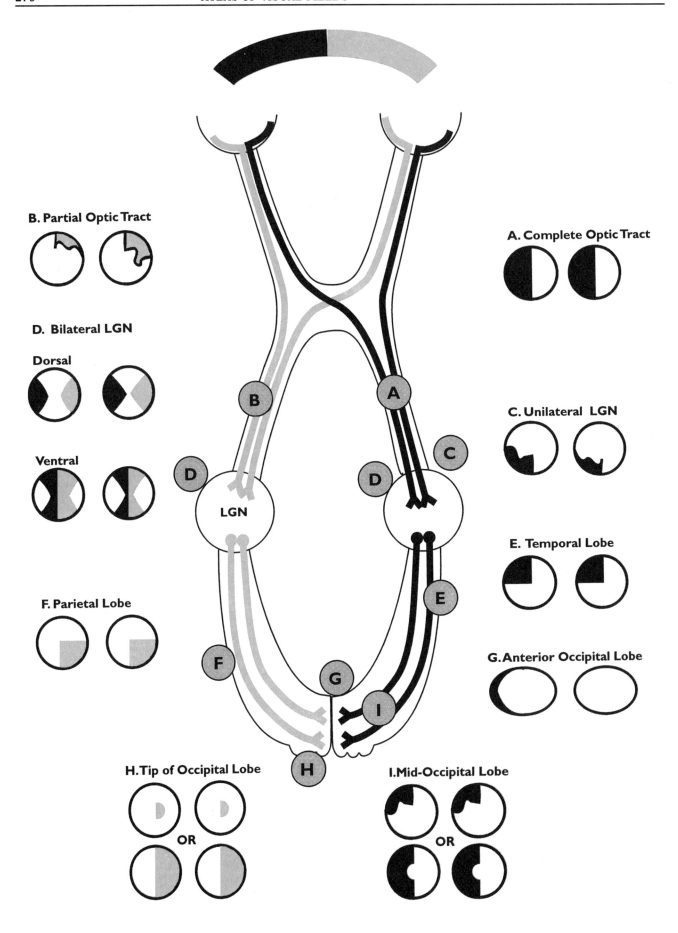

B. Partial Optic Tract

D. Bilateral LGN

Dorsal

Ventral

F. Parietal Lobe

A. Complete Optic Tract

C. Unilateral LGN

E. Temporal Lobe

G. Anterior Occipital Lobe

LGN

H. Tip of Occipital Lobe

OR

I. Mid-Occipital Lobe

OR

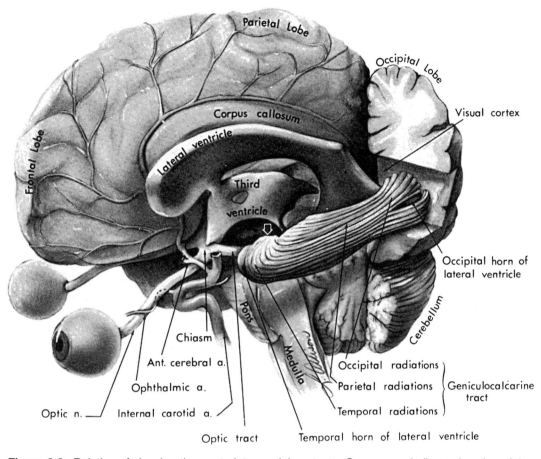

Figure 8-2. Relation of visual pathways to intracranial contents. Open arrow indicates location of the lateral geniculate nucleus, which is hidden by the optic radiations. (Used with permission from Glaser JS, Sadun AA. Anatomy of the visual sensory system. In: Glaser, JS, ed. Neuro-ophthalmology. 2nd ed. Philadelphia: Lippincott, 1990:62)

Figure 8-1. Anatomic basis of retrochiasmal visual field defects. Schematic representation of retrochiasmal visual pathways showing typical visual field patterns resulting from damage to fibers at each location. Complete interruption of the visual pathways on one side will result in a contralateral complete homonomous hemianopia, so this visual field pattern is nonlocalizing. Congruity of visual field defects increases as one moves more posteriorly in the posterior visual pathways.

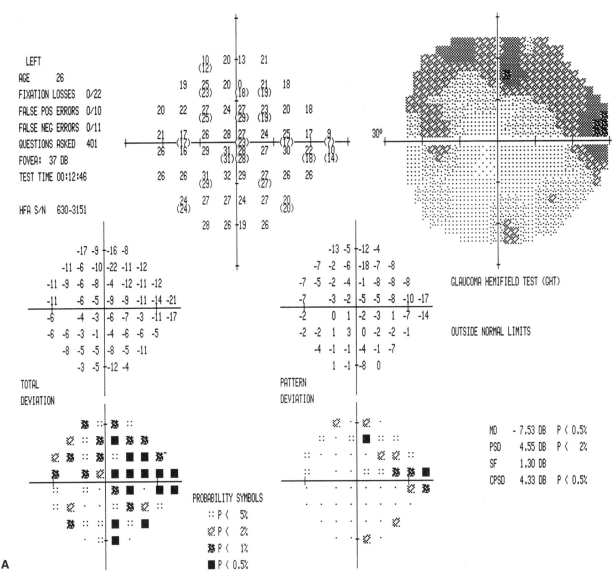

HFA S/N   630-3151

GLAUCOMA HEMIFIELD TEST (GHT)

OUTSIDE NORMAL LIMITS

MD   - 7.53 DB   P < 0.5%
PSD   4.55 DB   P < 2%
SF   1.30 DB
CPSD   4.33 DB   P < 0.5%

PROBABILITY SYMBOLS

:: P < 5%

% P < 2%

% P < 1%

■ P < 0.5%

A

Figure 8-3. Optic tract lesion. Visual fields of a 26-year-old man referred for evaluation of optic nerve pallor and visual field abnormalities. Fields,**(A)** left eye, **(B)** right eye, show an incongruous right homonymous hemianopia, worse in the superior quadrant, secondary to a large parasellar epidermoid tumor. The defect is worse superiorly because the inferior fibers of the optic tract, which are being compressed by the tumor, subserve the superior visual field. Optic disc pallor is a helpful clinical sign in patients with homonomous field defects, because it occurs only in patients with lesions involving the optic tract or lateral geniculate nucleus. Cases of transsynaptic degeneration producing optic atrophy from postgeniculate lesions are rare and occur only with lesions than are congenital or begin in very early childhood.

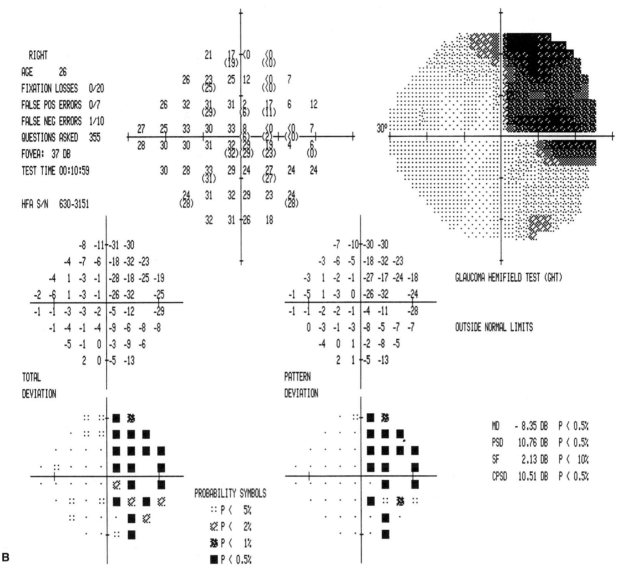

Figure 8-3. *Continued.*

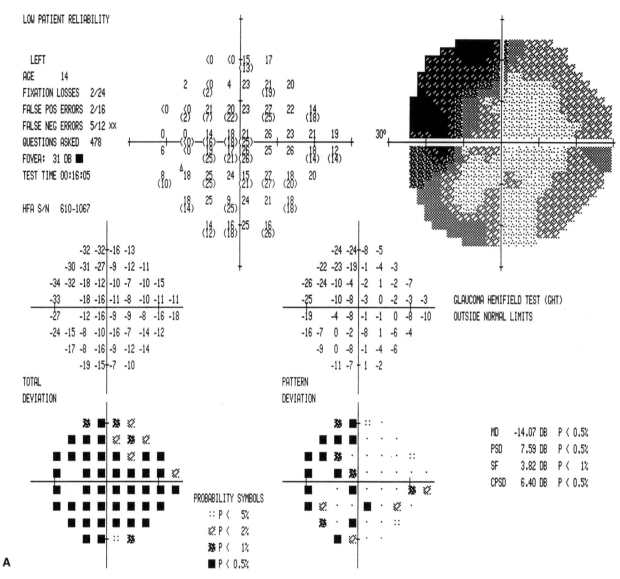

LOW PATIENT RELIABILITY

LEFT
AGE   14
FIXATION LOSSES 2/24
FALSE POS ERRORS 2/16
FALSE NEG ERRORS 5/12 xx
QUESTIONS ASKED 478
FOVEA: 31 DB ■
TEST TIME 00:16:05

HFA S/N 610-1067

30°

TOTAL
DEVIATION

PATTERN
DEVIATION

GLAUCOMA HEMIFIELD TEST (GHT)
OUTSIDE NORMAL LIMITS

PROBABILITY SYMBOLS
:: P < 5%
▨ P < 2%
▩ P < 1%
■ P < 0.5%

MD   -14.07 DB   P < 0.5%
PSD   7.59 DB   P < 0.5%
SF   3.82 DB   P < 1%
CPSD   6.40 DB   P < 0.5%

A

Figure 8-4. Optic tract lesion. Visual fields of a 14-year-old girl referred because of a 6-month history of blurry vision in the left eye, **(A)** left eye, **(B)** right eye. The visual acuity was 20/15 OS, but she had an afferent pupillary defect and red desaturation. Visual fields showed an incongruous left homonymous hemianopia. Neuroimaging demonstrated an intrinsic tumor of the right optic tract, just posterior to the optic chiasm. Histopathology confirmed an astrocytic hamartoma (optic glioma).

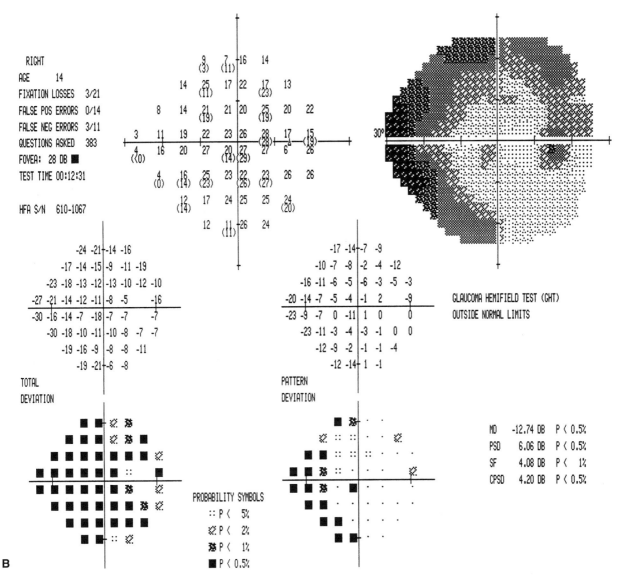

RIGHT

AGE   14
FIXATION LOSSES   3/21
FALSE POS ERRORS 0/14
FALSE NEG ERRORS 3/11
QUESTIONS ASKED   383
FOVEA: 28 DB ■
TEST TIME 00:12:31

HFA S/N   610-1067

```
                         9      7   16   14
                        (3)   (11)
                14     25    17  22   17    13
                      (11)              (23)
          8     14    21    21  20   25    20   22
                      (19)             (19)
    3    11    19    22    23  26   28    17   15
                                    (28)        (13)
    4    16    20    27    20  27   27     6    26
   (0)                    (14)(29)
    4    16    25    23    22  23   26     26
   (0)  (14)  (23)        (26)(27)
         12    17    24  25   25     24
        (14)                        (20)
               12    11   26   24
                    (11)
```

```
              -24 -21 -14 -16
          -17 -14 -15 -9 -11 -19
      -23 -18 -13 -12 -13 -10 -12 -10
  -27 -21 -14 -12 -11 -8 -5     -16
  -30 -16 -14 -7 -18 -7 -7      -7
      -30 -18 -10 -11 -10 -8 -7 -7
          -19 -16 -9 -8 -8 -11
              -19 -21 -6 -8
```

TOTAL
DEVIATION

```
              -17 -14 -7 -9
          -10 -7 -8 -2 -4 -12
      -16 -11 -6 -5 -6 -3 -5 -3
  -20 -14 -7 -5 -4 -1 2     -9
  -23 -9 -7 0 -11 1 0      0
      -23 -11 -3 -4 -3 -1 0 0
          -12 -9 -2 -1 -1 -4
              -12 -14 1 -1
```

PATTERN
DEVIATION

GLAUCOMA HEMIFIELD TEST (GHT)
OUTSIDE NORMAL LIMITS

PROBABILITY SYMBOLS

  ∷ P < 5%

  ▨ P < 2%

  ▩ P < 1%

  ■ P < 0.5%

MD   -12.74 DB   P < 0.5%
PSD   6.06 DB   P < 0.5%
SF   4.08 DB   P < 1%
CPSD   4.20 DB   P < 0.5%

B

Figure 8-4. *Continued.*

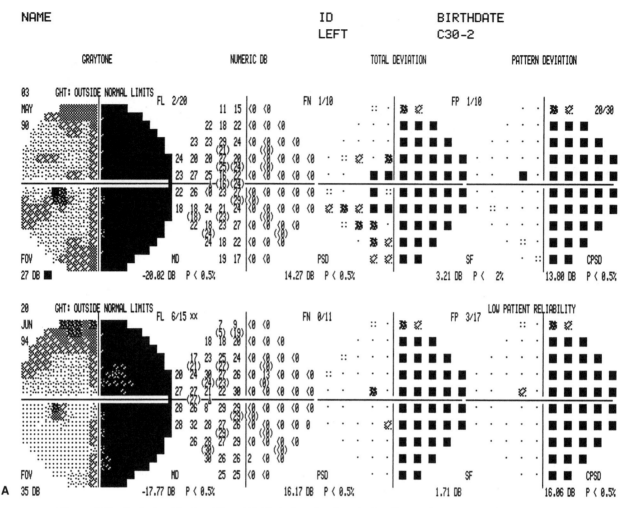

Figure 8-5. Optic tract lesion. Visual fields before (*top*) and after (*bottom*) resection of a large pituitary adenoma, which was compressing the left optic tract, **(A)** left eye, **(B)** right eye. Pituitary tumors may cause compression of the optic nerve, optic chiasm, or optic tract, depending on whether the chiasm is postfixed, normally fixed, or prefixed (Figure 7-2). In this case, a prefixed chiasm placed the optic tract superior to the sella turcica and allowed compression of the optic tract by the enlarging pituitary tumor.

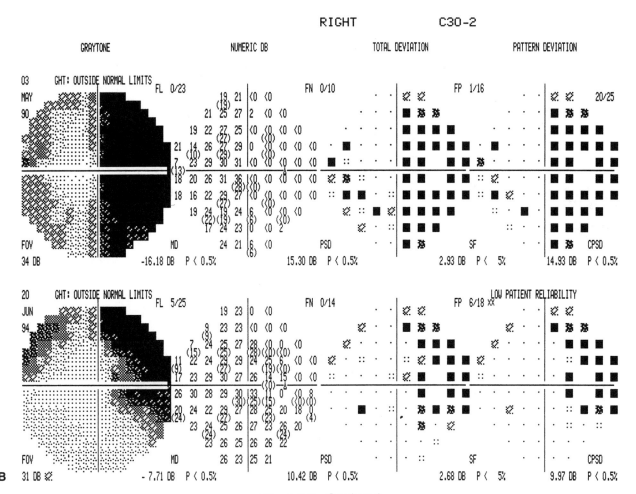

Figure 8-5. *Continued.*

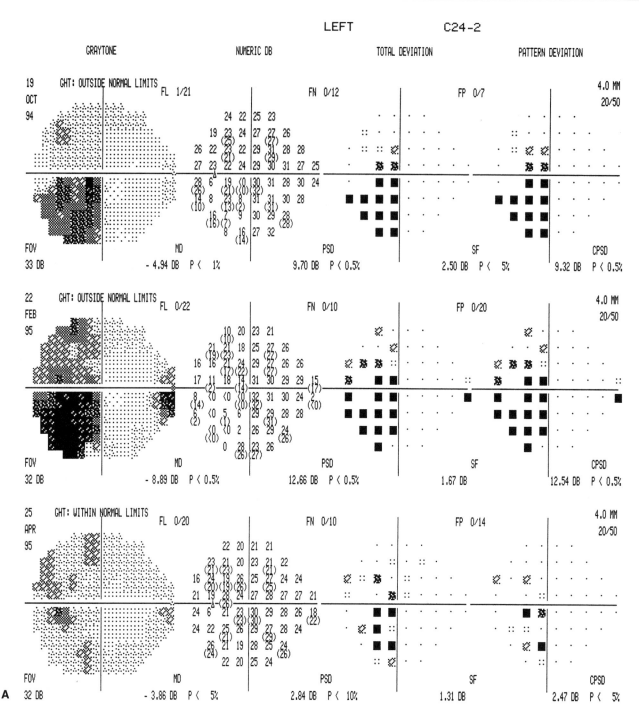

Figure 8-6. Optic tract lesion. Visual fields of a 73-year-old woman with unexplained poor central visual acuity following cataract surgery, **(A)** left eye, **(B)** right eye. A left incongruous hemianopia was noted, worse inferiorly than superiorly (*top*). The defects were originally attributed to an old occipital infarct, but such a lesion would be expected to produce a more congruous field defect. The follow-up field (*center*) demonstrated progression. Neuroimaging was performed, which demonstrated a craniopharyngioma compressing the right optic tract from above. The defect was initially worse inferiorly, which corresponds to the compression of the superior fibers of the optic tract. After surgical removal of the tumor, the visual fields improved (*bottom*). (Courtesy of Norman J. Schatz, M.D.)

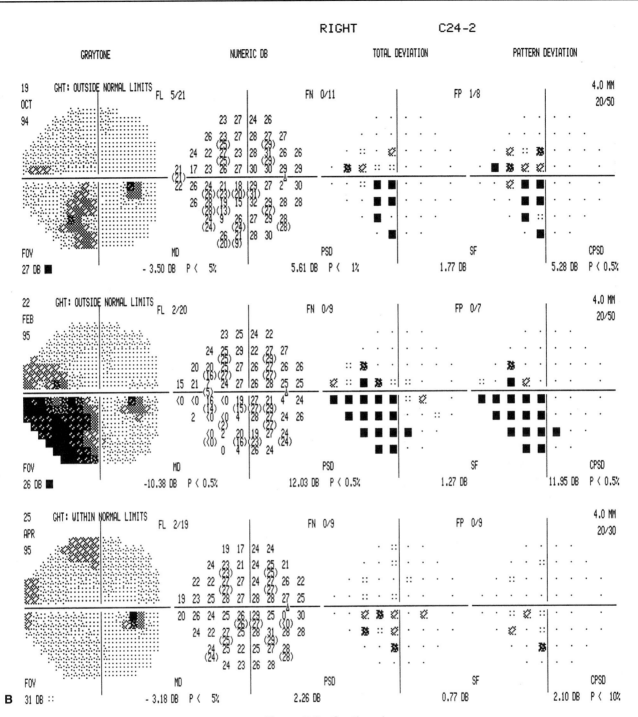

Figure 8-6. *Continued.*

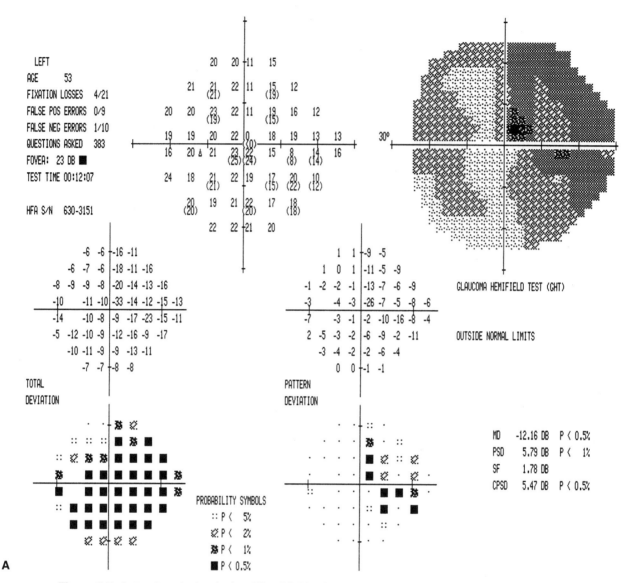

LEFT

AGE   53

FIXATION LOSSES   4/21

FALSE POS ERRORS   0/9

FALSE NEG ERRORS   1/10

QUESTIONS ASKED   383

FOVEA: 23 DB ■

TEST TIME 00:12:07

HFA S/N   630-3151

TOTAL DEVIATION

PATTERN DEVIATION

GLAUCOMA HEMIFIELD TEST (GHT)

OUTSIDE NORMAL LIMITS

MD   -12.16 DB   P < 0.5%

PSD   5.79 DB   P < 1%

SF   1.78 DB

CPSD   5.47 DB   P < 0.5%

PROBABILITY SYMBOLS

:: P < 5%

▨ P < 2%

▩ P < 1%

■ P < 0.5%

A

Figure 8-7. Lateral geniculate lesion. Visual fields of a 53-year-old man with a history of blurring of the right side of his vision. Visual fields, **(A)** left eye, **(B)** right eye, show an incongruous right homonymous hemianopia, and neuroimaging revealed a lacunar infarct of the left lateral geniculate nucleus.

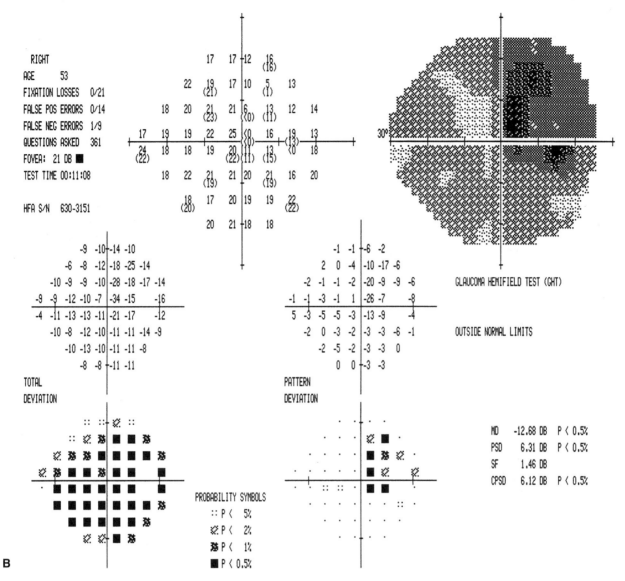

RIGHT
AGE 53
FIXATION LOSSES 0/21
FALSE POS ERRORS 0/14
FALSE NEG ERRORS 1/9
QUESTIONS ASKED 361
FOVEA: 21 DB ■
TEST TIME 00:11:08

HFA S/N 630-3151

GLAUCOMA HEMIFIELD TEST (GHT)

OUTSIDE NORMAL LIMITS

TOTAL
DEVIATION

PATTERN
DEVIATION

PROBABILITY SYMBOLS
∷ P < 5%
▨ P < 2%
▩ P < 1%
■ P < 0.5%

MD   -12.68 DB   P < 0.5%
PSD   6.31 DB   P < 0.5%
SF   1.46 DB
CPSD   6.12 DB   P < 0.5%

B

Figure 8-7. *Continued.*

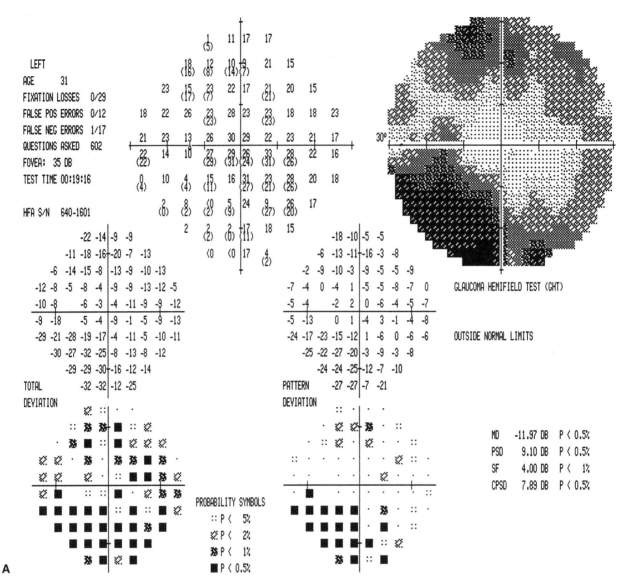

A

Figure 8-8. Lateral geniculate lesion. Visual fields of a 31-year-old man who complained of left inferior visual field loss, showing an incongruous left inferior quadrantanopia, **(A)** left eye, **(B)** right eye. Neuroimaging revealed a small enhancing lesion of the right lateral geniculate nucleus.

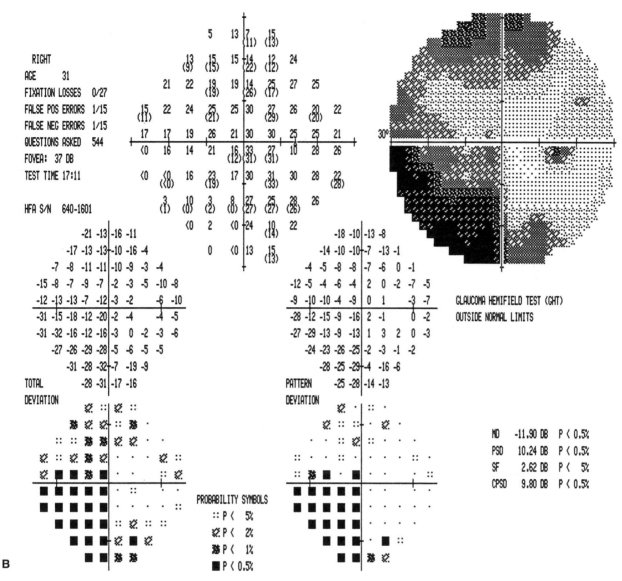

RIGHT

AGE 31

FIXATION LOSSES 0/27

FALSE POS ERRORS 1/15

FALSE NEG ERRORS 1/15

QUESTIONS ASKED 544

FOVEA: 37 DB

TEST TIME 17:11

HFA S/N 640-1601

TOTAL DEVIATION

PATTERN DEVIATION

GLAUCOMA HEMIFIELD TEST (GHT)
OUTSIDE NORMAL LIMITS

PROBABILITY SYMBOLS

∷ P < 5%

▨ P < 2%

▩ P < 1%

■ P < 0.5%

MD   -11.90 DB   P < 0.5%

PSD   10.24 DB   P < 0.5%

SF   2.62 DB   P < 5%

CPSD   9.80 DB   P < 0.5%

B

Figure 8-8. *Continued.*

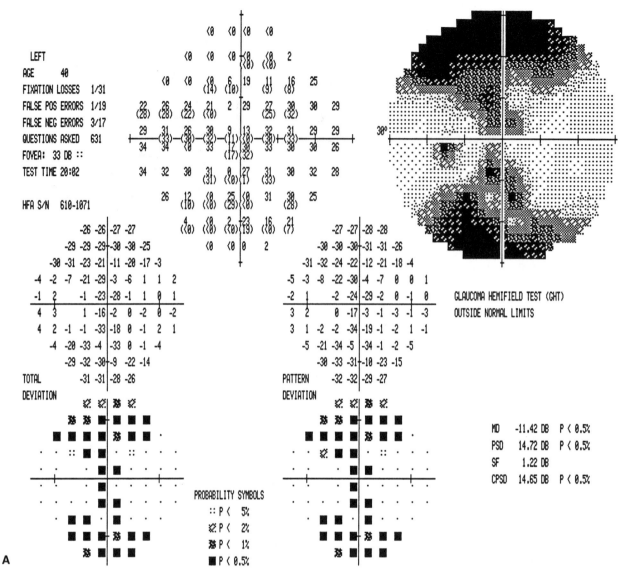

Figure 8-9. Bilateral lateral geniculate nucleus lesions. Visual fields of a 37-year-old woman who presented with bilateral visual loss, **(A)** left eye, **(B)** right eye. Visual acuities measured 20/25 in the right eye and 20/30 in the left eye and the ocular examination was otherwise normal. Visual fields showed congruous bilateral defects in an hourglass shape, suggestive of bilateral ventral involvement of the ventral lateral geniculate nuclei. Neuroimaging demonstrated bilateral enhancing geniculate lesions. (Adapted with permission from Donahue SP, Kardon RH, Thompson HS. Hourglass-shaped visual fields as a sign of bilateral lateral geniculate myelinosis. Am J Ophthalmol 1995;119:378)

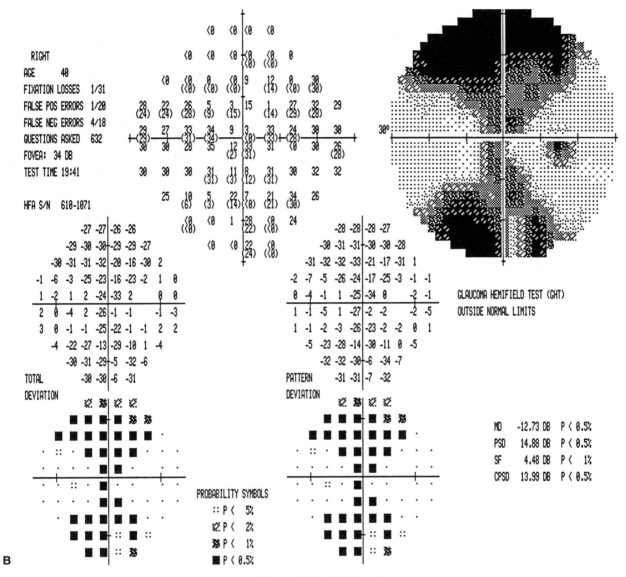

Figure 8-9. *Continued.*

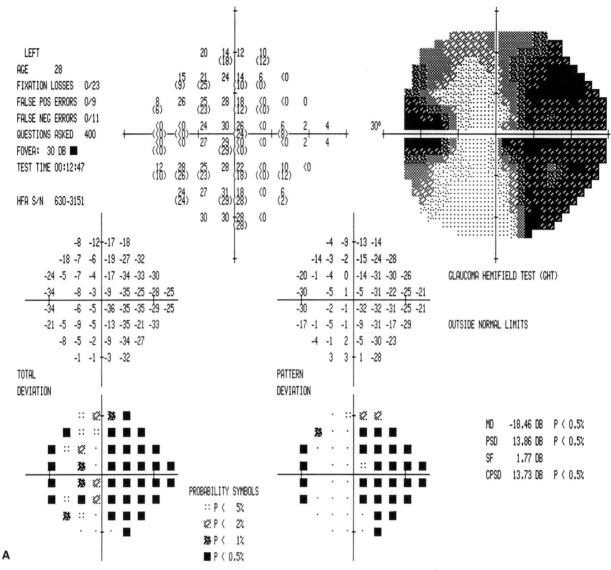

```
    LEFT                              20    14 12   10
                                        (18)      (12)
   AGE    28
   FIXATION LOSSES  0/23          15    21   24  14    6    <0
                                  (5)  (25)     (10) (0)
   FALSE POS ERRORS  0/9       8    26   25   28  18    8    <0   0
                              (6)      (23)     (12) (0)
   FALSE NEG ERRORS  0/11
                             (8) (8)  24   30  26   <0    6   2    4
   QUESTIONS ASKED   400      (0)(0)          (24)     (0)
   FOVEA:  30 DB ■           (0)(0)  27   29  (0)   <0    6   2    4
                              (0)          (23)(0)         (2)
   TEST TIME 00:12:47
                             12    28   25   28  22    8    10   <0
                            (10) (28) (23)    (18) (0) (12)
   HFA S/N   630-3151         24    27   31  18    <0    6
                             (24)     (25)(28)         (2)
                                  30    30  28   <0
                                         (28)
```

```
        -8  -12  -17  -18                    -4  -3  -13  -14

     -18  -7  -6  -19  -27  -32           -14  -3  -2  -15  -24  -28

  -24  -5  -7  -4  -17  -34  -33  -30   -20  -1  -4  0  -14  -31  -30  -26

   -34     -8  -3  -9  -35  -25  -28  -25   -30     -5  1  -5  -31  -22  -25  -21

   -34     -6  -5  -36  -35  -35  -29  -25   -30     -2  -1  -32  -32  -31  -25  -21

  -21  -5  -9  -5  -13  -35  -21  -33   -17  -1  -5  -1  -9  -31  -17  -29

     -8  -5  -2  -9  -34  -27              -4  -1  2  -5  -30  -23

           -1  -1  -3  -32                       3  3  1  -28
```

TOTAL   PATTERN
DEVIATION   DEVIATION

GLAUCOMA HEMIFIELD TEST (GHT)

OUTSIDE NORMAL LIMITS

PROBABILITY SYMBOLS

    :: P < 5%
    ▨ P < 2%
    ▩ P < 1%
    ■ P < 0.5%

MD   -18.46 DB   P < 0.5%
PSD   13.86 DB   P < 0.5%
SF   1.77 DB
CPSD   13.73 DB   P < 0.5%

A

Figure 8-10. Bilateral lateral geniculate nucleus lesions. Visual fields of a 28-year-old woman who presented with sudden painless visual loss in both eyes, **(A)** left eye, **(B)** right eye. Visual acuity, pupillary examination, and color testing were all normal, but visual field testing revealed incongruous bilateral homonymous field defects. Neuroimaging showed bilateral enhancing lesions of the lateral geniculate nuclei, which were attributed to parainfectious demyelinating disease. This pattern of visual field defect is from involvement of the dorsal lateral geniculate nucleus, as opposed to the previous case, which was from involvement of the ventral lateral geniculate nucleus. The orientation of visual fibers changes by 90° as they travel through the lateral geniculate to the optic radiations, thus producing different patterns of homonomous field defects depending on the location of the lesion. (Adapted from Greenfield D, Siatkowski RM, Schatz N, Glaser JS. Bilateral lateral geniculitis associated with traveler's diarrhea. Am J Ophthalmol, 122:280–81, 1996.)

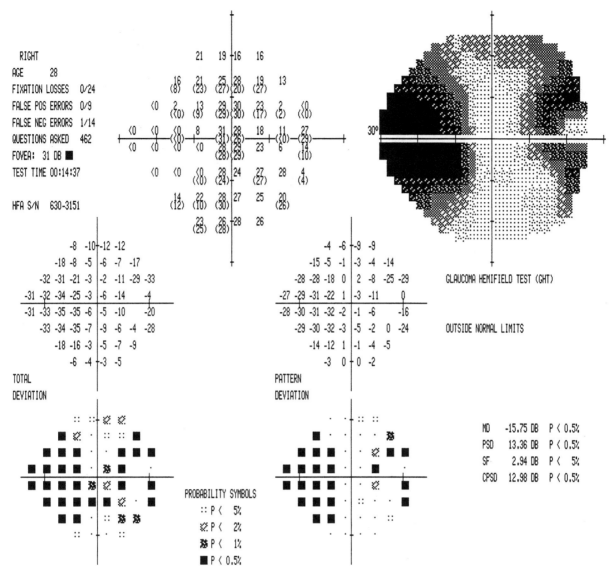

RIGHT

AGE 28

FIXATION LOSSES 0/24

FALSE POS ERRORS 0/9

FALSE NEG ERRORS 1/14

QUESTIONS ASKED 462

FOVEA: 31 DB ■

TEST TIME 00:14:37

HFA S/N 630-3151

GLAUCOMA HEMIFIELD TEST (GHT)

OUTSIDE NORMAL LIMITS

TOTAL DEVIATION

PATTERN DEVIATION

PROBABILITY SYMBOLS

:: P < 5%

⬚ P < 2%

▨ P < 1%

■ P < 0.5%

MD	-15.75 DB	P < 0.5%
PSD	13.36 DB	P < 0.5%
SF	2.94 DB	P < 5%
CPSD	12.98 DB	P < 0.5%

B

Figure 8-10. *Continued.*

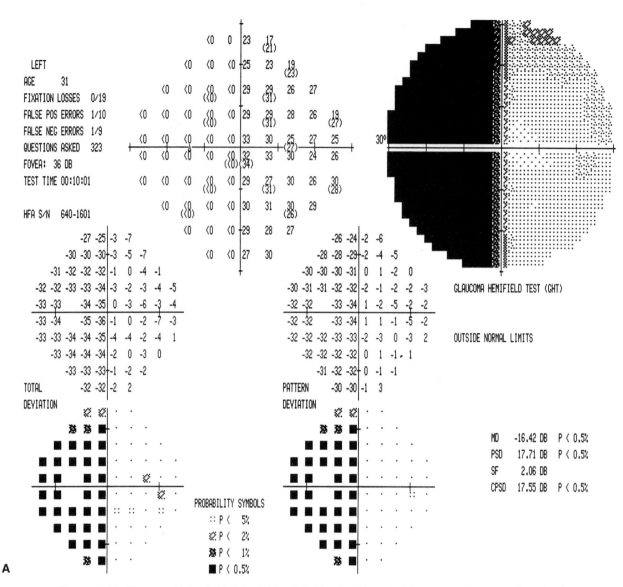

Figure 8-11. Temporal lobe field defect. Visual fields of a 31-year-old woman after resection of a right temporal lobe tumor, **(A)** left eye, **(B)** right eye. A complete left homonymous hemianopic defect is noted, indicating that the entire right optic radiation was affected, either by the tumor or the surgical resection. Complete homonymous hemianopic defects are nonlocalizing.

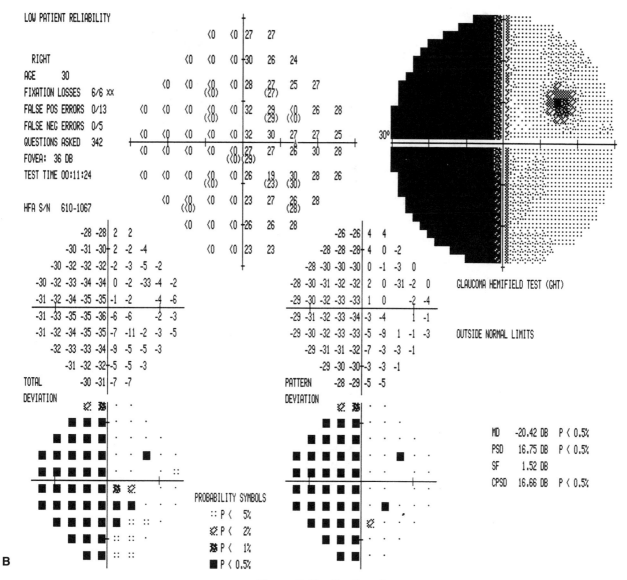

LOW PATIENT RELIABILITY

RIGHT

AGE   30
FIXATION LOSSES   6/6 xx
FALSE POS ERRORS   0/13
FALSE NEG ERRORS   0/5
QUESTIONS ASKED   342
FOVEA: 36 DB
TEST TIME 00:11:24

HFA S/N   610-1067

GLAUCOMA HEMIFIELD TEST (GHT)

OUTSIDE NORMAL LIMITS

MD	-20.42 DB	P < 0.5%
PSD	16.75 DB	P < 0.5%
SF	1.52 DB	
CPSD	16.66 DB	P < 0.5%

PROBABILITY SYMBOLS
∷ P < 5%
▨ P < 2%
▩ P < 1%
■ P < 0.5%

TOTAL DEVIATION

PATTERN DEVIATION

Figure 8-11. *Continued.*

B

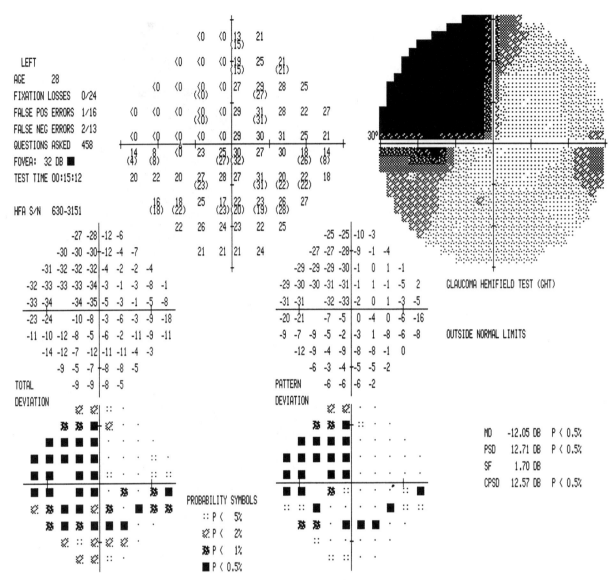

Figure 8-12. Temporo-occipital field defect. Visual fields of a 27-year-old man with a seizure disorder who had a homonymous field defect on confrontation testing, **(A)** left eye, **(B)** right eye. Automated perimetry revealed left superior quadrantanopias. Neuroimaging demonstrated a vascular malformation of the right temporo-occipital area. Such defects have been referred to as "pie in the sky."

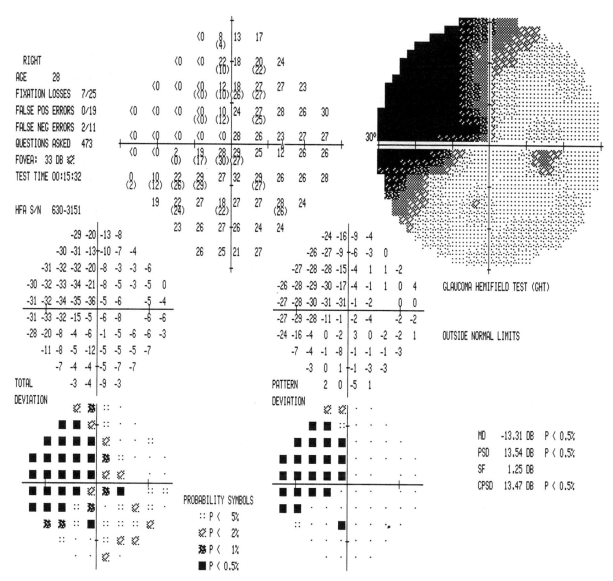

Figure 8-12. *Continued.*

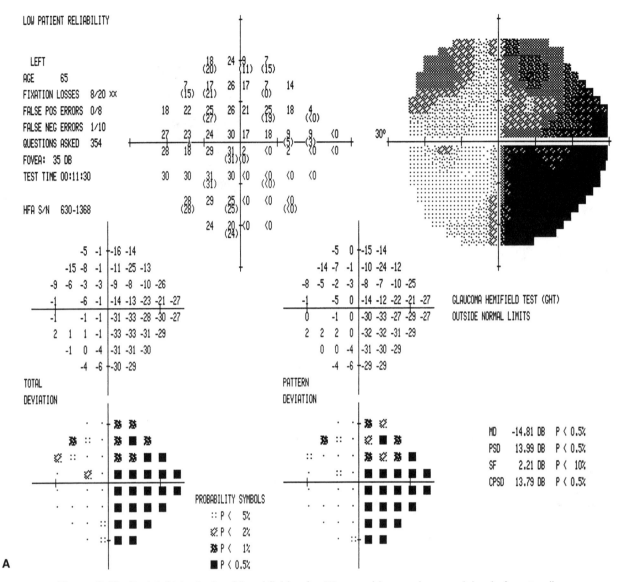

LOW PATIENT RELIABILITY

LEFT

AGE   65

FIXATION LOSSES   8/20 xx

FALSE POS ERRORS   0/8

FALSE NEG ERRORS   1/10

QUESTIONS ASKED   354

FOVEA: 35 DB

TEST TIME 00:11:30

HFA S/N   630-1368

GLAUCOMA HEMIFIELD TEST (GHT)

OUTSIDE NORMAL LIMITS

TOTAL DEVIATION

PATTERN DEVIATION

PROBABILITY SYMBOLS

:: P < 5%

⧄ P < 2%

❉ P < 1%

■ P < 0.5%

MD   -14.81 DB   P < 0.5%

PSD   13.99 DB   P < 0.5%

SF   2.21 DB   P < 10%

CPSD   13.79 DB   P < 0.5%

A

Figure 8-13. Parietal lobe lesion. Visual fields of a 65-year-old man who complained of unsteadiness 9 days following a hemorrhagic infarct of the left parietal lobe, **(A)** left eye, **(B)** right eye. Visual fields show a right homonymous hemianopia, worse inferiorly, which is characteristic of parietal lobe lesions. Such defects have been termed "pie on the floor."

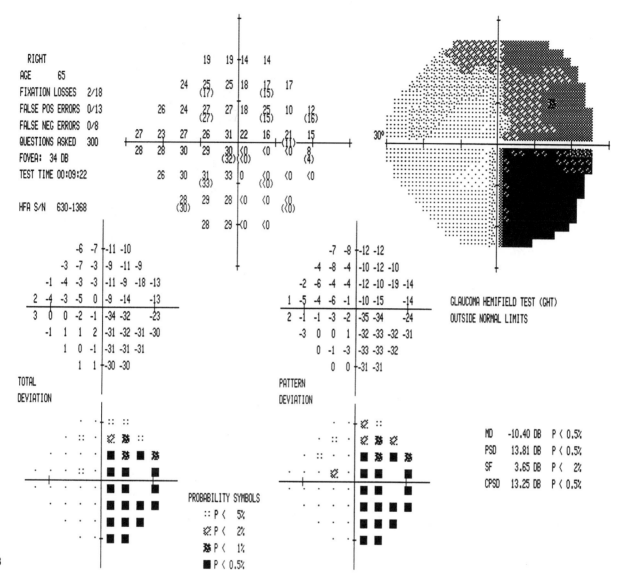

RIGHT

AGE   65
FIXATION LOSSES   2/18
FALSE POS ERRORS   0/13
FALSE NEG ERRORS   0/8
QUESTIONS ASKED   300
FOVEA: 34 DB
TEST TIME 00:09:22

HFA S/N   630-1368

TOTAL
DEVIATION

PATTERN
DEVIATION

GLAUCOMA HEMIFIELD TEST (GHT)
OUTSIDE NORMAL LIMITS

PROBABILITY SYMBOLS

:: P < 5%
▨ P < 2%
▩ P < 1%
■ P < 0.5%

MD	-10.40 DB	P < 0.5%
PSD	13.81 DB	P < 0.5%
SF	3.65 DB	P < 2%
CPSD	13.25 DB	P < 0.5%

B

Figure 8-13. *Continued.*

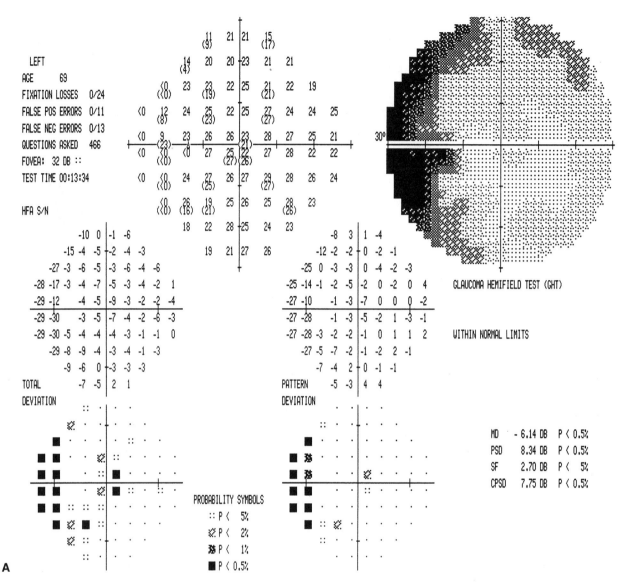

LEFT

AGE   69

FIXATION LOSSES   0/24

FALSE POS ERRORS 0/11

FALSE NEG ERRORS 0/13

QUESTIONS ASKED   466

FOVEA: 32 DB ::

TEST TIME 00:13:34

HFA S/N

GLAUCOMA HEMIFIELD TEST (GHT)

WITHIN NORMAL LIMITS

TOTAL
DEVIATION

PATTERN
DEVIATION

PROBABILITY SYMBOLS

:: P < 5%

▨ P < 2%

▩ P < 1%

■ P < 0.5%

MD   - 6.14 DB   P < 0.5%

PSD   8.34 DB   P < 0.5%

SF   2.70 DB   P < 5%

CPSD   7.75 DB   P < 0.5%

A

Figure 8-14. Occipital lobe infarct. Exquisitely congruous left homonomous hemianopia in a 69-year-old woman who had an ischemic infarct of the right anterior occipital lobe, **(A)** left eye, **(B)** right eye. (Courtesy of Douglas R. Anderson, MD)

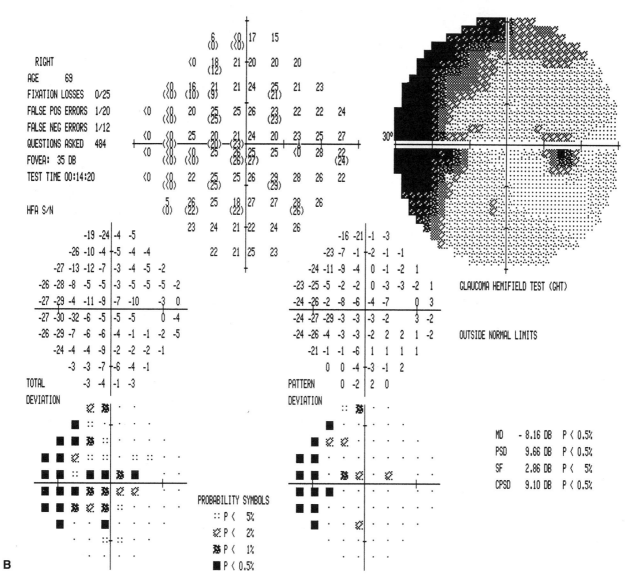

Figure 8-14. *Continued.*

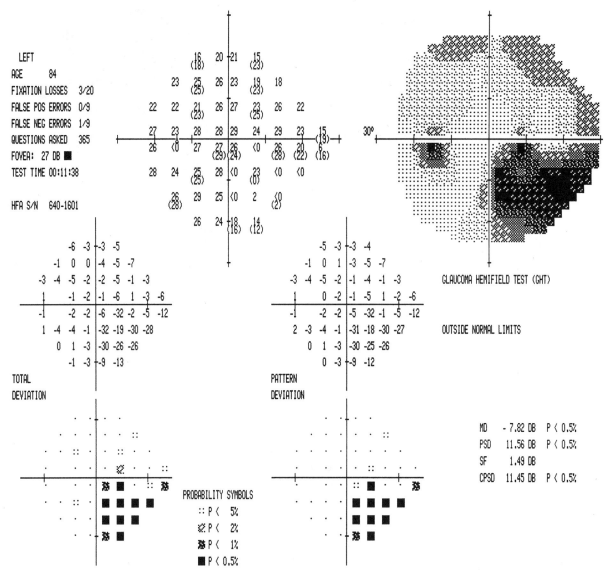

LEFT

AGE   84

FIXATION LOSSES 3/20

FALSE POS ERRORS 0/9

FALSE NEG ERRORS 1/9

QUESTIONS ASKED 365

FOVEA: 27 DB ■

TEST TIME 00:11:38

HFA S/N 640-1601

```
          16  20 21  15
         (18)       (23)
      23  25  26 23  19   18
         (25)       (23)
   22  22  21  26 27  23   26  22
         (23)       (25)
   27  23  28  28 29  24   29  23  15
                                 (19)
   26  <0  27  27 26  <0   26  20  6
             (29)(24)     (28)(22)(16)
   28  24  25  28 <0  23   <0  <0
         (25)       (0)
      26  29  25 <0  2    <0
      (28)                (2)
          26  24 18  14
             (16) (12)
```

30°

```
        -6  -3 -3  -5                    -5  -3 -3  -4
     -1   0  0 -4 -5 -7              -1   0  1 -3 -5 -7
  -3 -4 -5 -2 -2 -5 -1 -3         -3 -4 -5 -2 -1 -4 -1 -3
     -1 -2 -1 -6  1 -3 -6            0 -2 -1 -5  1 -2 -6
  -1   -2 -2 -6 -32 -2 -5 -12     -1   -2 -2 -5 -32 -1 -5 -12
   1 -4 -4 -1 -32 -19 -30 -28      2 -3 -4 -1 -31 -18 -30 -27
     0  1 -3 -30 -26 -26            0  1 -3 -30 -25 -26
     -1 -3 -9 -13                   0 -3 -9 -12
```

GLAUCOMA HEMIFIELD TEST (GHT)

OUTSIDE NORMAL LIMITS

TOTAL
DEVIATION

PATTERN
DEVIATION

MD   - 7.82 DB   P < 0.5%

PSD   11.56 DB   P < 0.5%

SF   1.49 DB

CPSD   11.45 DB   P < 0.5%

PROBABILITY SYMBOLS

:: P < 5%

▨ P < 2%

▩ P < 1%

■ P < 0.5%

A

Figure 8-15. Occipital pole infarct. Visual fields of an 84-year-old woman referred for glaucoma evaluation because of asymmetric cupping and visual field defects, **(A)** left eye, **(B)** right eye. The fields showed congruous right inferior quadrantanopias and MRI demonstrated an infarct of the left occipital pole, just above the calcarine fissure.

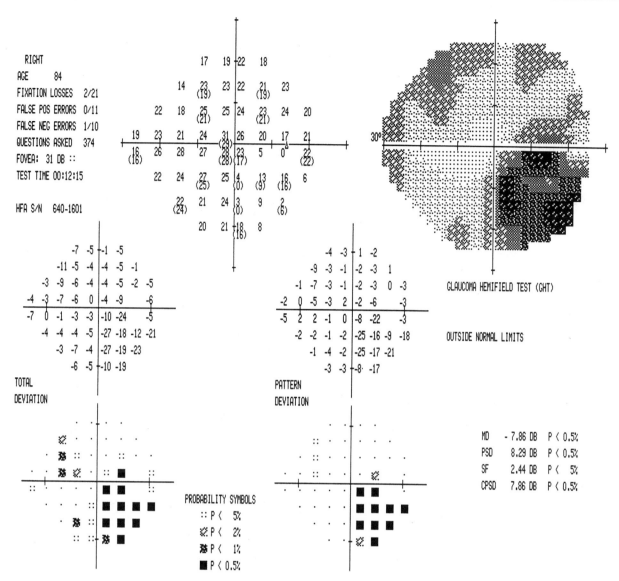

RIGHT

AGE   84
FIXATION LOSSES   2/21
FALSE POS ERRORS   0/11
FALSE NEG ERRORS   1/10
QUESTIONS ASKED   374
FOVEA: 31 DB ::
TEST TIME 00:12:15

HFA S/N   640-1601

TOTAL
DEVIATION

PATTERN
DEVIATION

PROBABILITY SYMBOLS
    :: P < 5%
    ▨ P < 2%
    ▩ P < 1%
    ■ P < 0.5%

GLAUCOMA HEMIFIELD TEST (GHT)

OUTSIDE NORMAL LIMITS

MD   - 7.86 DB   P < 0.5%
PSD   8.29 DB   P < 0.5%
SF   2.44 DB   P <   5%
CPSD   7.86 DB   P < 0.5%

B

Figure 8-15. *Continued.*

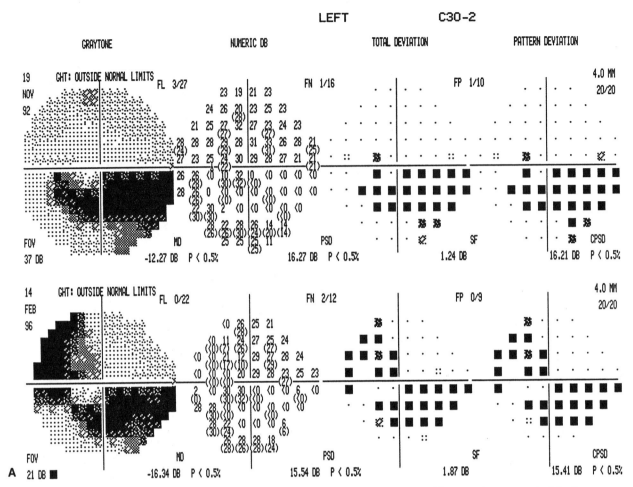

Figure 8-16. Occipital lobe infarct. Serial visual fields of an 86-year-old man who presented to the glaucoma service to rule out progressive normal pressure glaucoma. Fields in 1992 (*top*) show a dense inferior arcuate defect in the left eye **(A)** and early nasal step in the right **(B)**. Follow-up fields in 1996 (*bottom*) show a superimposed congruous left superior quadrantanopia. Because of the location, appearance, and exquisite congruity of the new defects, neuroimaging was performed which showed a right occipital lobe infarct.

RIGHT   C30-2

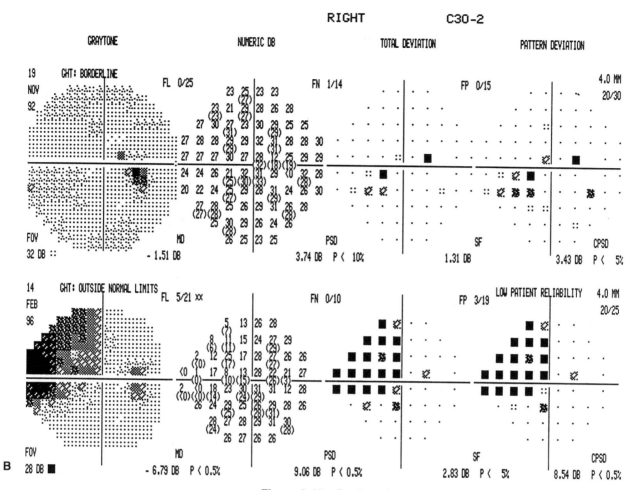

Figure 8-16. *Continued.*

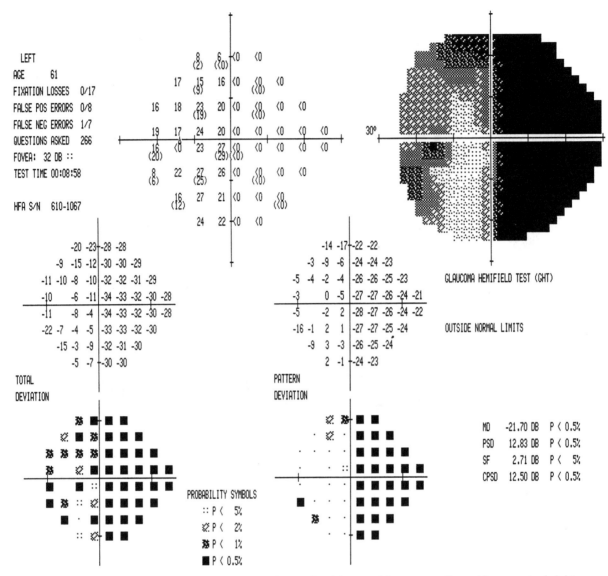

```
        LEFT                                  8   6  <0    <0
                                             (2) (<0)
        AGE      61                      17  15  16  <0  <8  <0
        FIXATION LOSSES  0/17                (9)         (8)
        FALSE POS ERRORS 0/8        16  18  23  20  <0  <8  <0
                                            (19)         (8)
        FALSE NEG ERRORS 1/7        19  17  24  20  <0  <0  <0  <0  <0
        QUESTIONS ASKED  266        16  <0  23  27 <(8 <0  <0  <0  <0
        FOVEA: 32 DB ::            (20)     (29)(<0)
        TEST TIME 00:08:58           8  22  27  26  <0  <8  <0  <0
                                    (6)    (25)         (8)
        HFA S/N   610-1067              16  27  21  <0  <0  <8
                                      (12)                 (8)
                                       24  22  <0  <0
```

```
        -20 -23 -28 -28                      -14 -17 -22 -22
      -9 -15 -12 -30 -30 -29               -3 -9 -6 -24 -24 -23
  -11 -10 -8 -10 -32 -32 -31 -29         -5 -4 -2 -4 -26 -26 -25 -23
    -10   -6 -11 -34 -33 -32 -30 -28       -3   0 -5 -27 -27 -26 -24 -21
    -11   -8 -4  -34 -33 -32 -30 -28       -5  -2  2 -28 -27 -26 -24 -22
  -22 -7 -4 -5  -33 -33 -32 -30        -16 -1  2  1 -27 -27 -25 -24
    -15 -3 -9  -32 -31 -30                 -9  3 -3 -26 -25 -24
      -5 -7 -30 -30                         2 -1 -24 -23
```

TOTAL   PATTERN
DEVIATION   DEVIATION

30°   GLAUCOMA HEMIFIELD TEST (GHT)

OUTSIDE NORMAL LIMITS

PROBABILITY SYMBOLS

:: P < 5%

⊠ P < 2%

▩ P < 1%

■ P < 0.5%

MD   -21.70 DB   P < 0.5%

PSD   12.83 DB   P < 0.5%

SF   2.71 DB   P < 5%

CPSD 12.50 DB   P < 0.5%

A

Figure 8-17. Occipital lobe infarct. Visual fields of a 61-year-old woman with sudden onset of right visual field loss, **(A)** left eye, **(B)** right eye. Fields show a complete right homonymous hemianopia, which appears to split the macula, localizing the lesion to the retrochiasmal portion of the visual pathways. Further localization required neuroimaging, which demonstrated an infarction of the left occipital lobe with sparing of the occipital tip. Macular sparing may be difficult to demonstrate with automated perimetry when the patient has significant fixation losses during examination. Also, if the degree of sparing is less than 6°, it will be missed on the 24-2 and 30-2 programs.

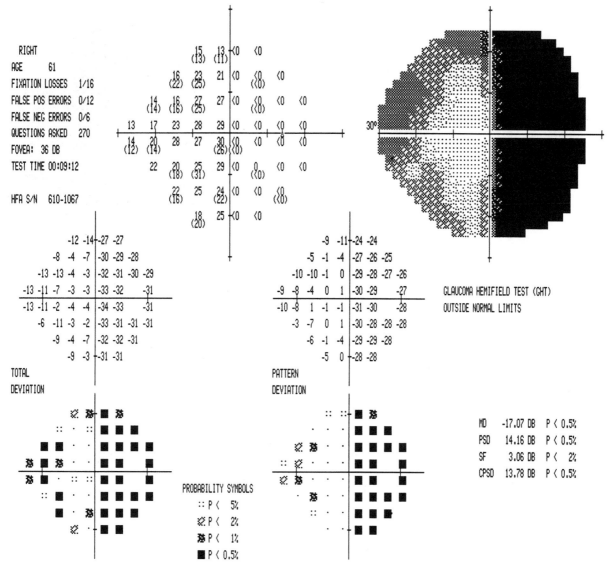

RIGHT

AGE   61

FIXATION LOSSES 1/16

FALSE POS ERRORS 0/12

FALSE NEG ERRORS 0/6

QUESTIONS ASKED 270

FOVEA: 36 DB

TEST TIME 00:09:12

HFA S/N 610-1067

```
            15   13  <0   <0
           (13) (11)
        16   23   21  <0   <0    <0
       (22) (25)        (<0)
     14  16   27   27  <0   <0    <0   <0
    (14)(18) (25)        (<0)
  13  17  23   28   29  <0   <0    <0   <0
  14  20   28   27   30 <0   <0    <0   <0
 (12)(14)          (26)(<0)
     22  20   25   29  <0   0    <0   <0
        (18)(31)        (<0)
        22   25   24  <0   <0    <0
       (16)      (22)        (<0)
            18   25  <0   <0
           (20)
```

30°

GLAUCOMA HEMIFIELD TEST (GHT)
OUTSIDE NORMAL LIMITS

```
     -12 -14 -27 -27                        -9 -11 -24 -24
  -8  -4  -7 -30 -29 -28                  -5  -1  -4 -27 -26 -25
-13 -13  -4  -3 -32 -31 -30 -29       -10 -10  -1   0 -29 -28 -27 -26
-13 -11  -7  -3  -3 -33 -32    -31     -9  -8  -4   0   1 -30 -29    -27
-13 -11  -2  -4  -4 -34 -33    -31    -10  -8   1  -1  -1 -31 -30    -28
 -6 -11  -3  -2 -33 -31 -31 -31        -3  -7   0   1 -30 -28 -28 -28
     -9  -4  -7 -32 -32 -31                -6  -1  -4 -29 -29 -28
     -9  -3 -31 -31                        -5   0 -28 -28
```

TOTAL
DEVIATION

PATTERN
DEVIATION

PROBABILITY SYMBOLS

:: P < 5%

▨ P < 2%

▩ P < 1%

■ P < 0.5%

MD	-17.07 DB	P < 0.5%
PSD	14.16 DB	P < 0.5%
SF	3.06 DB	P < 2%
CPSD	13.78 DB	P < 0.5%

B

Figure 8-17. *Continued.*

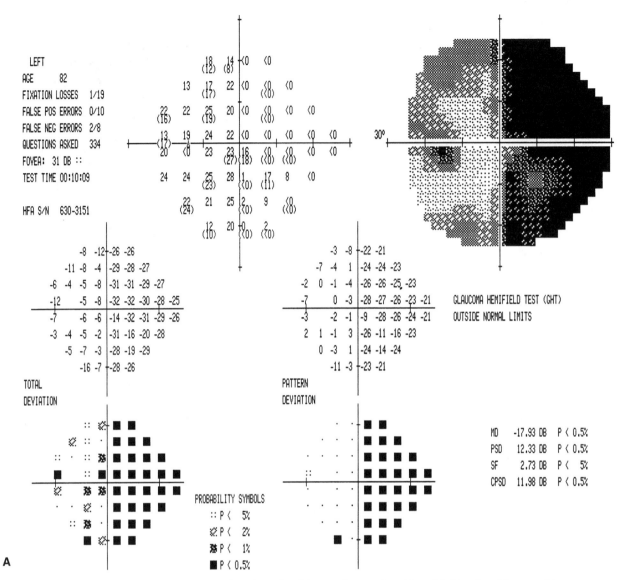

LEFT

AGE   82

FIXATION LOSSES   1/19

FALSE POS ERRORS 0/10

FALSE NEG ERRORS 2/8

QUESTIONS ASKED   334

FOVEA: 31 DB ::

TEST TIME 00:10:09

HFA S/N   630-3151

```
              18  14 <0   <0
             (12) (8)
        13   17  22 <0  <8  <0
            (17)       (8)
   22   22   25  20 <0  <8  <0  <0
  (16)      (19)        (8)
   13   19   24  22 <0  <0  <0  <0  <0
  (12)   8
   20  <0    23  23 16  <8  <8  <0  <0
                (27)(18)  (8) ((8))
   24   24   25  28  1  17   8  <0
            (23)   (0)(11)
        22   21  25  2   9  <8
       (24)        (0)     (0)
             12  20  0   2
            (10)    (0) ((0))
```

```
           -8  -12 -26 -26
      -11  -8   -4 -29 -28 -27
   -6  -4  -5   -8 -31 -31 -29 -27
  -12       -5  -8 -32 -32 -30 -28 -25
   -7       -6  -6 -14 -32 -31 -29 -26
   -3  -4   -5  -2 -31 -16 -20 -28
       -5  -7   -3 -28 -19 -29
          -16  -7 -28 -26
```

TOTAL
DEVIATION

```
              -3  -8 -22 -21
          -7  -4   1 -24 -24 -23
       -2   0  -1  -4 -26 -26 -25 -23
       -7       0  -3 -28 -27 -26 -23 -21
       -3      -2  -1 -9 -28 -26 -24 -21
        2   1  -1   3 -26 -11 -16 -23
            0  -3   1 -24 -14 -24
          -11  -3 -23 -21
```

PATTERN
DEVIATION

GLAUCOMA HEMIFIELD TEST (GHT)
OUTSIDE NORMAL LIMITS

[Total Deviation probability plot]

[Pattern Deviation probability plot]

PROBABILITY SYMBOLS

:: P < 5%

▨ P < 2%

▩ P < 1%

■ P < 0.5%

30°

MD   -17.93 DB   P < 0.5%

PSD   12.33 DB   P < 0.5%

SF   2.73 DB   P < 5%

CPSD   11.98 DB   P < 0.5%

A

Figure 8-18. Right homonymous hemianopia with macular sparing. Visual fields of an 82-year-old man who presented with difficulty reading, **(A)** left eye, **(B)** right eye. Examination led to performance of visual field testing, which showed a right homonymous hemianopia, worse superiorly, which spared the macula inferiorly, seen best on the graytone printout. Neuroimaging revealed a left temporo-occipital infarct.

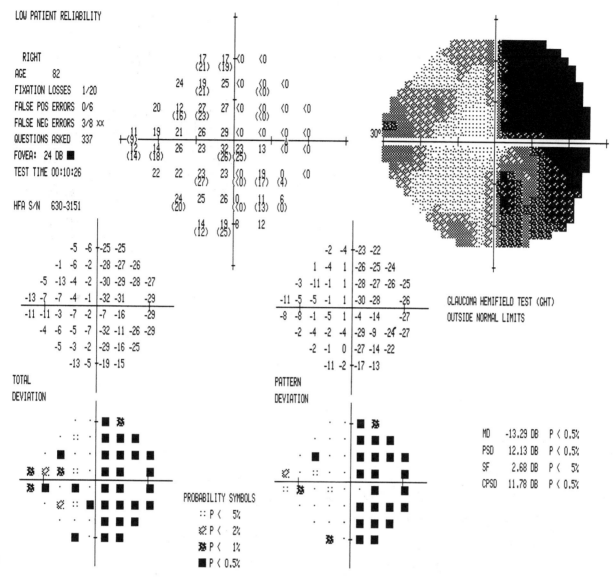

LOW PATIENT RELIABILITY

RIGHT

AGE   82

FIXATION LOSSES   1/20

FALSE POS ERRORS 0/6

FALSE NEG ERRORS 3/8 xx

QUESTIONS ASKED   337

FOVEA: 24 DB ■

TEST TIME 00:10:26

HFA S/N   630-3151

TOTAL
DEVIATION

PATTERN
DEVIATION

GLAUCOMA HEMIFIELD TEST (GHT)
OUTSIDE NORMAL LIMITS

PROBABILITY SYMBOLS

:: P < 5%

⨂ P < 2%

▨ P < 1%

■ P < 0.5%

MD   -13.29 DB   P < 0.5%

PSD   12.13 DB   P < 0.5%

SF   2.68 DB   P < 5%

CPSD 11.78 DB   P < 0.5%

B

Figure 8-18. *Continued.*

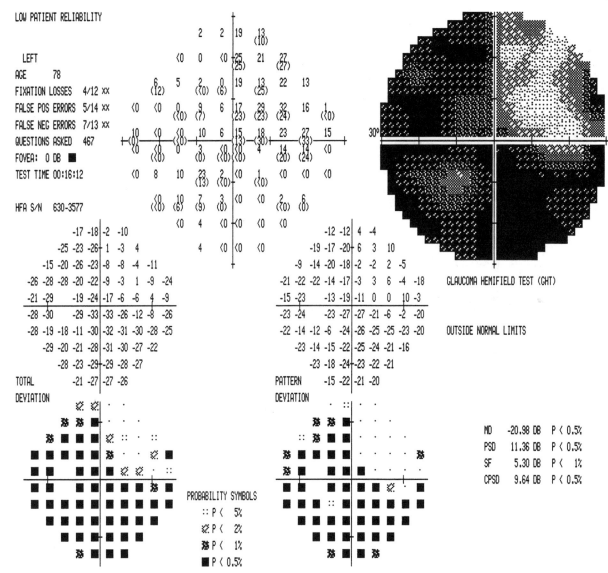

Figure 8-19. Left occipital infarct and chiasmal tumor. Visual fields of a patient with a bitemporal field defect from a pituitary tumor compressing the chiasm, **(A)** left eye, **(B)** right eye. This was resected but the patient developed a right inferior homonymous quadrantanopia 12 years later, secondary to a left occipital infarct. Because the temporal hemifield of the right eye already had a dense defect, the new quadrantanopia was only detectable on the visual field in the left eye.

A

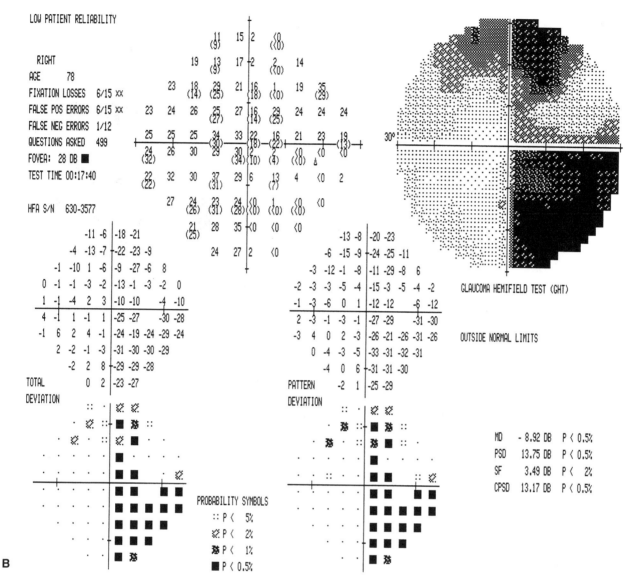

LOW PATIENT RELIABILITY

RIGHT

AGE 78

FIXATION LOSSES 6/15 xx

FALSE POS ERRORS 6/15 xx

FALSE NEG ERRORS 1/12

QUESTIONS ASKED 499

FOVEA: 28 DB ■

TEST TIME 00:17:40

HFA S/N 630-3577

30°

GLAUCOMA HEMIFIELD TEST (GHT)

OUTSIDE NORMAL LIMITS

TOTAL DEVIATION

PATTERN DEVIATION

PROBABILITY SYMBOLS

:: P < 5%

▨ P < 2%

▨ P < 1%

■ P < 0.5%

MD   - 8.92 DB   P < 0.5%

PSD   13.75 DB   P < 0.5%

SF   3.49 DB   P < 2%

CPSD   13.17 DB   P < 0.5%

B

Figure 8-19. *Continued.*

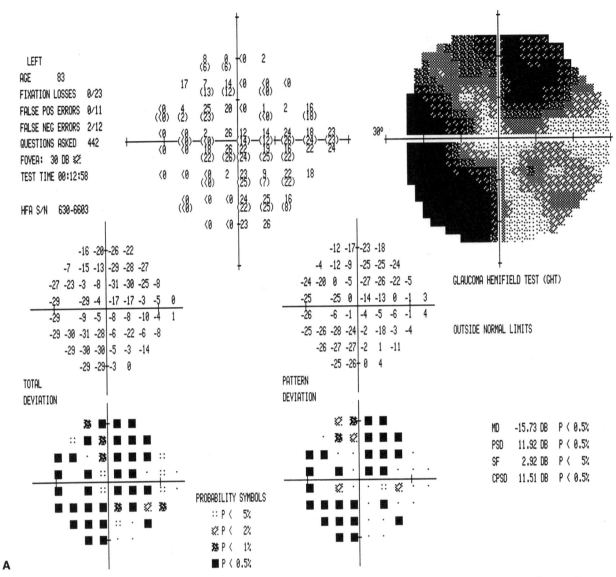

```
LEFT
AGE      83
FIXATION LOSSES   0/23
FALSE POS ERRORS  0/11
FALSE NEG ERRORS  2/12
QUESTIONS ASKED   442
FOVEA: 30 DB
TEST TIME 00:12:58

HFA S/N  630-6603
```

```
              8    8   <0   2
             (6)  (6)
        17    7   14   <0  <8    <0
             (13) (12)      (0)
     <8   4   25   20  <0   0    2    16
     (8) (2) (23)       (0)           (18)
     <0  <8    2   26  12  14   24   18   23
     (0) (8)  (0) (14)(12)(26) (24) (23)
     <0       9   5   8   8   10  4   1
     (0)     (22) (26)(24)(25) (22)
     <0  <0  <8   2  23   9   22   18
         (8)    (25)(7) (22)
         <8  <0  <0  24  25  16
         (8)        (22)(25)(8)
              <0  <0  23   26
```

```
        -16 -20 -26 -22
     -7  -15 -13 -29 -28 -27
  -27 -23  -3  -8 -31 -30 -25  -8
  -29      -29  -4 -17 -17  -3 -5   0
  -29       -9  -5  -8  -8 -10 -4   1
  -29 -30 -31 -28  -6 -22  -6  -8
     -29 -30 -30  -5  -3 -14
        -29 -29  -3   0

TOTAL
DEVIATION
```

```
        -12 -17 -23 -18
     -4  -12  -9 -25 -25 -24
  -24 -20   0  -5 -27 -26 -22  -5
  -25      -25   0 -14 -13  0 -1   3
  -26       -6  -1  -4  -5 -6 -1   4
  -25 -26 -28 -24  -2 -18 -3  -4
     -26 -27 -27  -2   1 -11
        -25 -26   0   4

PATTERN
DEVIATION
```

GLAUCOMA HEMIFIELD TEST (GHT)

OUTSIDE NORMAL LIMITS

```
MD   -15.73 DB   P < 0.5%
PSD   11.92 DB   P < 0.5%
SF     2.92 DB   P <  5%
CPSD  11.51 DB   P < 0.5%
```

```
PROBABILITY SYMBOLS
  :: P <  5%
  ⚟ P <  2%
  ▧ P <  1%
  ■ P < 0.5%
```

A

Figure 8-20. Bilateral occipital infarcts. Congruous defects in the left hemifield and right superior quadrants are seen on the visual fields of this 83-year-old man who sustained bilateral occipital infarcts.

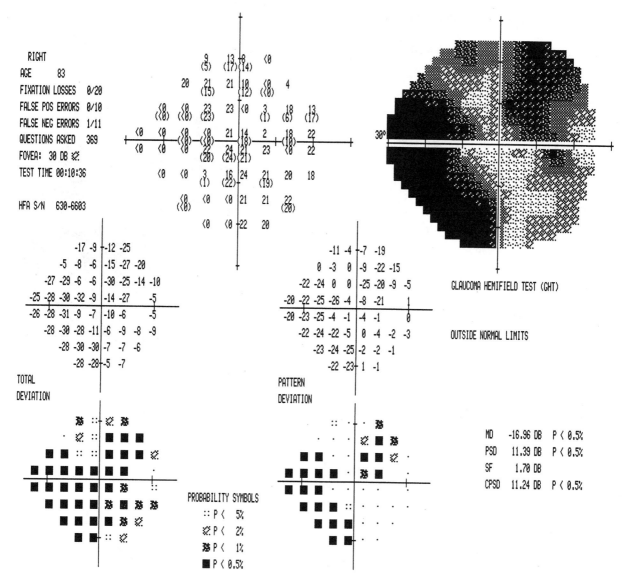

RIGHT

AGE 83

FIXATION LOSSES 0/20

FALSE POS ERRORS 0/10

FALSE NEG ERRORS 1/11

QUESTIONS ASKED 369

FOVEA: 30 DB

TEST TIME 00:10:36

HFA S/N 630-6603

GLAUCOMA HEMIFIELD TEST (GHT)

OUTSIDE NORMAL LIMITS

TOTAL DEVIATION

PATTERN DEVIATION

PROBABILITY SYMBOLS

:: P < 5%

P < 2%

P < 1%

■ P < 0.5%

MD -16.96 DB P < 0.5%

PSD 11.39 DB P < 0.5%

SF 1.70 DB

CPSD 11.24 DB P < 0.5%

B

Figure 8-20. *Continued.*

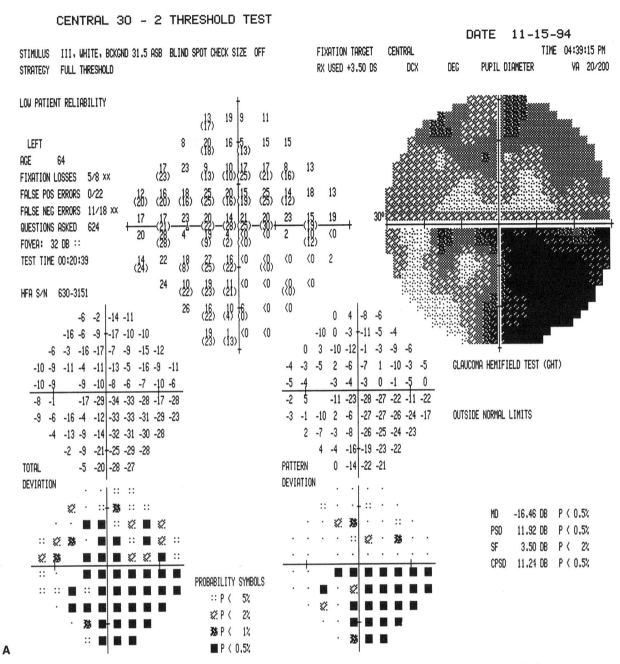

Figure 8-21. Bilateral occipital infarcts. Bilateral visual fields of a 64-year-old woman who had a hypoperfusion injury to the occipital lobe, **(A)** left eye, **(B)** right eye. MRI showed an infarct of the left occipital cortex, which caused the inferior congruous right homonymous defect. MRI also showed an infarct of the right occipital tip, which caused the central defect on the left involving fixation.

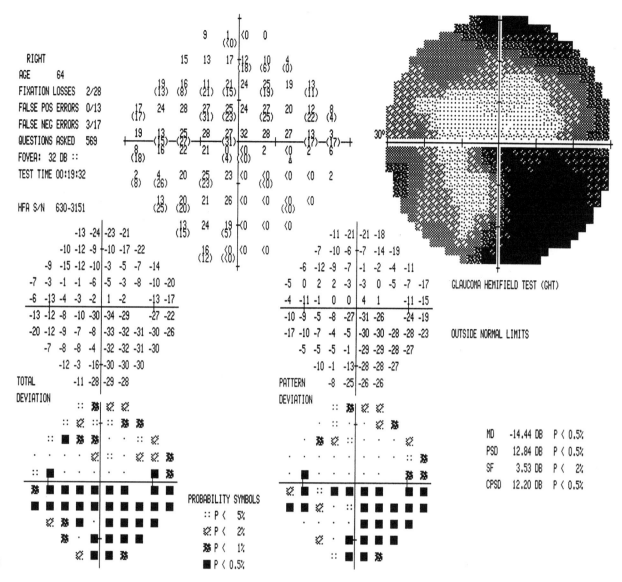

Figure 8-21. *Continued.*

References

1. Smith JL. Homonomous hemianopia: A review of 100 cases. Am J Ophthalmol 1962;54:616.
2. Miller NR. Clinical Neuro-ophthalmology. 4th ed. Baltimore: Williams and Wilkins, vol 1:1982:138.

9

Nonphysiologic Visual Field Loss

Donald A. Budenz

Visual fields associated with hysteria and malingering have been termed "nonphysiologic" or "functional" visual fields. In one large study, functional visual fields were the presenting problem in just over half of the patients presenting with functional visual loss.[1] Such a diagnosis is suspected when the visual field results are out of keeping with the clinical findings or if the pattern of field loss does not fit with any known pathologic process. Because the visual fields in these patients tend to be reliable,[2] means other than reliability parameters must be used to identify them as factitious, these include testing the field binocularly to determine if the defects are real or using tangent screen testing at various distances to detect nonexpanding visual fields.[3]

Figures 9.1–9.5 follow on pages 318–330.

References appear on page 331.

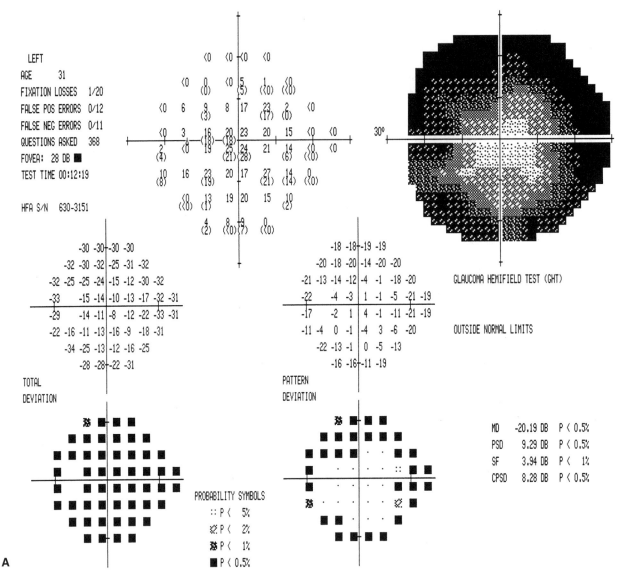

Figure 9-1. Constricted visual fields. Visual fields of a 31-year-old man who was involved in a motor vehicle accident that resulted in blunt head trauma, **(A)** left eye, **(B)** right eye. The patient presented with nonspecific visual complaints and was found to have severe constriction of both fields despite a normal ophthalmologic examination. The field was retested using the tangent screen and found to be tubular (ie, did not expand on doubling the test distance even though the size of the stimulus was also doubled). A diagnosis of nonorganic visual field loss was made.

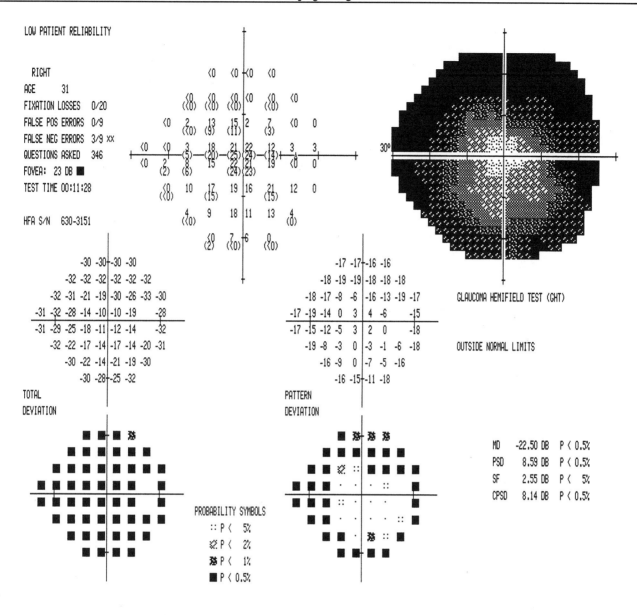

LOW PATIENT RELIABILITY

RIGHT
AGE 31
FIXATION LOSSES 0/20
FALSE POS ERRORS 0/9
FALSE NEG ERRORS 3/9 xx
QUESTIONS ASKED 346
FOVEA: 23 DB ■
TEST TIME 00:11:28

HFA S/N 630-3151

GLAUCOMA HEMIFIELD TEST (GHT)

OUTSIDE NORMAL LIMITS

TOTAL DEVIATION

PATTERN DEVIATION

PROBABILITY SYMBOLS
:: P < 5%
▨ P < 2%
▨ P < 1%
■ P < 0.5%

MD -22.50 DB P < 0.5%
PSD 8.59 DB P < 0.5%
SF 2.55 DB P < 5%
CPSD 8.14 DB P < 0.5%

REV BF X1

SYM										
ASB	.8 –.1	2.5 –1	8 –3.2	25 –10	79 –32	251 –100	794 –316	2512 –1000	7943 –3162	≥ 10000
DB	41 –50	36 –40	31 –35	26 –30	21 –25	16 –20	11 –15	6 –10	1 –5	≤0

B

Figure 9-1. *Continued.*

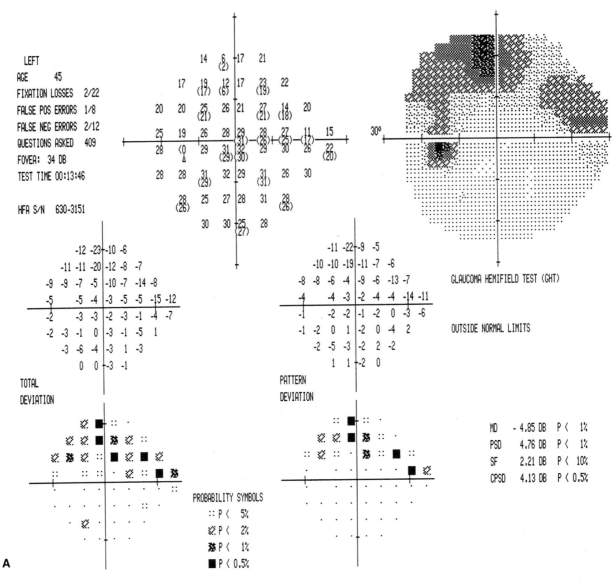

LEFT

AGE   45

FIXATION LOSSES   2/22

FALSE POS ERRORS 1/8

FALSE NEG ERRORS 2/12

QUESTIONS ASKED   409

FOVEA: 34 DB

TEST TIME 00:13:46

HFA S/N   630-3151

TOTAL
DEVIATION

PATTERN
DEVIATION

GLAUCOMA HEMIFIELD TEST (GHT)

OUTSIDE NORMAL LIMITS

MD   - 4.85 DB   P <   1%

PSD   4.76 DB   P <   1%

SF   2.21 DB   P < 10%

CPSD   4.13 DB   P < 0.5%

PROBABILITY SYMBOLS

:: P < 5%

⚏ P < 2%

⚌ P < 1%

■ P < 0.5%

A

Figure 9-2. Unilateral functional visual field loss. Visual fields of a 45-year-old woman who presented with nonspecific visual complaints. Complete eye examination was normal. Visual field testing showed nonspecific superior depression in the left eye **(A)** and a unilateral inferior quadrantanopia in the right eye **(B)**. Visual field testing performed with both eyes open **(C)** showed persistence of the inferior quadrantanopia, indicating that the defect was nonphysiologic in nature. When confronted with potentially fictitious visual field defects in only one eye, with normal areas in the same regions of the contralateral eye, recheck the field binocularly. If the defect persists on binocular testing, the diagnosis of functional visual field loss may be made.

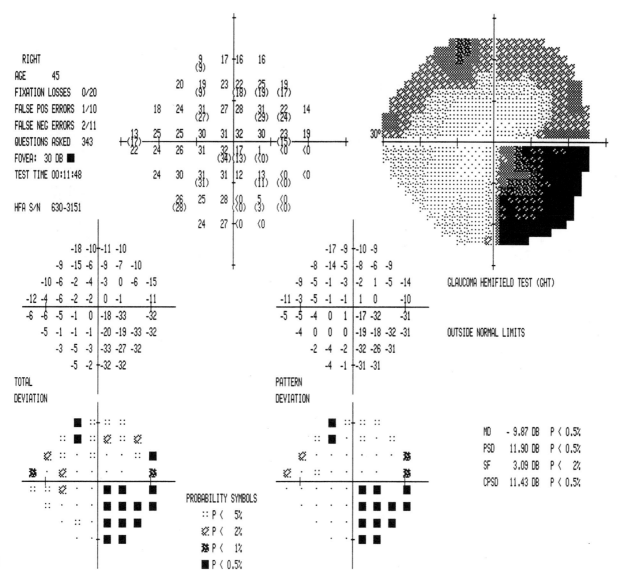

RIGHT

AGE 45

FIXATION LOSSES 0/20

FALSE POS ERRORS 1/10

FALSE NEG ERRORS 2/11

QUESTIONS ASKED 343

FOVEA: 30 DB ■

TEST TIME 00:11:48

HFA S/N 630-3151

```
                    8
                   (9)   17 +16   16
            20    19     23  22    25    19
                 (9)        (18)  (19)  (17)
         18  24  31     27  28    31    22    14
                 (27)             (29)  (24)
     13  25  25  30     31  32     30    23    19
    (17)                                (15)
     22  24  26  31     32 17      1    (0
                       (34)(13)   (0)
         24  30  31     31  12    13    (8    (0
                 (31)            (11)   (8)
            26   25     28  (8    5    (8
           (28)          (0)   (3)   (0)
            24   27    (0    (0
```

```
              -18 -10 +-11 -10
           -9 -15 -6 |-9  -7  -10
        -10 -6 -2 -4 |-3   0  -6  -15
     -12 -4  -6 -2 -2 |0  -1      -11
      -6 -6  -5 -1  0 |-18 -33     -32
         -5 -1 -1 -1 |-20 -19 -33 -32
            -3 -5 -3 |-33 -27 -32
               -5 -2 +-32 -32
```

TOTAL
DEVIATION

```
              -17 -9 +-10 -9
           -8 -14 -5 |-8  -6  -9
        -9 -5 -1 -3 |-2   1  -5  -14
     -11 -3 -5 -1 -1 |1   0      -10
      -5 -5 -4  0  1 |-17 -32    -31
         -4  0  0  0 |-19 -18 -32 -31
            -2 -4 -2 |-32 -26 -31
               -4 -1 +-31 -31
```

PATTERN
DEVIATION

GLAUCOMA HEMIFIELD TEST (GHT)

OUTSIDE NORMAL LIMITS

MD   - 9.87 DB   P < 0.5%

PSD   11.90 DB   P < 0.5%

SF   3.09 DB   P < 2%

CPSD   11.43 DB   P < 0.5%

PROBABILITY SYMBOLS

   :: P < 5%

   ▨ P < 2%

   ▩ P < 1%

   ■ P < 0.5%

B

Figure 9-2. *Continued.*

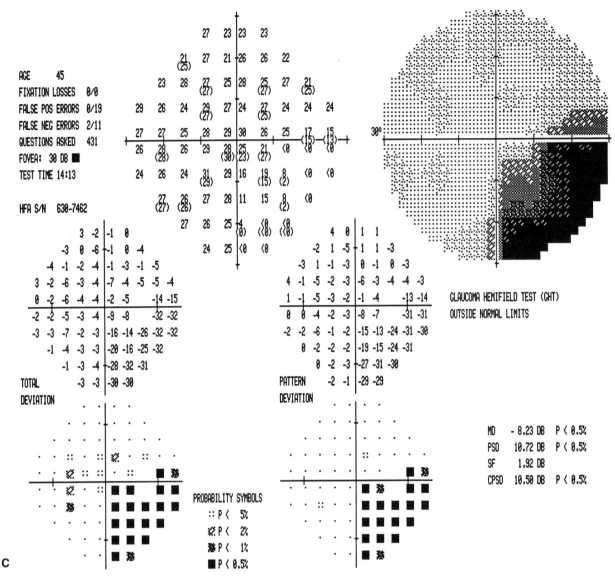

```
                              27   23  23   23

                                21   27   21  26   26   22
                               (25)
AGE      45                23   28    27   25  28    25   27   21
                                     (27)          (27)      (25)
FIXATION LOSSES  0/0
                         29   26   24    29   27  24    27  24    24   24
FALSE POS ERRORS  0/19                  (27)          (25)

FALSE NEG ERRORS  2/11    27   27   25    28   29  30    26   25  17   15
                                                              (15)  (13)
QUESTIONS ASKED   431     26    28   26   29    28  25    21    0
                              (28)           (30)(23)  (27)
FOVEA:  30 DB ■
                         24   26   24    31   29  16    19    8    0    0
TEST TIME 14:13                          (29)        (15)  (2)

                              27   26   27   28  11    15    8    0
HFA S/N   630-7462            (27) (26)                     (2)

                                    27   26   25  4    0    0
                                                 (0)  (0)  (0)
                                         24   25  0    0
```

```
              3  -2 |-1   0                                    4   0 | 1   1
          -3   0  -6 |-1   0  -4                          -2   1  -5 | 1   1  -3
       -4  -1  -2  -4 |-1  -3  -1  -5                  -3   1  -1  -3 | 0  -1   0  -3
    3  -2  -6  -3  -4 |-7  -4  -5  -5  -4           4  -1  -5  -2  -3 |-6  -3  -4  -4  -3
    0  -2  -6  -4  -4 |-2  -5      -14 -15          1  -1  -5  -3  -2 |-1  -4     -13 -14
   -2  -2  -5  -3  -4 |-9  -8      -32 -32          0   0  -4  -2  -3 |-8  -7     -31 -31
   -3  -3  -7  -2  -3 |-16 -14 -26 -32 -32         -2  -2  -6  -1  -2 |-15 -13 -24 -31 -30
      -1  -4  -3  -3 |-20 -16 -25 -32                  0  -2  -2  -2 |-19 -15 -24 -31
         -1  -3  -4 |-28 -32 -31                          0  -2  -3 |-27 -31 -30
TOTAL        -3  -3 |-30 -30                 PATTERN       -2  -1 |-29 -29
DEVIATION                                    DEVIATION
```

GLAUCOMA HEMIFIELD TEST (GHT)

OUTSIDE NORMAL LIMITS

MD   - 8.23 DB   P < 0.5%

PSD   10.72 DB   P < 0.5%

SF   1.92 DB

CPSD   10.50 DB   P < 0.5%

PROBABILITY SYMBOLS

:: P < 5%

▨ P < 2%

▩ P < 1%

■ P < 0.5%

C

Figure 9-2. *Continued.*

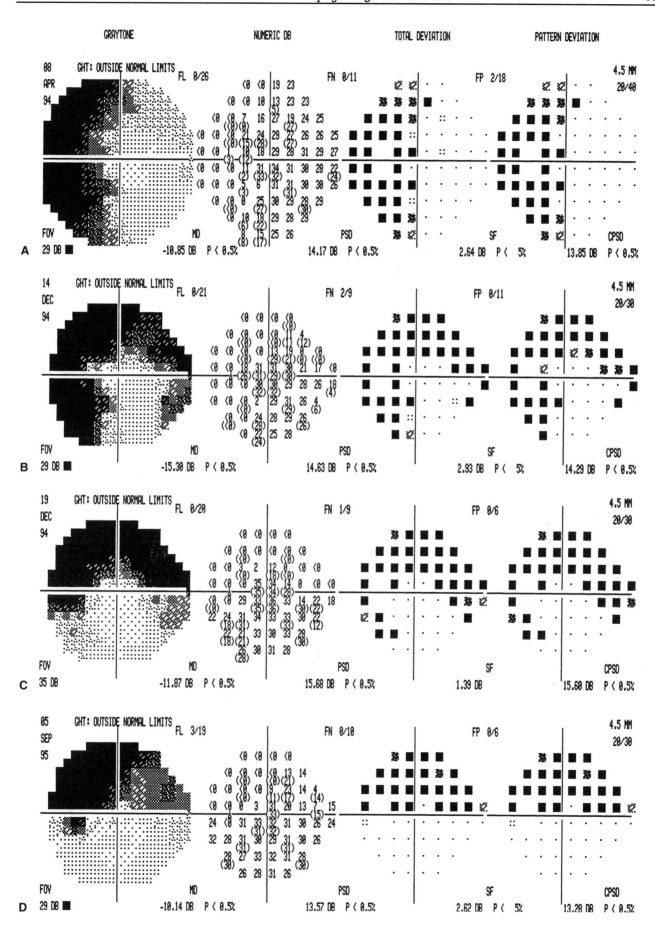

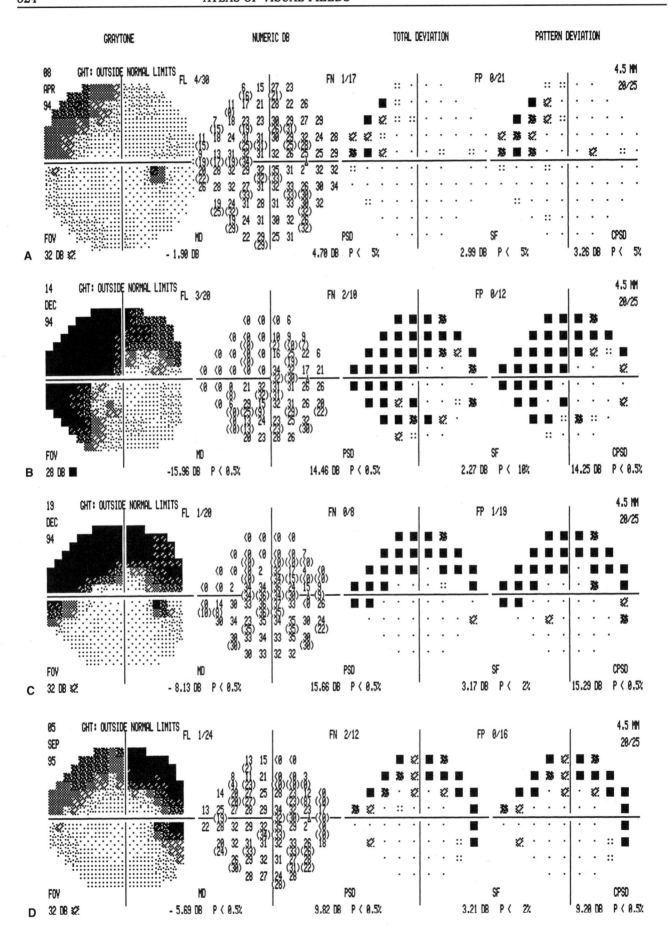

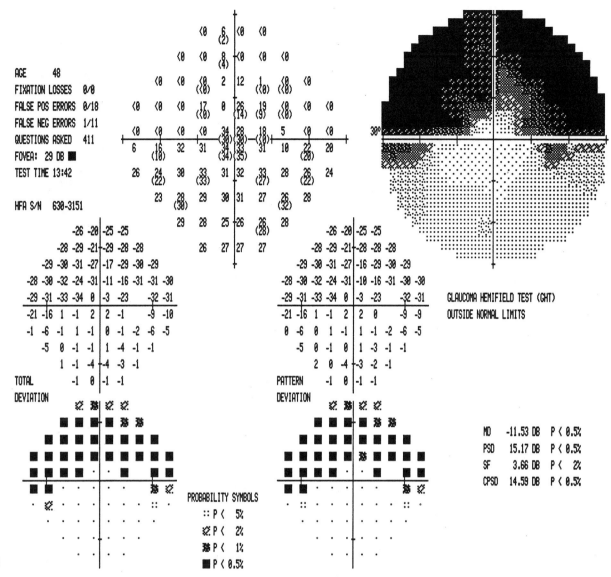

AGE 48
FIXATION LOSSES 0/0
FALSE POS ERRORS 0/18
FALSE NEG ERRORS 1/11
QUESTIONS ASKED 411
FOVEA: 29 DB ■
TEST TIME 13:42

HFA S/N 630-3151

GLAUCOMA HEMIFIELD TEST (GHT)
OUTSIDE NORMAL LIMITS

TOTAL
DEVIATION

PATTERN
DEVIATION

PROBABILITY SYMBOLS
:: P < 5%
▨ P < 2%
▩ P < 1%
■ P < 0.5%

MD   -11.53 DB   P < 0.5%
PSD   15.17 DB   P < 0.5%
SF   3.66 DB   P < 2%
CPSD 14.59 DB   P < 0.5%

E

Figure 9-3. Bilateral functional visual field loss. Fluctuating visual fields in a 47-year-old woman who had undergone surgery in the left eye for glaucoma. Fields numbered 1 are from the left eye, fields numbered 2 are from the right eye. Fields **A1 A2** suggested an incongruous left hemianopia, prompting an MRI, which was normal. Fields **B1 B2** showed a superior defect that crossed the vertical meridian. The field was repeated with the eyelids taped to rule out lid artifact (Fields **C1 C2**), and improved, but mostly inferiorly and were inconsistent with previous findings. Fields **D1 D2** were different from all previous fields. Binocular field testing was performed (Field **E**), which confirmed the suspicion of functional visual field loss since a dense superior defects persisted despite having both eyes open. Inconsistency in visual field results over time should raise the perimetrist's suspicion of functional field loss, particularly if the visual fields do not correlate with clinical findings. Although the patient had a history of elevated intraocular pressures, there was insufficient cupping to explain the field loss.

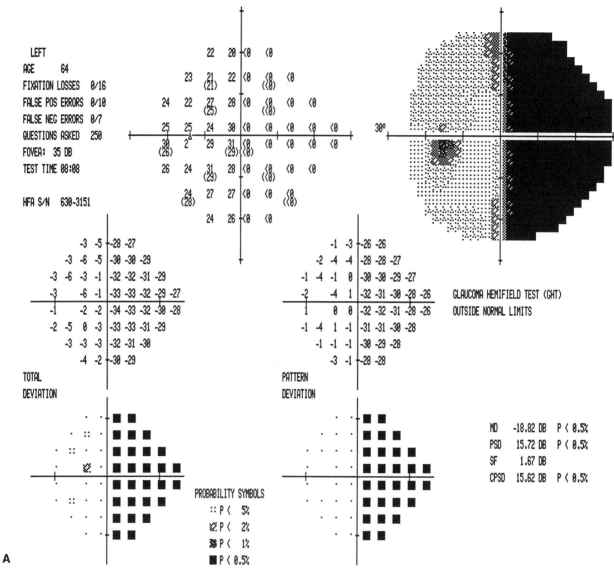

Figure 9-4. Functional visual field loss. Visual fields of a 64-year-old woman referred for neuro-ophthalmic consultation because of binasal hemianopic field defects, **(A)** left eye, **(B)** right eye. Examination, including confrontation visual fields, was entirely normal. Binasal hemianopia respecting the vertical meridian would be an exceedingly rare finding related to simultaneous compression of both lateral aspects of the optic chiasm. This patient did not have any abnormality of the optic nerves, which excludes this diagnosis. Other diagnoses that can cause binasal field defects include retinoschisis, sector retinitis pigmentosa, glaucomatous, and nonglaucomatous optic neuropathies. However, none of these disorders, which would be apparent ophthalmoscopically, would cause defects that respect the vertical meridian in both eyes.

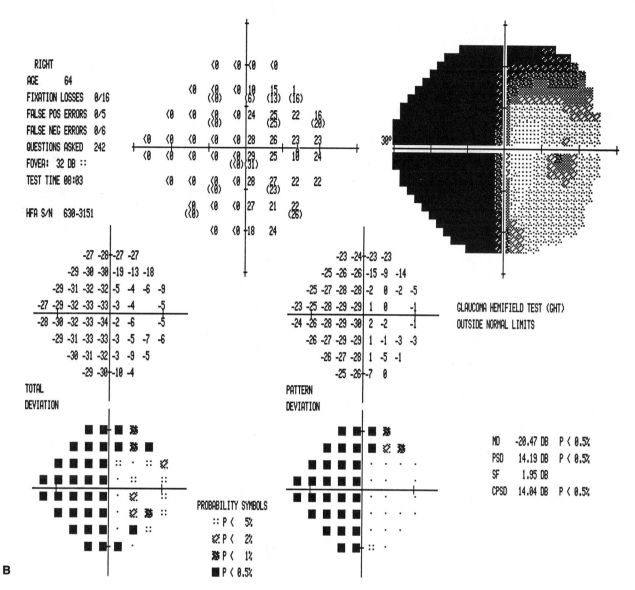

Figure 9-4. *Continued.*

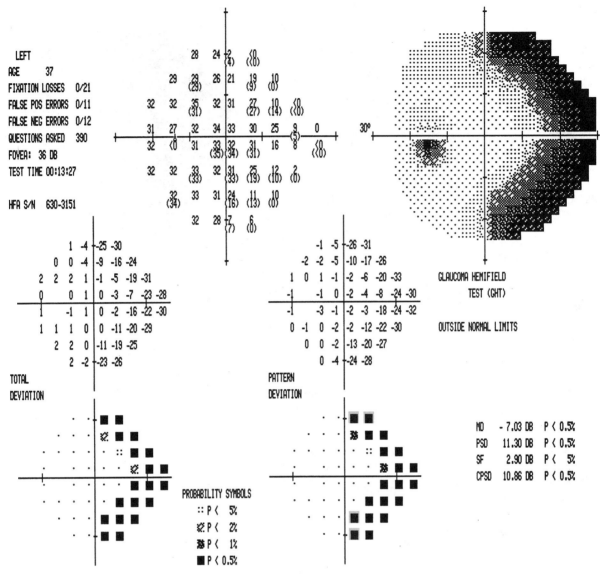

LEFT

AGE   37
FIXATION LOSSES   0/21
FALSE POS ERRORS 0/11
FALSE NEG ERRORS 0/12
QUESTIONS ASKED   390
FOVEA: 36 DB
TEST TIME 00:13:27

HFA S/N   630-3151

```
            28  24  2   (8
                    (4)  (8)
        29  29  26  21  19  10
            (29)        (9) (0)
    32  32  35  32  31  27  10  (8
            (31)        (27)(14) (8)
    31  27  32  34  33  30  25  9   0
    32  (0  31  33  32  31  16  8
            (35)(34)(31)          (8)
    32  32  33  32  31  25  12  2
            (33)    (33)(19)(10) (0)
        32  33  31  24  11  10
        (34)        (16)(13) (0)
            32  28  7   6
                    (7) (0)
```

```
        1  -4 -25 -30           -1  -5 -26 -31
     0  0  -4 -9 -16 -24     -2 -2 -5 -10 -17 -26
  2  2  2  1 -1  -5 -19 -31  1  0  1 -1 -2 -6 -20 -33
  0     0  1  0  -3  -7 -23 -28  -1    -1  0 -2 -4 -8 -24 -30
  1    -1  1  0  -2 -16 -22 -30  -1    -3 -1 -2 -3 -18 -24 -32
  1  1  1  0  0 -11 -20 -29  0 -1  0 -2 -2 -12 -22 -30
     2  2  0 -11 -19 -25       0  0 -2 -13 -20 -27
        2 -2 -23 -26              0  -4 -24 -28
```

30°

GLAUCOMA HEMIFIELD
TEST (GHT)

OUTSIDE NORMAL LIMITS

TOTAL
DEVIATION

PATTERN
DEVIATION

PROBABILITY SYMBOLS
:: P < 5%
▨ P < 2%
▩ P < 1%
■ P < 0.5%

MD   - 7.03 DB P < 0.5%
PSD   11.30 DB P < 0.5%
SF   2.90 DB P < 5%
CPSD 10.86 DB P < 0.5%

A

Figure 9-5. Functional visual field loss. Bilateral central 24° visual fields of a 37-year-old woman suspected of malingering, **(A)** left eye, **(B)** right eye. The visual field pattern looks like a right homonymous hemianopia with macular sparing. Several repeat fields performed over several months showed persistent, but slightly dissimilar, defects on each occasion. Magnetic resonance imaging was normal. A central 30° field performed with both eyes open **(C)** shows a defect that does not come up to the vertical meridian. The points adjacent to the vertical meridian (*highlighted*) should be abnormal in the bilateral field since they are abnormal in both eyes in the monocular fields at corresponding points. In addition, binocular visual field testing using a tangent screen failed to confirm the defect. (Courtesy of R. Michael Siatowski, M.D.).

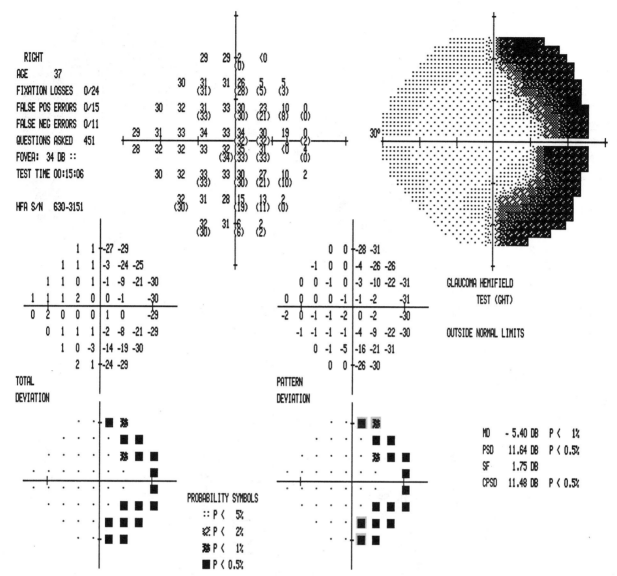

Figure 9-5. *Continued.*

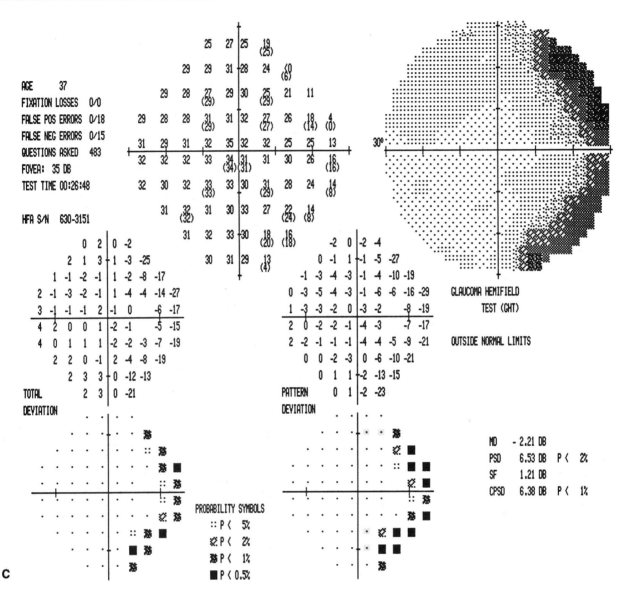

Figure 9-5. *Continued.*

References

1. Keltner JL, May WN, Johnson CA, Post RB. The California syndrome: functional visual loss with potential economic impact. Ophthalmology 1985;92:427.
2. Smith TJ, Baker RS. Perimetric findings in functional disorders using automated testing. Ophthalmology 1987;94:1562.
3. Glaser J. S. Neuro-ophthalmic examination: The visual sensory system. In: Glaser, JS, ed. Neuro-ophthalmology. 2nd ed. Philadelphia: Lippincott, 1990:30.

10

Blepharoptosis

Donald L. Budenz

Upper eyelid ptosis has been shown to decrease the superior visual field by 8° per millimeter of ptosis.[1] We have already examined how eyelid or eyebrow ptosis can cause artifactual visual field defects (Chapter 2, figures 2-7 and 2-8). Measurement of the superior visual field using visual field testing has become an essential part of the preoperative work-up of the patient with ptosis. Ptosis surgery has been shown to improve the superior visual field, both in primary gaze and while reading.[2] Prior to surgery, the superior visual field is measured in primary gaze without the upper eyelid taped to determine the amount of disability due to the ptosis and with the upper eyelid taped to determine the amount of improvement expected after surgery.[3]

Suprathreshold testing using automated perimetry is a fast and accurate way to quantitate the amount of superior visual field loss from ptosis as well as to approximate the amount of expected improvement. The Humphrey and Octopus perimeters both have "blepharoptosis" programs designed for this purpose. The Humphrey blepharoptosis program presents suprathreshold stimuli (10 dB) in the superior field from 20° to 60° in the vertical meridian and from 10° to 40° in both horizontal meridians. An example is shown in Figure 10-1.

References appear on page 336.

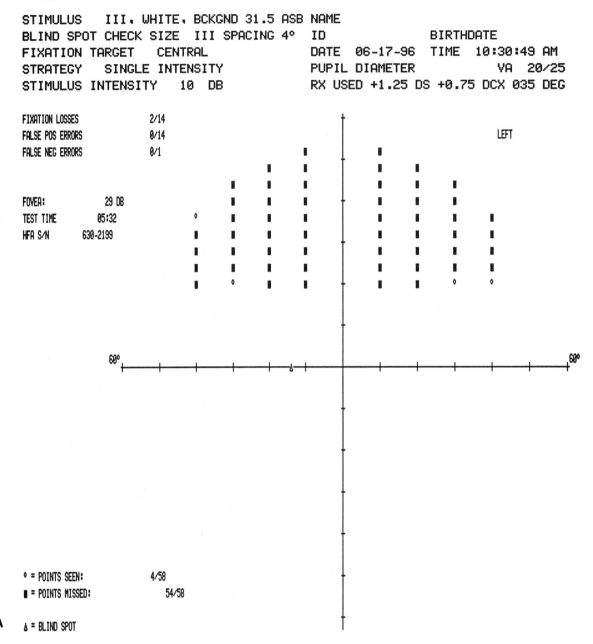

BLEPH SCREENING TEST

STIMULUS   III. WHITE. BCKGND 31.5 ASB NAME
BLIND SPOT CHECK SIZE   III SPACING 4°   ID   BIRTHDATE
FIXATION TARGET   CENTRAL   DATE 06-17-96 TIME 10:30:49 AM
STRATEGY   SINGLE INTENSITY   PUPIL DIAMETER   VA 20/25
STIMULUS INTENSITY   10 DB   RX USED +1.25 DS +0.75 DCX 035 DEG

FIXATION LOSSES   2/14
FALSE POS ERRORS   0/14   LEFT
FALSE NEG ERRORS   0/1

FOVEA: 29 DB
TEST TIME   05:32
HFA S/N   630-2199

                60°   60°

° = POINTS SEEN: 4/58
■ = POINTS MISSED: 54/58

A   ▲ = BLIND SPOT

Figure 10-1. Blepharoptosis fields. Suprathreshold visual field testing of the left eye of a patient with ptosis of the left upper eyelid. Visual field **A** was performed with the patient in the relaxed state without eyelid taping. Locations where the stimuli were seen are recorded as open circles and those that were not are recorded as solid rectangles. The patient missed 54 of the 58 suprathreshold stimuli presented in the superior field.

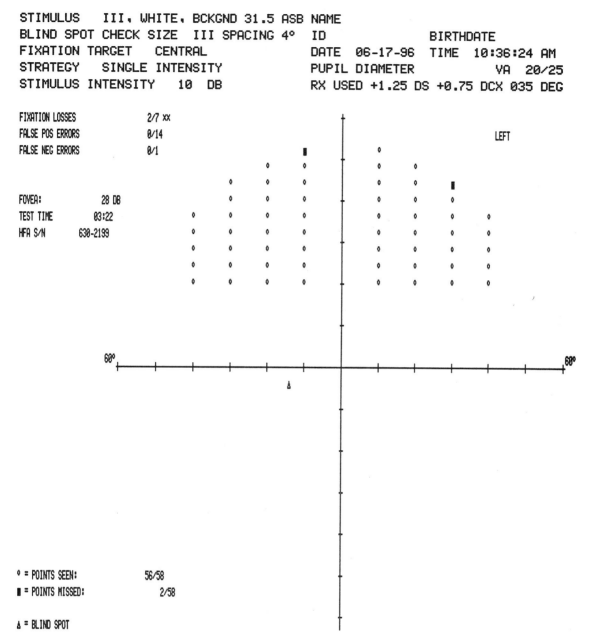

BLEPH SCREENING TEST

STIMULUS   III, WHITE, BCKGND 31.5 ASB NAME
BLIND SPOT CHECK SIZE   III SPACING 4°   ID   BIRTHDATE
FIXATION TARGET   CENTRAL   DATE 06-17-96 TIME 10:36:24 AM
STRATEGY   SINGLE INTENSITY   PUPIL DIAMETER   VA 20/25
STIMULUS INTENSITY   10 DB   RX USED +1.25 DS +0.75 DCX 035 DEG

FIXATION LOSSES   2/7 xx
FALSE POS ERRORS   0/14   LEFT
FALSE NEG ERRORS   0/1

FOVEA: 28 DB
TEST TIME   03:22
HFA S/N   630-2199

60°   60°

Δ

° = POINTS SEEN: 56/58
■ = POINTS MISSED: 2/58

B   Δ = BLIND SPOT

Figure 10-1. *Continued.* **(B)** After the upper eyelid was taped, the patient only missed 2 of the 58 stimuli presented.

References

1. Meyer DR, Linberg JV, Powell SR, Odom JV. Quantitating the superior visual field loss associated with ptosis. Arch Ophthalmol 1989;107:840.
2. Patipa M. Visual field loss in primary gaze and reading gaze due to acquired blepharoptosis and visual field improvement following ptosis surgery. Arch Ophthalmol 1992;110:63.
3. Putnam JR, Nunery WR, Tanenbaum M, McCord CD. Blepharoptosis. In: McCord CD, Tanenbaum M, Nunery WR, eds. Oculoplastic surgery. 3rd ed. New York: Raven Press, 1995:175.

11

Assessing Visual Disability

Donald L. Budenz and Steven J. Gedde

Previous chapters have dealt with the assessment of the monocular visual field in the diagnosis and follow-up of disorders affecting the visual pathways. Binocular suprathreshold screening testing with the automated perimeter is a fast and effective way to assess visual field function. Esterman has developed a binocular field test for the automated static perimeter[1] to measure visual field disability.

The Esterman test, available on most automated perimeters, is based on the principal that some regions of the visual field are functionally more important than others. The binocular version of the test presents suprathreshold stimuli equivalent to a III4e (10 dB) target on the Goldmann perimeter at 120 loci throughout the visual field, including 150° in the horizontal meridian (75° in each direction) and 100° in the vertical meridian (40° superiorly and 60° inferiorly). More stimuli are presented centrally, inferiorly, and along the horizontal meridian than at other locations as these areas of the visual field are thought to be the most important functionally. (Figure 11-1) Points that are missed are retested once before a miss is recorded. The percentage of points seen by the patient comprises the Esterman efficiency score.

The Esterman test has been used to assess visual field disability in workers' compensation patients, motor vehicle license applicants, and patients with severe visual field loss due to glaucoma. The Esterman scoring system has been adopted by the American Medical Association as a standard for rating visual disability[2] Visual standards for driving vary from state to state[3] but usually include a component of visual field. The visual field requirement typically consists of the ability to see for at least 120° to 140° in the horizontal meridian with both eyes together. The Esterman test can be used to document the extent of the binocular horizontal field for drivers license requirements. In addition, the Esterman test has been used to assess functional disability in patients with glaucoma[4].

Figures 11.1–11.2 follow on pages 338–341.

References appear on page 342.

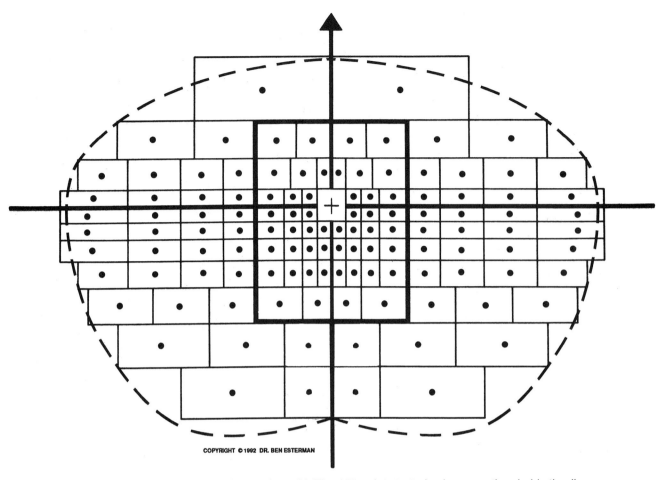

COPYRIGHT © 1992 DR. BEN ESTERMAN

Figure 11-1. Esterman binocular scoring grid. The 120 points tested using suprathreshold stimuli are shown . Each point is assigned a value of 1. Points are more highly concentrated centrally, inferiorly, and along the horizontal meridian. The number of points seen is multiplied by 5/6 to obtain the Esterman efficiency score. A score of 100 means that the patient saw all 120 stimuli presented.

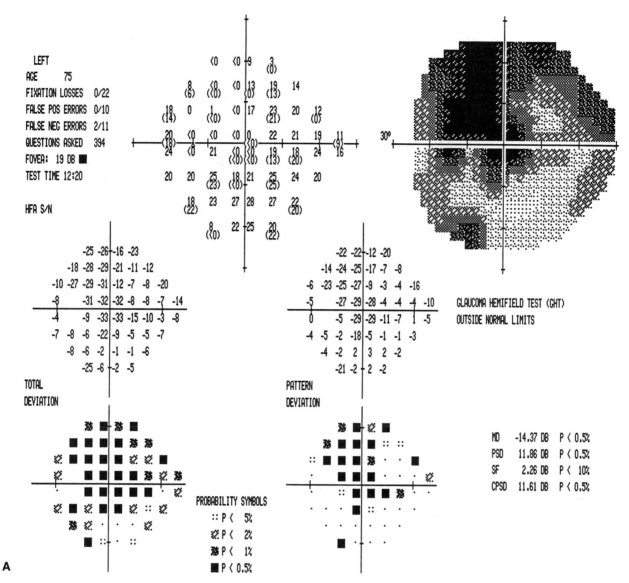

LEFT

AGE   75

FIXATION LOSSES   0/22

FALSE POS ERRORS   0/10

FALSE NEG ERRORS   2/11

QUESTIONS ASKED   394

FOVEA: 19 DB ■

TEST TIME 12:20

HFA S/N

```
              <0  <0 +9   3
                           (0)
         8    (8) <0  13  19  14
        (8)           (0) (13)
   18    0    1   <0  17  23  20  12
  (14)       (<0)         (21)    (0)
   20  <0   <0   <0  0   22  21  19  11
  (18) <0       21 <0 <8 (19) (18) 24 (9)
   24          (<0)(<0)(13)(20)    16
   20  20   25  18  21  25  24  20
            (23)(<0)    (25)
         18  23  27  28  27  22
        (22)                (20)
          8    22 +25  20
         (0)              (22)
```

```
        -25 -26 -16 -23
      -18 -28 -29 -21 -11 -12
   -10 -27 -29 -31 -12 -7 -8 -20
     -8     -31 -32 -32 -8 -8 -7 -14
     -4     -9 -33 -33 -15 -10 -3 -8
    -7 -8 -6 -22 -9 -5 -5 -7
      -8 -6 -2 -1 -1 -6
      -25 -6  -2 -5
```

TOTAL
DEVIATION

```
         -22 -22 -12 -20
       -14 -24 -25 -17 -7 -8
     -6 -23 -25 -27 -9 -3 -4 -16
     -5     -27 -29 -28 -4 -4 -4 -10
      0     -5 -29 -29 -11 -7  1 -5
    -4 -5 -2 -18 -5 -1 -1 -3
      -4 -2 2  3  2 -2
      -21 -2  2 -2
```

GLAUCOMA HEMIFIELD TEST (GHT)
OUTSIDE NORMAL LIMITS

PATTERN
DEVIATION

PROBABILITY SYMBOLS

∷ P < 5%

▨ P < 2%

▩ P < 1%

■ P < 0.5%

MD	-14.37 DB	P < 0.5%
PSD	11.86 DB	P < 0.5%
SF	2.26 DB	P < 10%
CPSD	11.61 DB	P < 0.5%

A

Figure 11-2. Comparison of central monocular fields and Esterman binocular fields in severe glaucoma. The central 30° fields both meet criteria for severe visual field defects according to criteria outlined in Table 5-4. Note that the areas of the visual field that are lost in the right eye **(B)** are almost the opposite of those in the left eye **(A)**. When the field is measure binocularly using the Esterman test **(C)**, normal areas in each eye compensate for affected areas in the contralateral eye and the Esterman efficiency score is 91% (out of a total possible score of 100%). If one were to base eligibility for driver's license on the monocular central 30° fields, this patient would inappropriately be denied a license in most states, which use a total field of 140° as the requirement. Binocular Esterman testing demonstrates excellent horizontal field capability.

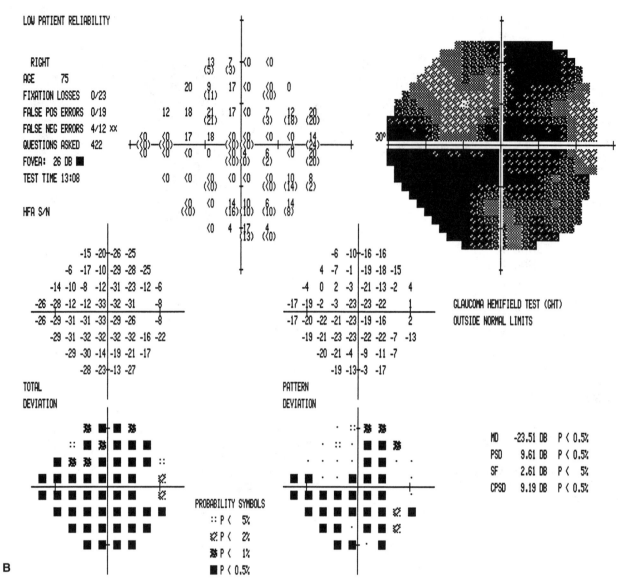

LOW PATIENT RELIABILITY

RIGHT
AGE   75
FIXATION LOSSES   0/23
FALSE POS ERRORS 0/19
FALSE NEG ERRORS 4/12 xx
QUESTIONS ASKED   422
FOVEA: 26 DB ■
TEST TIME 13:08

HFA S/N

```
              13   7  <0   <0
              (5) (3)
          20   9  17  <0   <8   0
              (11)         (8)
      12  18  21  17  <0    7   12  20
              (21)        (3) (18) (20)
  <8   <8  17  18  <8  <8  <0   <0   14
              <0   0    4    6       (24)
                       (0)  (2)      (20)
      <0   <0  <8  <0  <0      <8   10    8
                  (8)              (14)  (2)
          <8   <0  14  10   6   14
          (8)      (16)(10)(10)  (8)
              <0   4  17   4
                      (13) (0)
```

```
      -15 -20 -26 -25                   -6 -10 -16 -16
   -6 -17 -10 -29 -28 -25             4  -7  -1 -19 -18 -15
 -14 -10 -8 -12 -31 -23 -12 -6      -4  0   2  -3 -21 -13 -2  4
-26 -28 -12 -12 -33 -32 -31    -8  -17 -19 -2  -3 -23 -23 -22    1
-26 -29 -31 -31 -33 -29 -26    -8  -17 -20 -22 -21 -23 -19 -16   2
   -29 -31 -32 -32 -32 -32 -16 -22   -19 -21 -23 -23 -22 -22 -7 -13
      -29 -30 -14 -19 -21 -17          -20 -21 -4 -9 -11 -7
         -28 -23 -13 -27                 -19 -13 -3 -17
```

TOTAL
DEVIATION

PATTERN
DEVIATION

GLAUCOMA HEMIFIELD TEST (GHT)
OUTSIDE NORMAL LIMITS

PROBABILITY SYMBOLS
:: P < 5%
▨ P < 2%
▩ P < 1%
■ P < 0.5%

MD   -23.51 DB   P < 0.5%
PSD   9.61 DB   P < 0.5%
SF   2.61 DB   P < 5%
CPSD   9.19 DB   P < 0.5%

B

Figure 11-2. *Continued.*

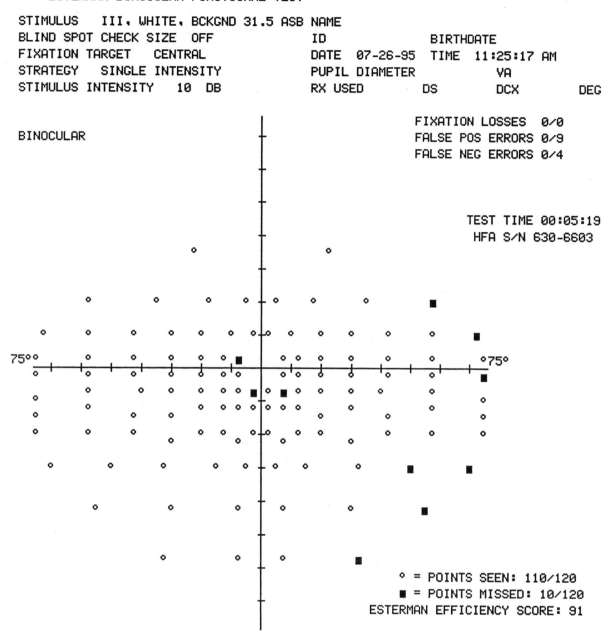

Figure 11-2. *Continued.*

References

1. Esterman B. Functional scoring of the binocular field. Ophthalmology 1982;89:1234.
2. American Medical Association. Guides to the evaluation of permanent impairment. 4th ed. Chicago: American Medical Association, 1994:209.
3. Mahlman HE. Handbook of federal vision requirements and information. 2nd ed. Chicago: Professional Press, 1982:121.
4. Mills RP, Drance SM. Esterman disability rating in severe glaucoma. Ophthalmology 1986;93:371.

Appendix

Test Strategies of the Humphrey Visual Field Analyzer

The following descriptions of the test strategies most commonly used by the Humphrey Visual Field Analyzer is provided for the interested reader. Figures have been redrawn, with permission, from the Humphrey Field Analyzer Manual, Allergan Humphrey, San Leandro, California, 1991.

An alternate strategy for determining threshold values, currently called the Swedish Interactive Thresholding Algorithm, is being released soon. This test begins by determining thresholds at the 4 primary points using the standard 4/2 dB staircase strategy described in Figure APX-1. As the test progresses to neighboring points, the results obtained at the 4 primary points are used as starting points for determining thresholds at the remaining points. However, instead of performing a staircase threshold determination on the remainder of the points, information regarding the expected values in normal and pathologic fields for the patient's age at each location are taken into account, as well as the results of surrounding points. A continuous calculation of threshold estimates based on these factors allows for more precise, and therefore faster, determination of threshold values.

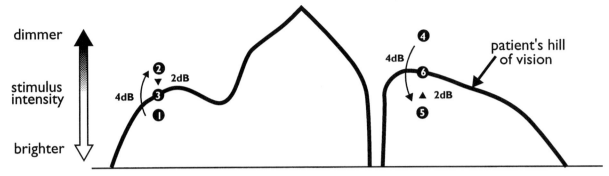

Figure APX-1. Full threshold strategy. Most detailed strategy for determining threshold using a 4/2 dB staircase strategy that crosses threshold twice. A presumed suprathreshold stimulus (based on values obtained for the four primary points as well as surrounding values) is presented (*1*) and, if the subject responds as expected, the stimulus intensity is decreased by 4 dB intervals until the subject does not respond (*2*). When the subject does not respond, the stimulus is increased in intensity by 2 dB intervals until the subject responds (*3*). This stimulus is recorded as the threshold. If the subject does not respond to the initial presumed suprathreshold stimulus (*4*), the stimulus intensity is increased by 4 dB until the subject responds (*5*). When the subject responds, the stimulus intensity is decreased in 2 dB intervals until the subject does not respond. The last stimulus seen (*6*) is recorded as the threshold. The ten points used in the calculation of short-term fluctuation are determined twice using this strategy and the second value is placed in parentheses under the first. In addition, any value that differs by more than 4 dB from that expected in age-matched control subjects is double-determined and the second value appears under the first in parentheses.

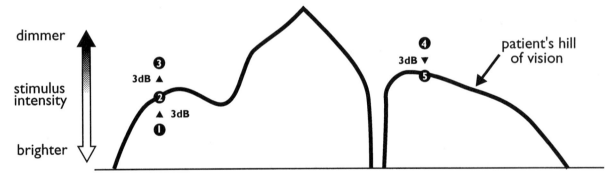

Figure APX-2. FASTPAC. Alternate (faster) strategy for determining threshold values using a 3 dB strategy that crosses threshold only once. In this strategy, a presumed suprathreshold stimulus is presented and, if the subject responds as expected (*1*), the stimulus intensity is decreased by 3 dB intervals until the subject does not respond (*3*). The last seen stimulus is recorded as the threshold (*2*). If the subject does not respond to the initial presumed suprathreshold stimulus (*4*), the stimulus is increased by 3 dB until the subject responds. The first stimulus seen (*5*) is recorded as the threshold. Double determination is performed for the ten locations used to determine short-term fluctuation and at any locations that differ more than 4 dB from expected in age-matched normal control subjects.

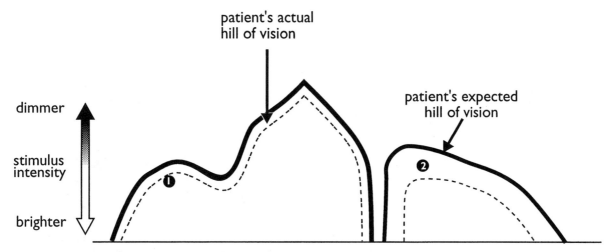

Figure APX-3. Threshold-related suprathreshold screening strategy. In this strategy, the four primary points are determined using the full-threshold strategy described above. Subsequent points are assigned expected values according to a central reference level (CRL), which is derived from the second highest (least intense) threshold at the four primary points or 26 dB, whichever is greater. The perimeter then presents stimuli 6 dB more intense than the expected value. If the patient responds to the presumed suprathreshold stimulus, the point is reported as normal. If it is not seen, the same suprathreshold stimulus is presented again. If not seen a second time, the point is recorded as abnormal. A more useful variation of this test uses a CRL based on data collected from a normal age-adjusted population. Expected values are generated based on this CRL and suprathreshold stimuli 2 dB lower (more intense) than the expected value are projected. If the stimulus is seen (*1*), the location is considered normal. If the suprathreshold point is not seen (*2*), the stimulus is presented a second time. If it is still not seen, the point is recorded as abnormal.

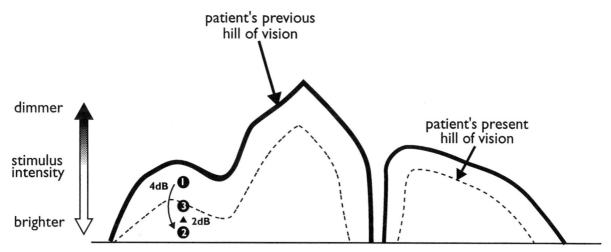

Figure APX-4. Full-threshold from prior data. Instead of determining the sensitivities de novo on a follow-up test, this strategy uses the information from the previous test as a starting point for determining threshold values. The threshold is determined using the full 4/2 dB staircase strategy, but the starting point is closer to the subject's threshold, thus reducing test taking time in most cases. In the above example, a presumed suprathreshold stimulus, based on the subject's previous hill of vision, is presented (*1*). If it is not seen, the stimulus intensity is increased in 4 dB increments until it is seen (*2*). The stimulus intensity is then decreased in 2 dB increments until it is seen for the last time (*3*), and this value is recorded as the threshold.

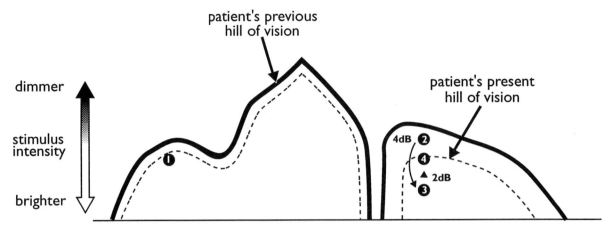

Figure APX-5. Fast threshold. A visual field test used to determine nonprogression from a previous field. In this strategy, the computer presents a stimulus 2 dB brighter than that obtained from a previous baseline test or set of tests (called a master file). If the stimulus is seen (*1*), the point is recorded as unchanged. If the stimulus is not seen after two presentations (*2*), full thresholding is performed as described above (*3, 4*) using the 4/2 dB staircase strategy.

Glossary of Terms

Absolute scotoma: A depression in the visual field in which the largest, brightest stimulus that the perimeter is capable of presenting cannot be seen. The physiologic blind spot is an example of an absolute scotoma.

Apostilb (asb): A measure of luminance, or light intensity. The higher the apostilb value, the more intense the stimulus. The Goldmann and Octopus perimeters can generate a maximal stimulus of 1,000 asb (4e and 0 dB, respectively). The Humphrey perimeter can generate a maximal stimulus of 10,000 asb (0 dB).

Artifact: An abnormality in the visual field caused by anything other than physiologic abnormalities. Common artifacts in visual field testing include inexperience, poor reliability, long-term fluctuation, trial frame lens rim, edge artifact, prominent eyebrow, ptosis, fatigue, small pupil, incorrect refraction, incorrect fixation, and dim projector bulb.

Central reference level (CRL): A value used to calculate a subject's expected hill of vision for threshold-related screening strategies. This value is determined by measuring the threshold at the four primary points, using the full threshold strategy (see Appendix) or may be assigned a value based on the age-matched normal population.

Corrected pattern standard deviation (CPSD): The corrected pattern standard deviation is a measure of the amount of localized depression (as opposed to diffuse depression) of the visual field corrected for the patient's age and short-term fluctuation. A low CPSD indicates that the hill of vision is smooth and a high CPSD indicates that there are localized irregularities in the hill of vision.

Decibel (dB): A measure of attenuation of light. The higher the decibels, the dimmer the stimulus intensity. Because different perimeters have different maximal stimuli (see apostilb), the decibel values are not the same from perimeter to perimeter.

Fixation losses (FL): The fixation loss rate is quantified to get a rough estimate of the percentage of the time the patient fails to look at the central fixation light. It is determined by projecting approximately 5% of the stimuli within the patient's blind spot. Alternate explanations for high fixation losses are described in Chapter 1.

False negatives (FN): A reliability parameter on the Humphrey perimeter. The false negative rate is the percentage of times the patient fails to respond to a presumed suprathreshold stimulus. Alternate explanations for high false negative rates are described in Chapter 1.

False positives (FP):   Number of times the subject presses the response button when a stimulus was not presented. False positive errors are determined by the analyzer setting up to project a stimulus (with all the accompanying mechanical noises and appropriate time delay) but then not projecting one. If the patient presses the response button in this situation, a false positive response is counted. Alternate explanations for high false positive rates are described in Chapter 1.

Homonymous defect: Visual field defect that occurs on the same side of the vertical meridian of the visual field in both eyes.

Hemianopic defect: Visual field defect that occurs on one half of the visual field, generally respecting either the horizontal or vertical meridian.

Mean deviation (MD):   One of the global indices in Humphrey perimetry, the mean deviation is the average difference between the patient's overall sensitivity and that of age-matched controls. It is a weighted arithmetic mean of the values contained in the total deviation printout.

Meridian: Lines of longitude and latitude on the visual field. The key meridians in visual field testing are the horizontal and vertical meridians. Scotomas that respect these meridians have particular anatomic correlates.

Pattern standard deviation (PSD):   The pattern standard deviation is a measure of the amount of localized depression (as opposed to diffuse depression) in the patient's visual field as compared with that of the expected age-matched control population. A low PSD indicates that the hill of vision is smooth and a high PSD indicates that there are localized irregularities in the hill of vision. The PSD does not take into account the effect of short-term fluctuation, so is not thought to be as useful a measure of localized visual field irregularity as the corrected pattern standard deviation.

Primary points: Four points in the visual field which lie 9° from the horizontal and vertical meridians in each of the four quadrants. These four points are tested first and the results used as a starting point for surrounding locations. They are double-determined and the variation between the values is used in the determination of short-term fluctuation (along with six other points, all of which are shown in Chapter 1, Figure 1-15).

Relative scotoma: A depression in the visual field that is not absolute. That is, there is some stimulus size or intensity that the perimeter can generate that can be seen.

Scotoma: A depression in the visual field.

Short-term fluctuation: Short-term fluctuation is a measure of normal physiologic variation and intratest reliability. It is measured when the analyzer double-determines 10 preselected points during the course of the test session.

Suprathreshold stimulus: A stimulus that is presumed to be more intense than a predetermined value.

Threshold: Dimmest stimulus seen by a subject, 50% of the time. Measured in decibels in automated perimetry.

Statpac: Statistical program that accompanies the Humphrey perimeter, which allows for comparison of threshold values obtained from testing to age-matched control data. The program also factors out overall depression of the field, and calculates information that helps judge progression of the visual field over time.

Subject Index